ELLIS P. LEONARD, B.S., D.V.M.

Professor of Small Animal Surgery,
Head of the Department of Small Animal Medicine and Surgery,
Director of the Small Animal Clinic
New York State Veterinary College, Cornell University

DRAWINGS BY MARION NEWSON

1968

FUNDAMENTALS OF

SMALL ANIMAL SURGERY

W. B. Saunders Company

PHILADELPHIA · LONDON · TORONTO

W. B. Saunders Company: West Washington Square
Philadelphia, Pa. 19105

12 Dyott Street
London W.C.1

1835 Yonge Street
Toronto 7, Ontario
Canada

Fundamentals of Small Animal Surgery

 Press of W. B. Saunders Company. Library of Congress catalog card number 68–10402.

Preface

There is an old proverb which goes something like this–"You must learn to creep before you walk and learn to walk before you run." To become a good surgeon you must not only possess good manual dexterity; you must learn by practice and experience the fundamentals which support the surgical treatment of disease. In order to excel, a surgeon must constantly rehearse, not for the sake of a great operating room performance, but to improve his ability to preserve life. This book is written for the student of surgery, whether undergraduate or graduate, who wants to improve himself for the sake of his patient.

Having taught a course in operative surgery for many years, the author has felt the need of a treatise dealing with the detail involved in all common surgical procedures. All of the surgery contained here has been written about many times before, but often without the minutia required by the student who is attempting to acquire basic surgical skills. An effort has been made to include all of the elements and principles of good surgery without becoming too monotonous and repetitious and without attempting to cover the entire field of general small animal surgery.

A number of good books have been published which deal with the subject of small animal surgery. The reader is referred to these books. They cover the fields of anesthesia, general surgery, neurosurgery, ophthalmic surgery, and orthopedic surgery. It is not the purpose of this book to intrude upon these disciplines in detail but rather to present the basic ideas and techniques along with the surgical exercises of common operations. Once the student of surgery has mastered these principles, he is prepared for more specialized surgery.

Much of the material presented on these pages is the result of experience in performing surgery on dogs and cats for over thirty years. During that time, many procedures were tried; some were adopted and some were discarded. The distillate provided here is the product of many minds and much testing. For further ideas and methods, one is referred to the list of references at the end of each chapter. These are provided for the student of surgery who is interested in pursuing the subject further and are not necessarily documentary.

With the exception of certain illustrations modified from Miller,

Christensen, and Evans' *Anatomy of the Dog*, the line drawings and photographs are all original and were prepared from factual material. Emphasis has been placed on the illustrative aspects of the book so that the reader can more readily visualize each step of a procedure.

The author is grateful for the assistance given him by colleagues and friends. Without their help the book could not have been written. My colleague Dr. George E. Ross, Jr., gave much time to the illustrative material and offered sound advice in the presentation.

Miss Marion Newson, Medical Illustrator, was responsible for the excellent line drawings, all of which were made from original sketches.

Dean George C. Poppensiek encouraged the work and made facilities of the New York State Veterinary College available.

Miss Mia Reinap and her staff at the Flower Library provided the necessary assistance with reference research.

Mrs. Louise Dedlow meticulously carried out the onerous task of typing the manuscript.

Most of the photographs were made by Mr. Martin Bingham of the Photo Science Studios at Cornell University. The remainder were prepared by Mr. John Brock, photographer for the New York State Veterinary College. Mrs. Olga Reidemanis, Miss Susan Quick, and Mr. A. E. Scheld assisted in the preparation of photographic material.

My wife was of great assistance with the proofreading and indexing.

The staff at W. B. Saunders Company provided outstanding assistance, as usual, in the editing and publishing of this work.

ELLIS P. LEONARD, D.V.M.

Contents

Chapter 1

INTRODUCTION

All soft tissue repair is essentially the same whether the nature of the wound be accidental or intentional. The principal difference lies in the preparation of the site for surgery. In one case, preparation is made in advance of the wound, while in the other, preparation must be made in the presence of the wound.

For the most part we shall be concerned with planned surgery, but some understanding of the management of soft tissue damage should furnish insight into the healing processes so vital to successful operative surgery.

In the general consideration of wound healing there are certain factors that should be taken into account which have a direct bearing on the progress of healing. These factors can quite conveniently be divided into two groups: those affecting the body as a whole, and those which exert an influence on the specific tissues involved in the wound.

General factors which influence wound healing include such things as the nutritional state of the patient, the age of the patient, and any disease affecting the body as a whole. Hypoproteinemia and dehydration also bring about bodily changes which may interfere with wound healing. Vitamin deficiencies may enter into the picture, with vitamin A playing a very important role in the healing of mucous membranes. It is believed that vitamin C deficiency is less likely to occur in the dog although this is a common cause of poor wound healing in humans.

It has been fairly well established that cortisone and ACTH delay wound healing in animals. There seems to be some difference of opinion, however, as to the exact mechanism of the cortical hormones in relation to wound healing. Some workers feel that wound healing is only delayed in those patients that have been on cortisone therapy for a long time. Others believe that there is a delay in the formation of granulation tissue and fibroplasia whether cortisone is used prior to the wound or subsequent to it. In view of the experimental findings, perhaps it is best that one not use the corticosteroids during the early healing of fresh wounds, whether they be of a surgical type or the result of an accident.

One certainly has no direct control over these general factors, but they should be given careful consideration in assessing a wound, making a prognosis, and undertaking treatment.

The local factors influencing wound healing include the type of incision, the extent of the trauma, the presence of infection, the degree of hemostasis, the amount of drainage required, the kind of suture material, the presence of foreign bodies, the adequacy of blood supply, the presence of devitalized tissue, the amount of edema, and the accuracy of approximation. Minor wounds of the skin and subcutaneous tissue are frequently allowed to heal by granulation, particularly if they occur on the torso of long-haired dogs, where the hair coat will obscure any subsequent scar formation. However, if such wounds are left to heal by granulation in short-haired dogs, or if they occur in exposed places such as the face and lower appendages or in areas where there is considerable movement such as the skin over joints, they may result in unsightly scarring. Closure of even small wounds will shorten the healing time and give a more presentable result. Such wounds must be both mechanically and bacteriologically clean, and the edges must be smooth. The use of any type of cautery will delay the healing and in most instances will not result in first intention repair. Any procedure which traumatizes the tissues, whether it be cauterization, rough handling, or careless clamping with forceps, will delay and jeopardize healing.

While it is virtually impossible to have an accidental wound that is absolutely free from contamination, a reasonably clean wound may be obtained by proper cleansing. The use of strong antiseptics produces cellular damage and usually tends to retard healing. Thorough cleansing with surgical soaps or hexachlorophene gives a far superior result, especially when coupled with systemic use of antibiotics. All damaged tissue should be carefully removed from the wound, and good hemostasis should be practiced. Blood clots form an excellent media in which to propagate bacteria.

An accidental wound is packed with sterile sponges, and the surrounding area cleared of hair and debris by clipping. A vacuum is used to remove the loose hair. The sponges are removed, and the wound and the adjacent skin are thoroughly cleaned with soap and water. The skin should also be defatted with ether and disinfected with 70 per cent isopropyl alcohol.

Surgical scissors are used to incise the skin at a point about 3 mm. from the edge of the wound so that the wound is circumscribed. The free skin is held with forceps while the incision is continued until the surface of the wound is entirely undermined and can be lifted from the spot intact. It will contain all the contaminated material as well as any mutilated or necrotic tissue.

Such a procedure is not always possible, and it may be necessary to remove the contaminated and necrotic tissue piecemeal. If this is the case, one should be careful not to recontaminate the wound. In any event, the debridement should be radical enough to remove all foreign material as well as all damaged and devitalized tissue. When the wound is absolutely clean and the edges appear fresh and healthy, it is ready for closure.

Closure of wounds should be carried out under strict asepsis, particularly in those wounds which involve the deeper structures such as fascia, muscle, blood vessels, tendons, and bone. Suture materials should be selected with care so that maximum tensile strength will be obtained while at the same time tissue reaction will be minimized. Chromic catgut rapidly loses its strength in the presence of serum, blood, inflammatory exudate, and any of the secretions of the body. This suture material can therefore only be used in areas where the tissue fluids are at a normal level. The use of catgut in edematous tissues or where there is a rapid collection of blood or serum will lead to early disintegration of the gut and subsequent disruption of the wound. Catgut also disintegrates rapidly when used in mucous membranes because of its contact with secretions.

During the first four or five days, very little holding power other than fibrinous adhesions is produced within the tissues themselves. During this time the patency of the wound depends largely upon the stability of the catgut. By suturing the fascial layers with an adequate number of interrupted sutures and using small sizes of catgut (2-0 and 4-0), we have found that we can maintain good stability in the average wound. Since catgut produces some tissue reaction, an excessive number of sutures should not be placed, but there should be a sufficient number to obtain adequate closure without the interposition of fat or muscle tissue. Continuous sutures with catgut are usually hazardous. It is also true that catgut picks up fluid more readily than silk, cotton, or stainless steel and that it is more likely to become contaminated.

Both cotton and silk are acceptable and actually cause less tissue reaction than catgut. However, these substances are foreign materials which must be encapsulated by the body. Frequently, in the presence of contamination, they will gradually migrate to the surface. Ordinary sewing cotton or mercerized cotton has been found acceptable and usually maintains its tensile strength for a longer period of time than catgut or silk. The sizes commonly used are number 30 for fascial closures and number 60 for ligatures. While mercerized cotton is slightly stronger than plain cotton, neither of these products is as strong as silk or catgut when compared size for size.

In order to minimize the amount of foreign body placed within the wound by suturing, it is recommended that *both* silk and cotton be used in interrupted sutures, that the knots be kept simple, and that the ends be cut extremely short.

In recent years, stainless steel wire has come into wide use as a suture material for wound repair. Both monofilament and multifilament wire are used for this purpose. Stainless steel wire is especially useful in those areas of the body where great tension is placed on the repaired tissues. It is extremely useful in the repair of muscle attachments, tendons, and joint injuries. If properly placed, it works exceedingly well. Interrupted sutures should be used whenever possible, and these sutures should be well buried in the tissues. Wire should not be used in the dermal layer of the skin, but should be buried beneath the subcutaneous tissues so that it will not work to the surface. Needless to say, the ends must be cut short and turned in toward the knot so that the sharp edges will not irritate the tissues. When using the larger sizes of wire, one may secure the sutures either by twisting or tying. This material adds great strength to the wound and will remain in position indefinitely without causing tissue reaction.

These then are the principal materials in common use for wound closure within the body. There is even a wider choice of materials that may be used externally for skin closure. Since sutures placed in the skin are subsequently removed, they do not require such a critical evaluation. A wide selection of suture materials for the skin is available. The materials vary from metal skin clips to glass thread. Since the tensile strength of skin is very poor as compared with fascia, it is important that the underlying tissues, including the subcutaneous tissues, be securely closed so that the skin edges are nearly approximated when skin closure is begun. Skin sutures should not be under tension, since their principal purpose is simply to hold the edges in approximation during the healing period. Tension on the skin will do little to hold the underlying tissues in apposition. It is both fruitless and detrimental to have the skin sutures too tight. If skin sutures are properly placed, they need not and should not be removed before 10 days have elapsed and sufficient healing has taken place to assure nondisruption of the wound.

REPAIR OF SPECIALIZED SOFT TISSUE

FASCIA

Fascia is the strongest soft tissue in the body and has great tensile strength. Because of this, it is usually quite easy to repair, even when it is badly lacerated. In the average wound, only the free tag ends of torn fascia need to be removed before suturing is begun. Fascia holds sutures well and is frequently used as replacement tissue where muscle or tendon has been lost because of injury. It can easily be transplanted from one part of the body to another, but it must be kept moistened during the interchange and not allowed to dry excessively. Wherever possible the fascial layers of a wound should be closed, because doing so adds greatly to the strength of the wound. If one were to compare the strength of various soft tissues using a tensile index of 10 for fascia, the other tissues would fall into the following order: skin 5, peritoneum 1, muscle 1/4, and fat 0. One can readily see from this the importance of fascia repair in every wound.

MUSCLE

Simple muscle repair can usually be brought about by closure of the sheath, but where large masses of muscle have been lost or the tendinous end has been disrupted, it may be necessary to make more extensive repairs. Muscle tissue in itself has very little holding power for suturing and therefore must have the support of a stronger tissue. Occasionally, when the tissue loss is not great, one may be able to draw small muscles together by the use of mattress sutures, but many times it is necessary to further support this repair by applying strips of fascia over the muscle and suturing from side to side so that the fascia forms a supporting covering for the injury. When the tendinous end of the muscle has been ruptured, the repair can be made with fascia. This is done by placing a sleeve of fascia around the muscle so that mattress sutures may be placed through both fascia and muscle from side to side. When the fascial sleeve has been securely fastened to the muscle belly, the tendinous end is brought into position and sutured in a like manner. This requires manipulation of the limb so that the muscle is not under undue tension. The suture material used in this case should be cotton, silk, or stainless steel.

SKIN

Except in the lower parts of the extremities, the skin lends itself very easily to correction and repair. Usually closure of the skin over most of the body presents no problem. One should bear in mind, however, that skin closure does not have to follow a straight line; wherever possible it should follow the general contour lines of the body. The biggest problems in skin closure occur distal to the elbows and stifles. Many times, however, these difficult repairs can be made by simple skin transfers. In many instances round or irregularly shaped lesions must be reshaped into either a circle, triangle, square, or rectangle. From these basic forms, one can make several types of skin transfers, for the skin can be moved in a longitudinal direction along the leg even though there is a scarcity of skin in the circumferential direction.

One should always attempt to use the simplest method possible and economize on the amount of undercut skin. The layer of skin should be deep enough to include the subcutaneous tissues, and the skin should be undercut sufficiently so that there is no tension on the sutures. Small interrupted stitches placed quite close together should be used, and a fairly snug bandage with adequate padding should be placed over the finished operation. This bandage should go undisturbed for at least four days before the wound is inspected.

One of the difficult decisions to make whenever wounds of the legs are repaired is whether or not to restrict movement. A good general rule to follow in this respect is to restrict movement in all those cases in which movement will create extra tension on the suture line. In all other cases, unrestricted movement is beneficial, and bandaging should be kept to a minimum. We usually follow the practice of applying patch bandages whenever movement is not a factor.

In all soft tissue repair, there are certain basic principles that must be followed, but beyond this one must use his own ingenuity in bringing about a satisfactory result.

REFERENCES

Archibald, J. *Canine Surgery*. 1st ed. Santa Barbara, California: American Veterinary Publications Inc., 1965.

Armistead, W. W. *J.A.V.M.A.* 117:301, 1950.

Caulfield, P. A., and Madigan, H. S. *Amer. J. Surg.* 86:249–254, 1953.

Hampton, P. P., Jr. *J.A.M.A.* 154:1326, 1954.

Chapter 2

SURGICAL ACCOUTERMENTS

A basic knowledge of the materials used in the operating room, such as apparel, instruments, sutures and drapes, is essential if one is to master the technique of good aseptic surgical procedure. A well-trained surgeon should be familiar with the materials available, their usefulness, and the methods used in preparing them for surgery. All these things play an important role in the final surgical result.

DRAPES

Various types of draping material can be used with good results. The material most commonly used is heavy unbleached muslin. This can be dyed to improve its appearance and reduce the amount of light reflected into the surgeon's eyes. Colors frequently used are blue, green, and gray. Most commercial laundries will dye the cloth, but in order to get a uniform color, the bolt of muslin should be separated into short lengths. Each length should be sufficiently long to make three or four large drapes.

The dyed cloth should be torn (not cut) into pieces of the desired size and the torn edges hemmed. The selvage edge does not require hemming. An average size drape should be about 36 inches by 60 inches. With this as a standard size for all drapes, a system of multiple drapes or single drapes with various openings can be used. Three drapes of identical overall size but with different size openings are illustrated (Fig. 2–1). This type of drape can be used for simple procedures, but a multiple-drape system is preferable for major surgery.

Other materials, such as plastic and rubber, are used less frequently than cloth drapes. These materials are easily cleaned but present some problems in sterilizing. Disposable plastic drapes for draping to the incision are also available. This material is very thin and is used only for draping the immediate surgical area. It is used in conjunction with conventional drapes. Adhesive is used to anchor it to the skin. One form requires the application of adhesive to the skin; another form is adhesive backed. They are best applied to flat surfaces such as the abdomen.

Folding of the cloth drapes is the first important step toward preparing them for the surgery (Fig. 2–2). The first fold is lengthwise, thereby reducing the width to half (Fig. 2–3). The long edges are then turned back on either side to the line of the original fold (Fig. 2–4). This reduces the width to one-quarter and leaves the free edges on the outside (Fig. 2–5). An accordion fold is then started at one end of the folded material and continued to the opposite end by making folds about 4 inches wide (Fig. 2–6).

Since small bundles are easier to sterilize, it is best to wrap various items such as drapes, gowns, and instruments in separate bundles. Single drapes are wrapped separately, and multiple drapes are wrapped four or six to a bundle. The folded drapes are wrapped by placing them in the center of a double thickness of muslin approximately 30 inches square (Fig. 2–7). They should be placed diagonally so that the corners of the wrapper are opposite the sides and ends of the stacked drapes. The first corner of the wrapper is folded over the drapes, the tip folded outward (Fig. 2–8). This is followed by folding the opposite corner in the same way snugly over the first (Fig. 2–9). The third (far) corner is then folded over the pack, with the end folded inward (Fig. 2–10). Finally, the fourth (near) corner is folded similar to the third, and the bundle is fastened with a safety pin or tape (Figs. 2–11 and 2–12). The bundle should be tight enough so that it will not loosen or open when handled roughly. If it is fastened with a safety pin, the pin should not penetrate all the layers of the wrapper, because the bundle could be contaminated when the pin is removed. A single wrap of pressure-sensitive indicator tape is preferable to the safety pin because it serves as a sterilizing indicator as well as a binding. There is also no danger of contaminating the bundle.

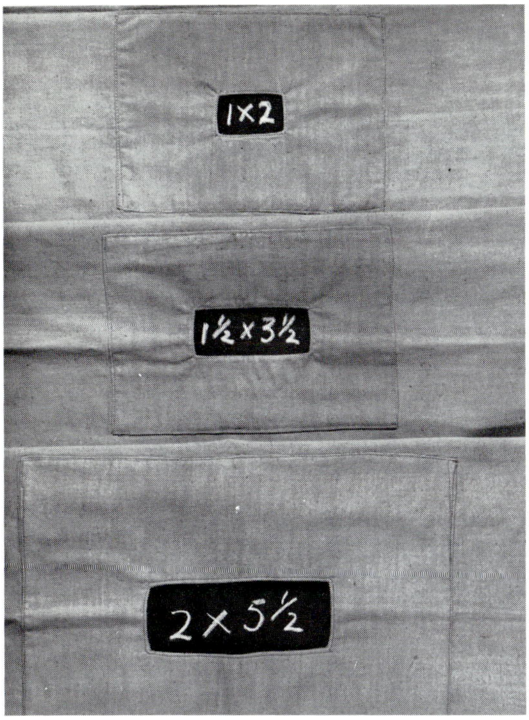

FIGURE 2–1.

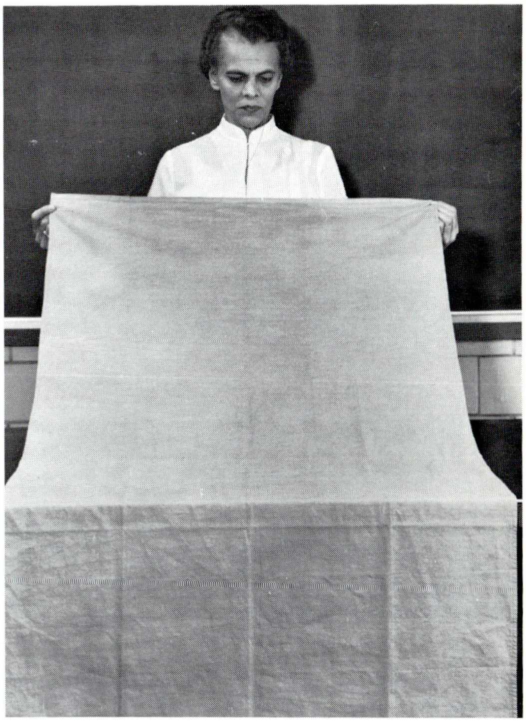

FIGURE 2–2.

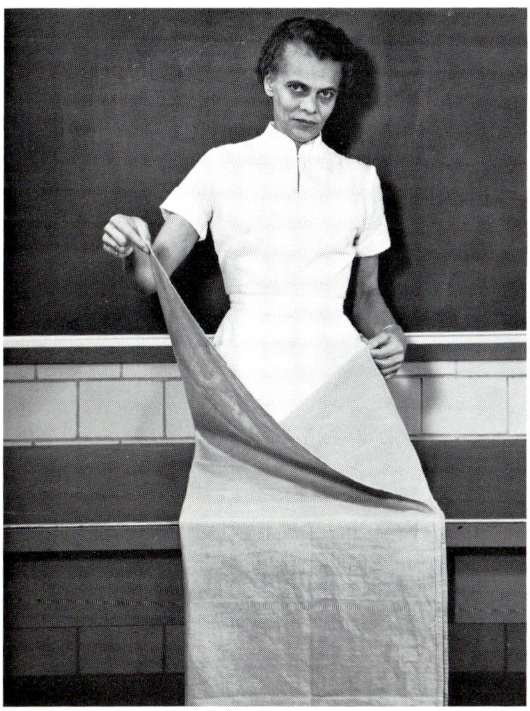

FIGURE 2–3.

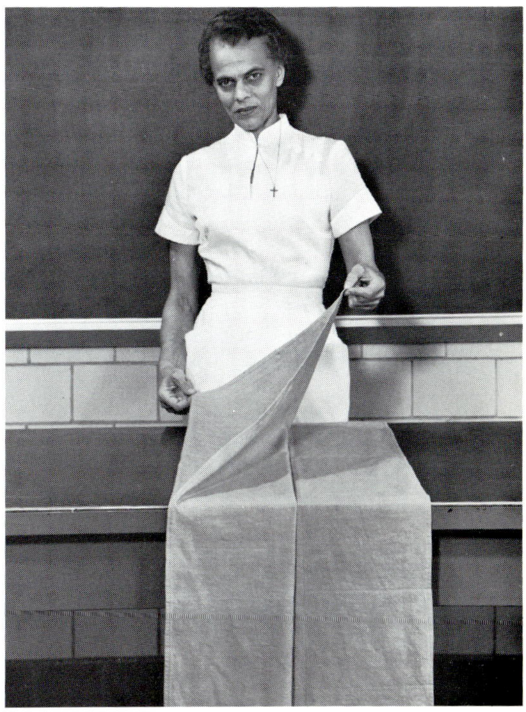

FIGURE 2–4.

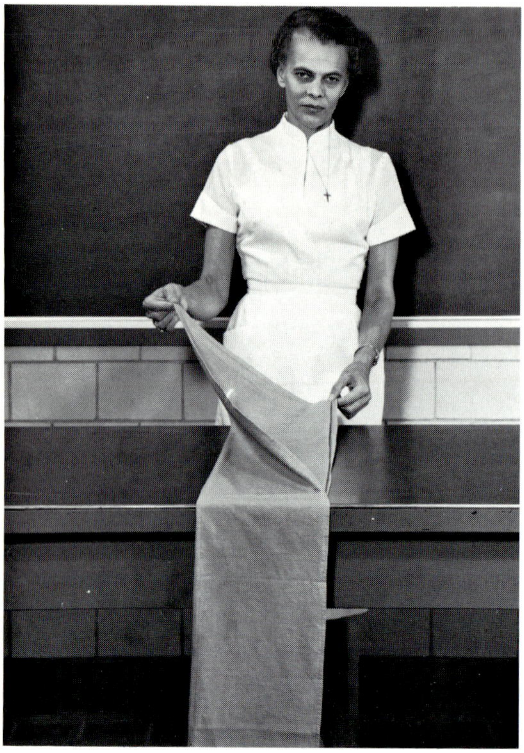

FIGURE 2–5.

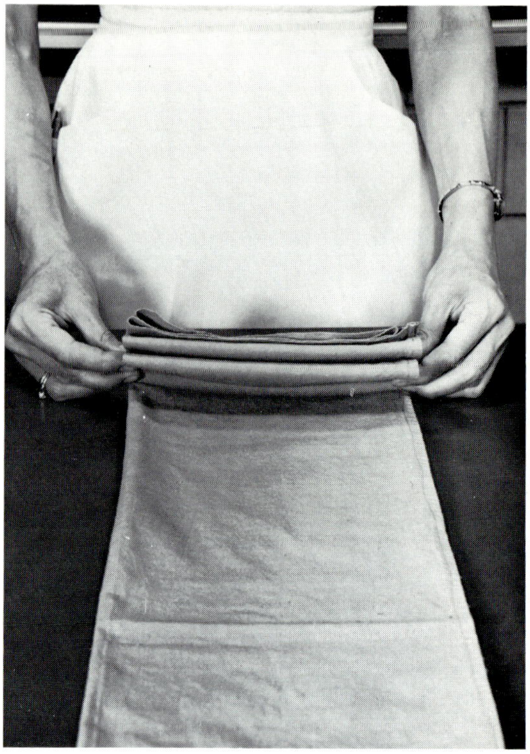

FIGURE 2–6.

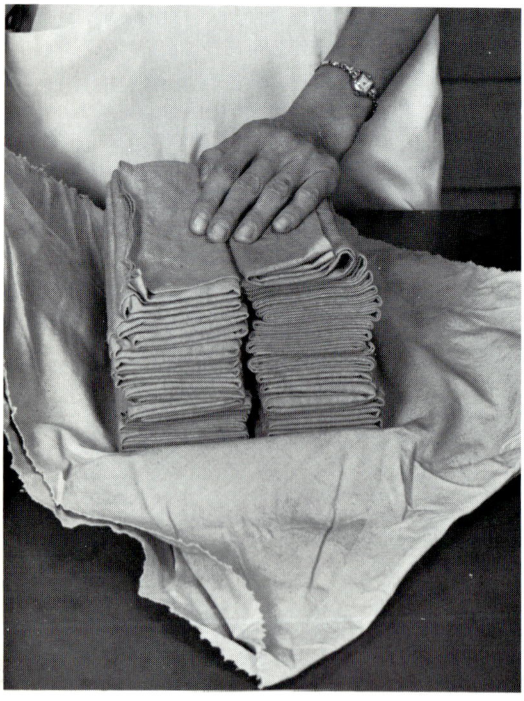

FIGURE 2–7.

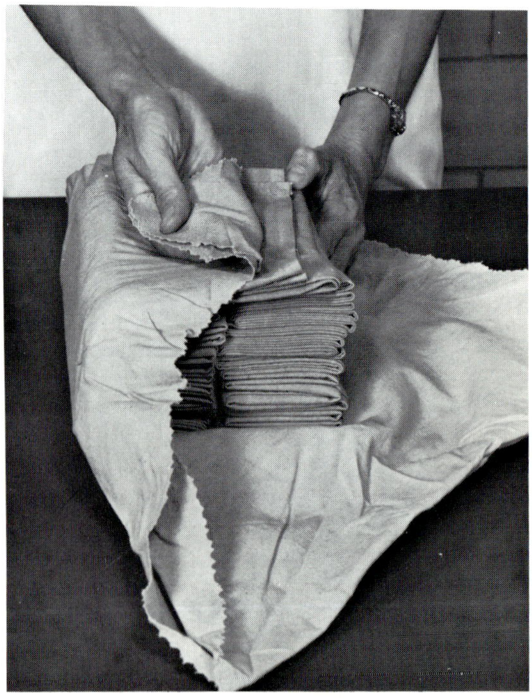

FIGURE 2–8.

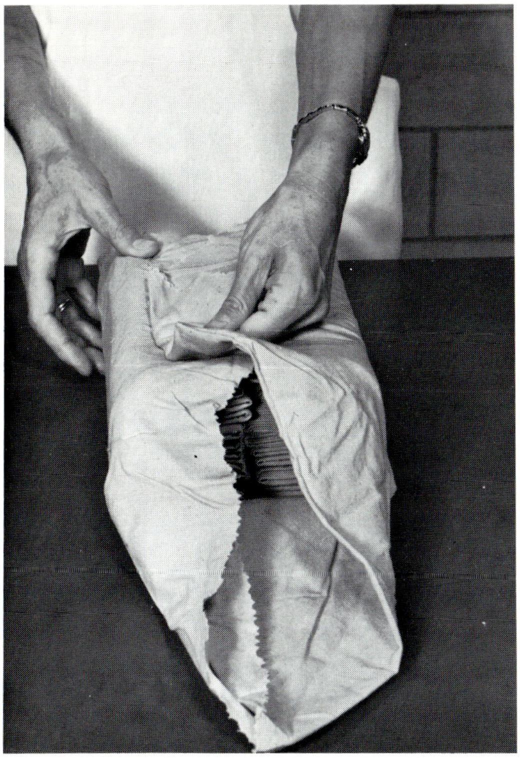

FIGURE 2–9.

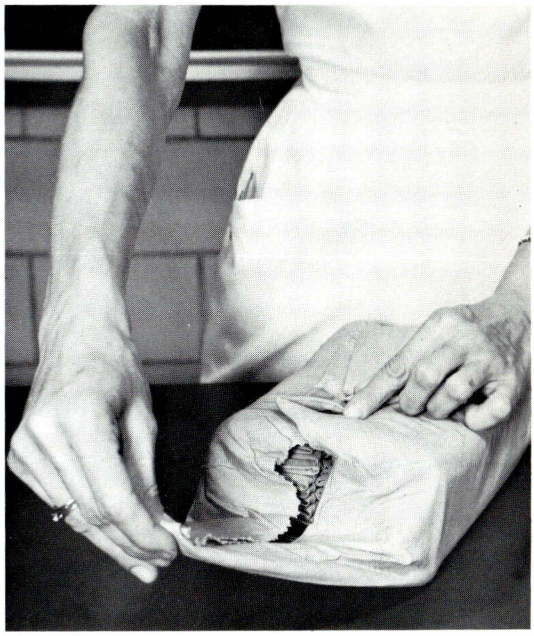

FIGURE 2–10.

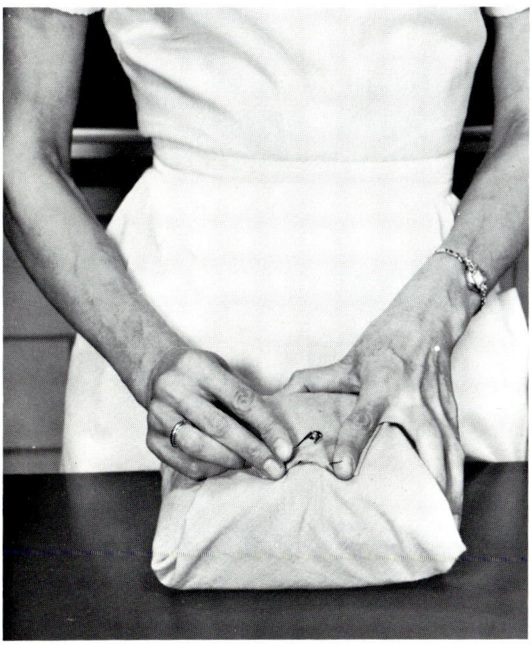

FIGURE 2–11.

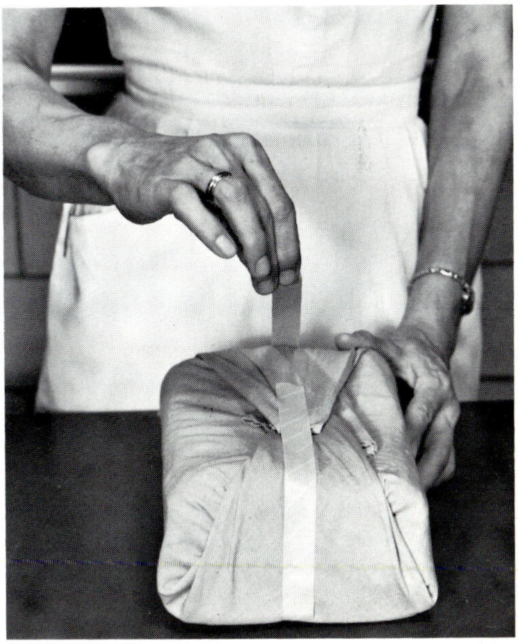

FIGURE 2–12.

GOWN

The ideal operating gown is full length with an opening in the back and has long sleeves that terminate in stockinet cuffs. Other forms of apparel, such as short-sleeved gowns, pullovers, and two-piece uniforms, are designed primarily for scrub-up or treatment-room work.

The gown is prepared for sterilization by folding it in a manner similar to that used in folding a suit coat. The sleeves are pulled straight and smoothed (Fig. 2–13). The ends of the collar are turned outward and brought together. This turns the gown inside out with a fold running lengthwise through the middle and the sleeves inside the fold (Fig. 2–14). It is again folded lengthwise down the middle, wrinkles are smoothed, and the edges are brought together (Fig. 2–15). A third lengthwise fold is made after the gown is laid on a flat surface (Fig. 2–16). With the width of the folded gown now reduced to about 8 inches, an accordion fold about 4 inches wide is started at the bottom hem and continued to the collar (Fig. 2–17 and 2–18). The folded gown is placed diagonally in the center of the wrapper, with the collar up and the ties on top (Fig. 2–19). A gown wrapper is made of double-thickness muslin about 20 inches square.

A folded towel is placed on top of the gown (Fig. 2–20). A disposable professional towel is quite adequate. The bundle is then wrapped by folding opposite corners of the wrapper over the bundle, with the ends turned outward (Fig. 2–21). This is followed by folding the two remaining corners, the ends of which are turned inward, and fastening the bundle by passing a single strip of indicator tape around it (Figs. 2–22, 2–23, and 2–24).

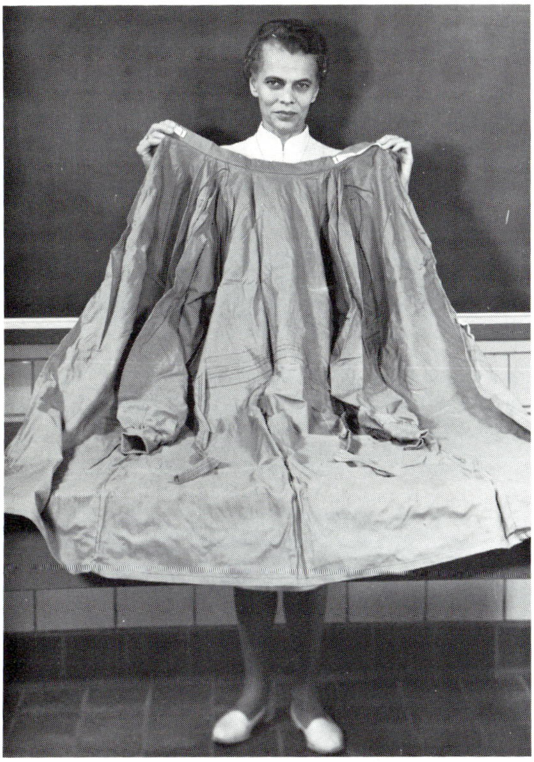

FIGURE 2–13.

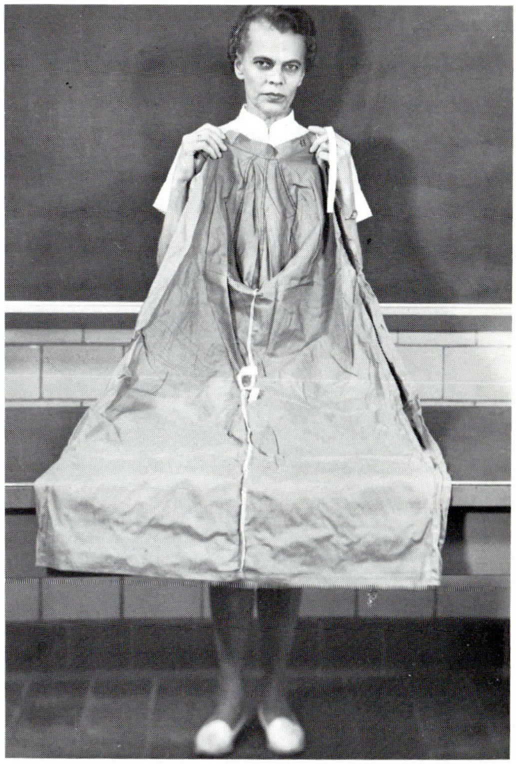

FIGURE 2–14.

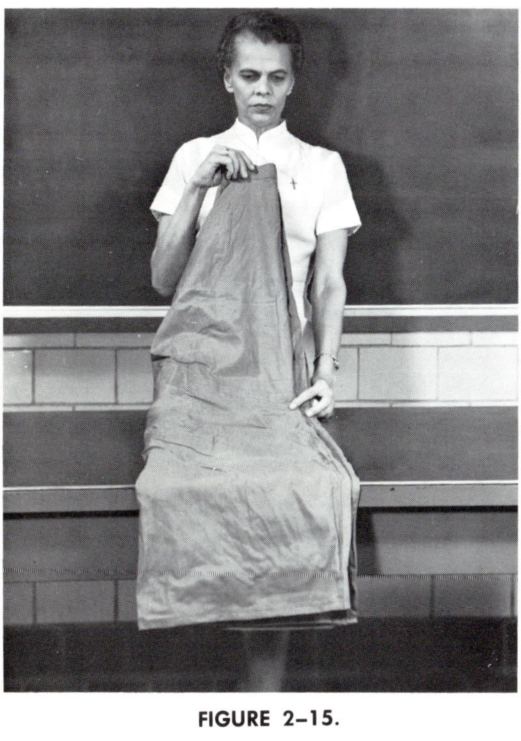

FIGURE 2–15.

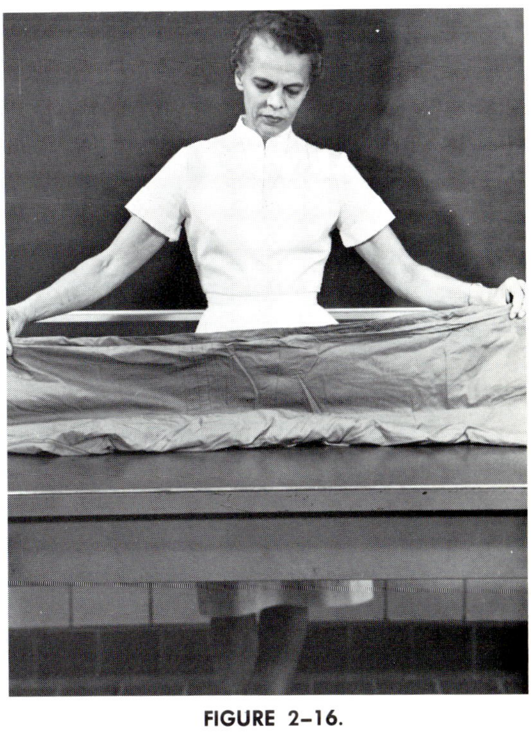

FIGURE 2–16.

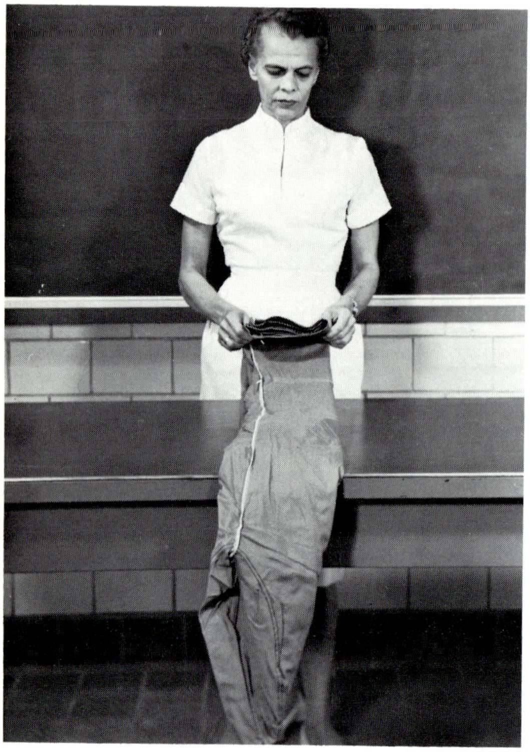

FIGURE 2–17.

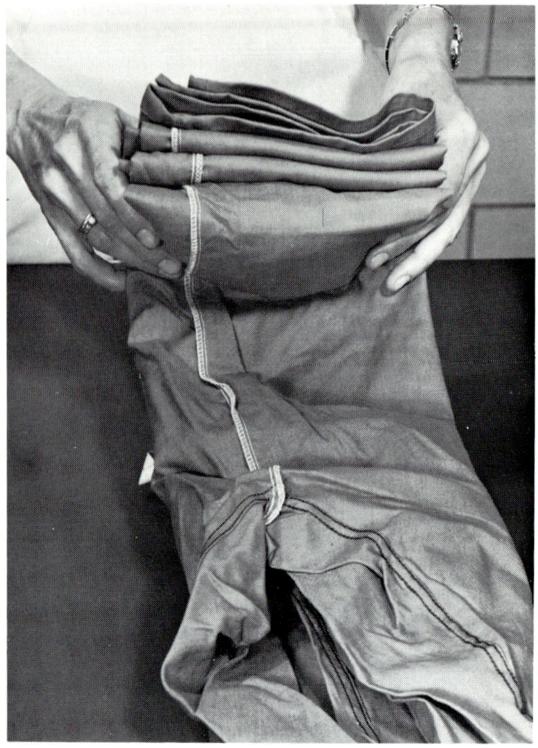

FIGURE 2–18.

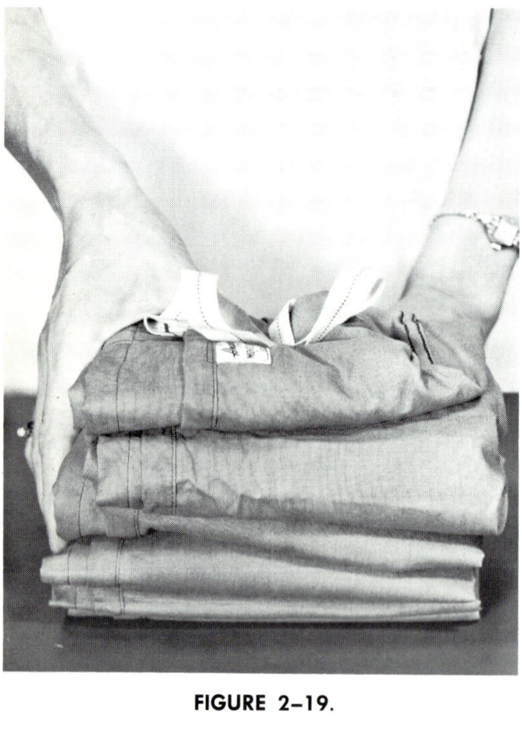

FIGURE 2–19.

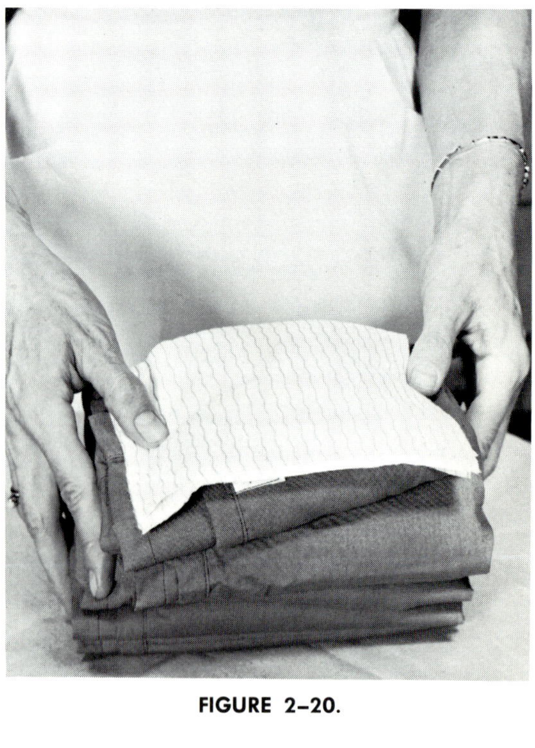

FIGURE 2–20.

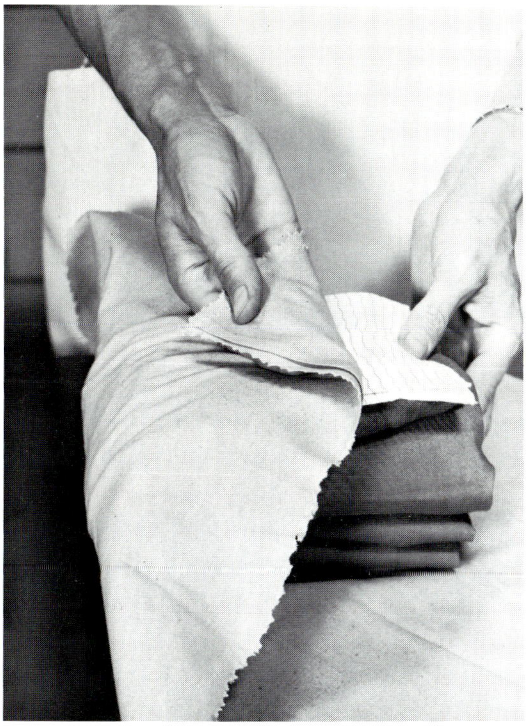

FIGURE 2–21.

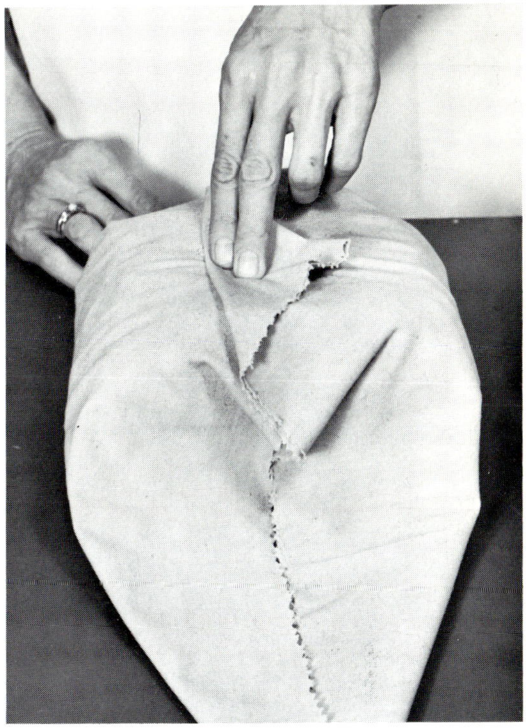

FIGURE 2–22.

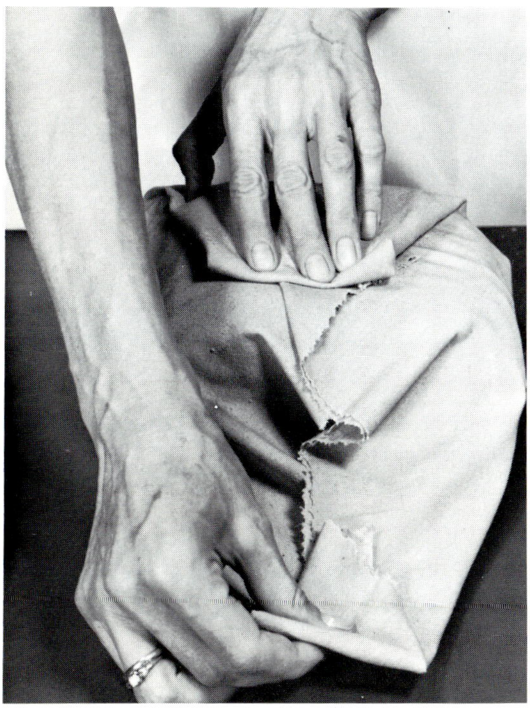

FIGURE 2–23.

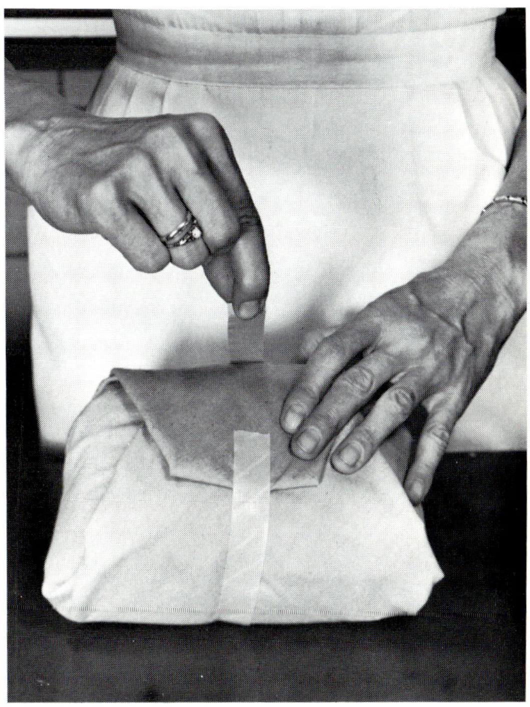

FIGURE 2–24.

GLOVES

The gloves must be prepared for surgery with care. They must be clean, and in this respect the surgeon can assist by thoroughly washing them before removal. Testing for holes can be done by shaking the glove to full length, stretching the cuff with both hands, and twirling it to entrap and compress the air inside. The glove can then be examined for leaks either by holding it to the ear or immersing it in water.

After the gloves are washed and air dried, they are powdered. The best material for dusting is a treated corn starch preparation (Biosorb). It does not have the irritating properties of talc. A pair of gloves can be placed in a discarded glove carton and sprinkled lightly with powder (Fig. 2–25). The lid is closed and the box shaken (Fig. 2–26). The gloves are then turned inside out and shaken again. A second sprinkling of powder is unnecessary.

After the gloves are dusted, they should be checked to see that they are right side out. This can be determined by examining the trademark and glove size stamped on the cuff. This is always on the outside. The cuffs are everted and a gauze sponge inserted to keep the glove open, thereby allowing steam to enter during sterilization (Fig. 2–27). The amount of cuff everted should always be adequate. The tendency is to allow too little cuff for grasping during the gloving procedure.

The gloves are inserted into a glove envelope palm side up. One glove is put in each pocket, with the thumb to the inside of the pocket (Fig. 2–28). The gloves are then correctly positioned for donning. A packet of powder is placed on the outside of the pocket, and the envelope is folded between the pockets (Figs. 2–29 and 2–30). This is unnecessary when cream is used. A second envelope can be folded over the first from the opposite direction and fastened with a paper clip, or the pack can be wrapped with double-thickness muslin.

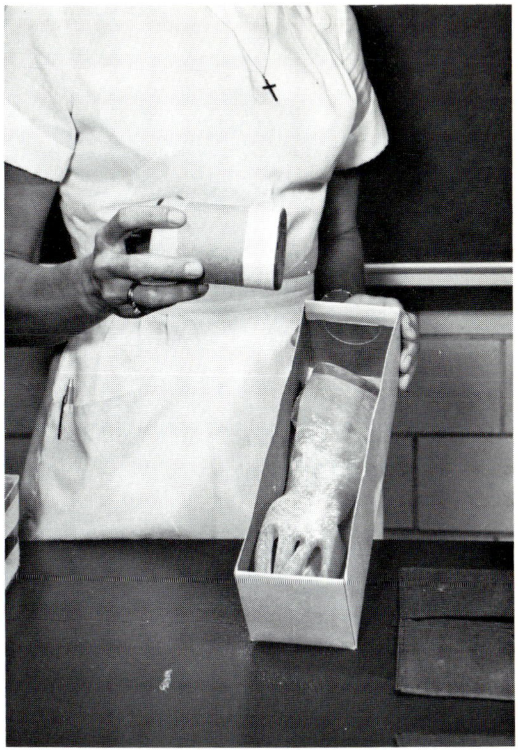

FIGURE 2-25.

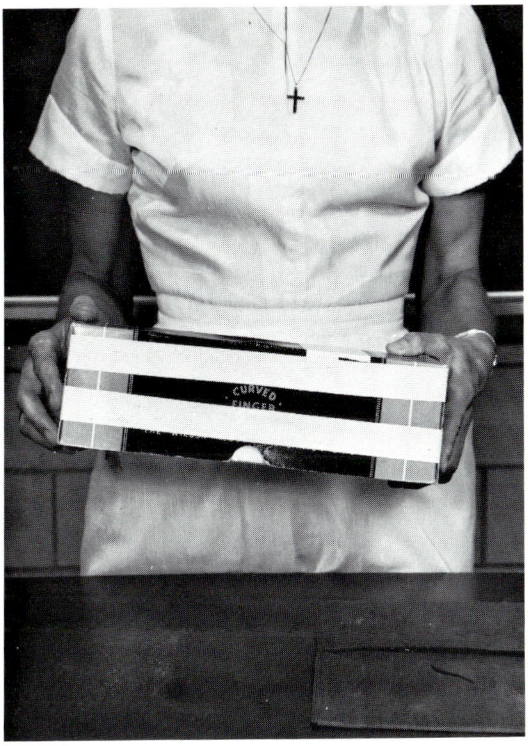

FIGURE 2-26.

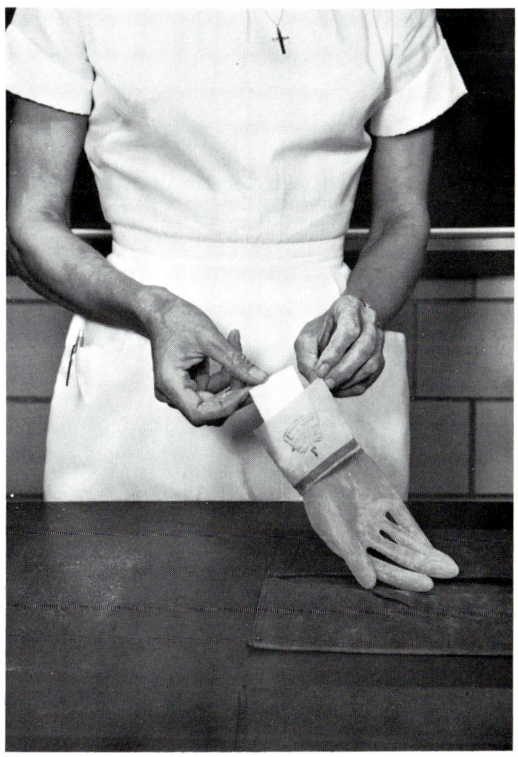

FIGURE 2-27.

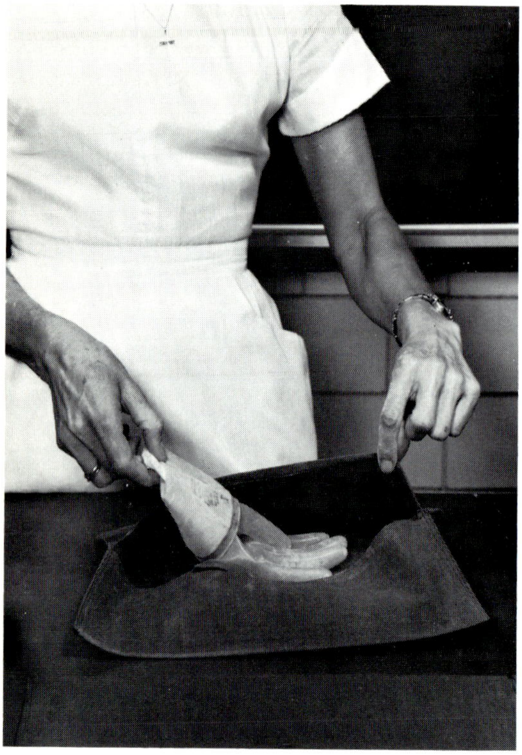

FIGURE 2–28.

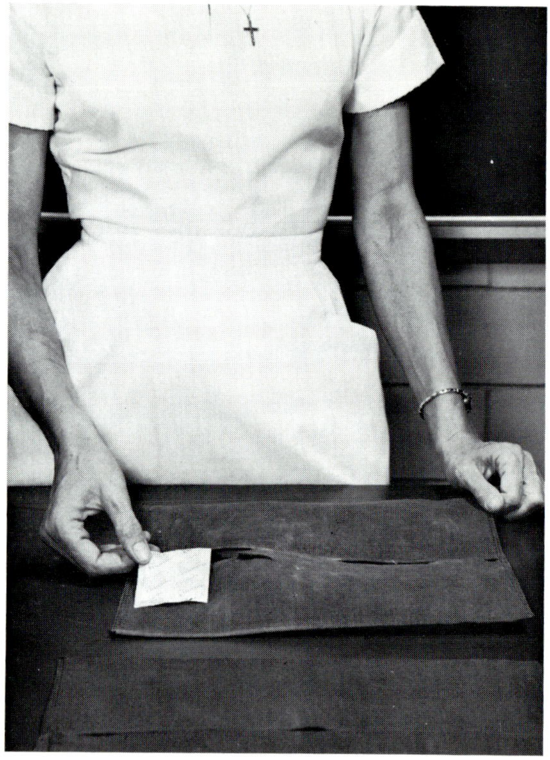

FIGURE 2–29.

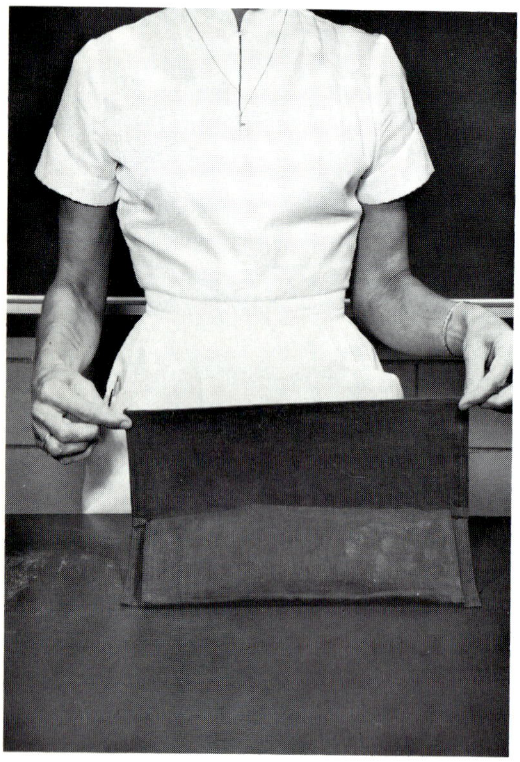

FIGURE 2–30.

INSTRUMENTS

There is an abundance of surgical instruments of all kinds. There are many varieties of some of the simplest instruments. For this reason selection of the proper instruments sometimes presents problems to the young surgeon. Actually most surgery is done with a few simple instruments, and only an occasional operation requires special instruments. The beginner should thoroughly acquaint himself with basic instruments and their use. As surgical experience is gained, knowledge concerning specialized instruments is gradually accumulated.

THUMB FORCEPS

The thumb forceps, sometimes referred to as the tissue forceps, is used to hold tissue during surgical dissection and during wound closure (Fig. 2–31). Sometimes it is used to grasp a needle during suturing. These forceps are made in 30 or 40 different forms to fit individual tastes, but on the average, a 6 inch forceps with three to four teeth on one prong and four to five teeth on the other is quite satisfactory. This type of forceps should not be used on internal organs or the eye. This instrument should be held between the thumb and index finger and supported by the middle finger. This ensures a light touch and is less awkward than clutching it in the clenched fist.

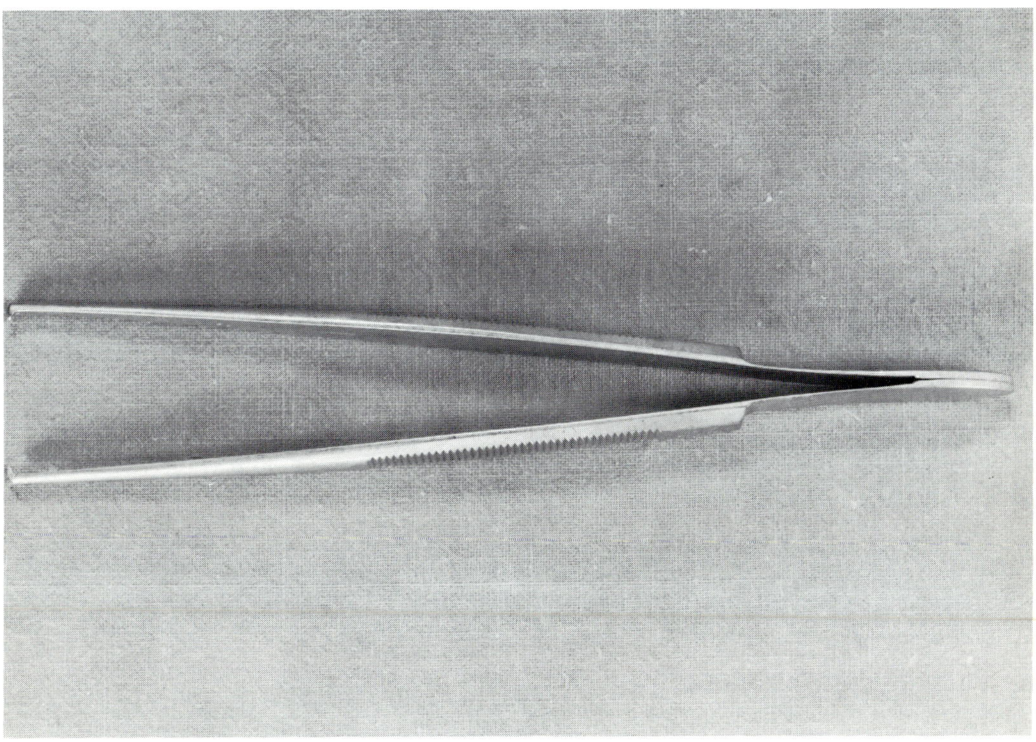

FIGURE 2–31.

KNIFE

Surgical knives with changeable blades are most commonly used. The knife shown in Figure 2–32 is a Bard-Parker with a No. 3 handle and a No. 10 blade. Both the handle and the blade may be obtained in a variety of sizes and shapes. Blades may be purchased in individual sterile wraps or nonsterile, in which case they must be stored in a sterilizing solution before being used. Any form of heat sterilization damages the cutting edge. A blade changer or blade forceps should be used for attaching or removing blades. An old hemostat will also serve, but a good hemostat should never be used for this purpose. Blades should be changed frequently.

Since the knife is a cutting instrument, it should be held firmly in the hand and the index finger should be placed on the rib of the blade. This makes for absolute control of the blade both as to direction and depth.

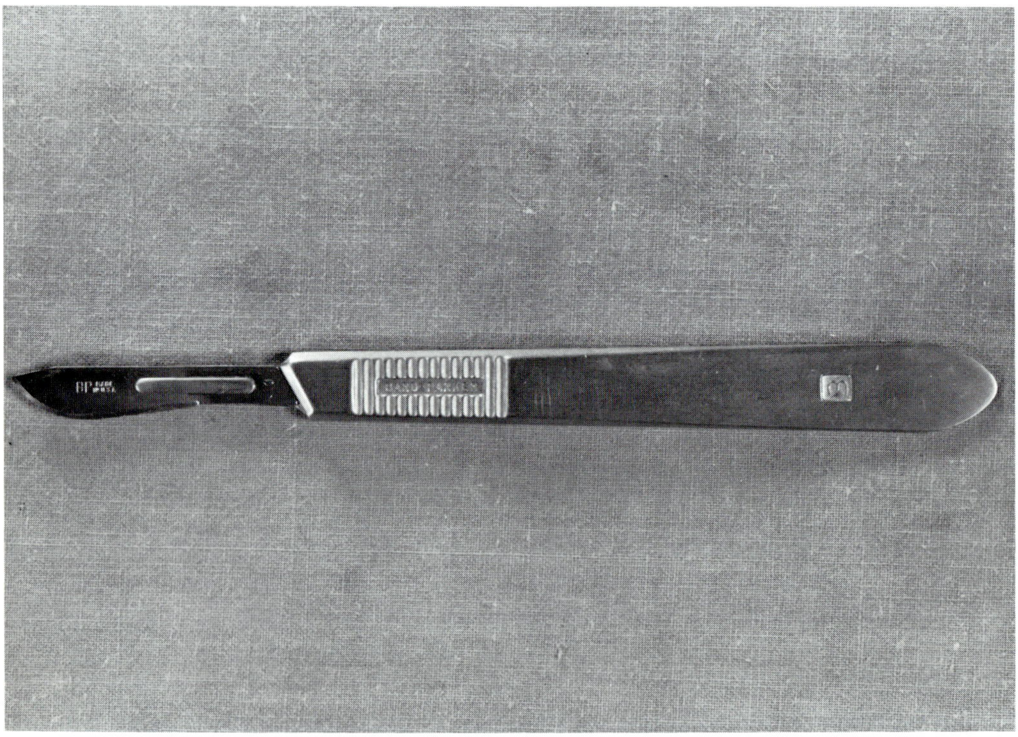

FIGURE 2–32.

SCISSORS

Surgical scissors of various types are available, but for general surgery the Metzenbaum type serves well as an all purpose scissors (Fig. 2–33). The shanks are long, and the blades short and slim. Both blunt and sharp dissection can be done with this type of scissors, but they should only be used on tissue. The cutting of sutures should be performed with suture scissors (Fig. 2–34). These are small scissors with short stubby serrated blades made especially for cutting cotton, silk, nylon and wire.

In order to avoid dulling the cutting edges, surgical scissors should be kept in a cold sterilizing solution (Pentacresol). If a pair of scissors has been contaminated by spore-forming organisms they should be heat sterilized, but fortunately this situation seldom arises in canine surgery.

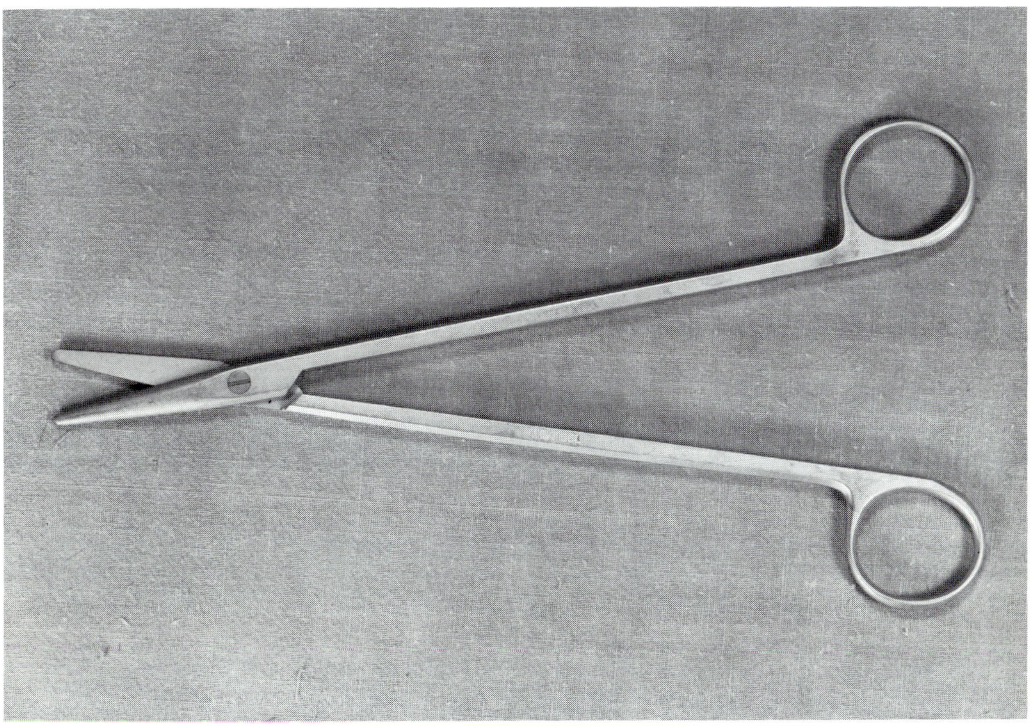

FIGURE 2–33.

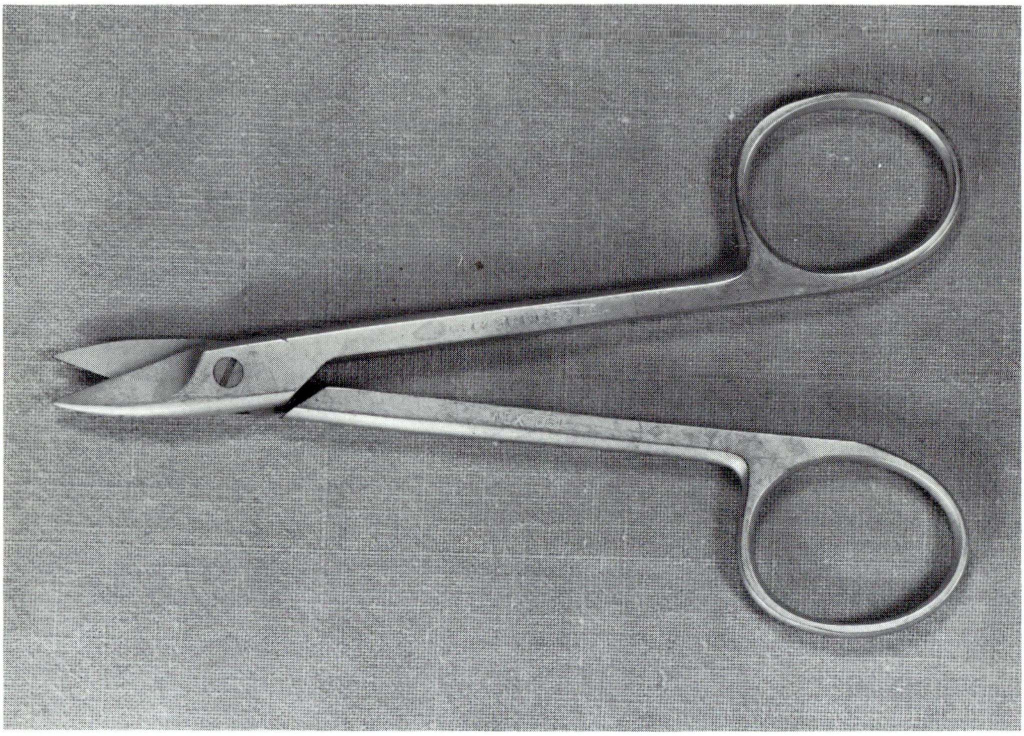

FIGURE 2–34.

HEMOSTATIC FORCEPS

HALSTEAD MOSQUITO HEMOSTAT. The hemostat most frequently used in general surgery is the Halstead mosquito forceps (Fig. 2–35). Once the proper use of this hemostat is mastered, one may wish to use other types for special situations. The jaws may be straight or curved, but the serrations should fit exactly. Teeth are not necessary; in fact, they are likely to cause excessive damage by tearing the clamped vessel. The mosquito hemostat is used when one wishes to clamp small blood vessels without damaging surrounding tissue; therefore, the tips of the jaws should close firmly, and the shanks should spring sufficiently to apply pressure with minimum trauma. They should not be used for clamping large masses of tissue.

A good hemostat is a priceless instrument and is designed to control hemorrhage. It should not be abused by being used to pry or clamp hard materials. The box lock should be kept clean so that the jaws work smoothly and easily. More will be said about cleaning later.

CARMALT FORCEPS. The Carmalt forceps is 6 to 8 inches in length and has serrations running lengthwise along the jaws (Fig. 2–36). The tips have cross-serrations as well. This forceps is used in crushing bands of tissue and in oversewing. The jaw blade is easily withdrawn after the oversewing is completed.

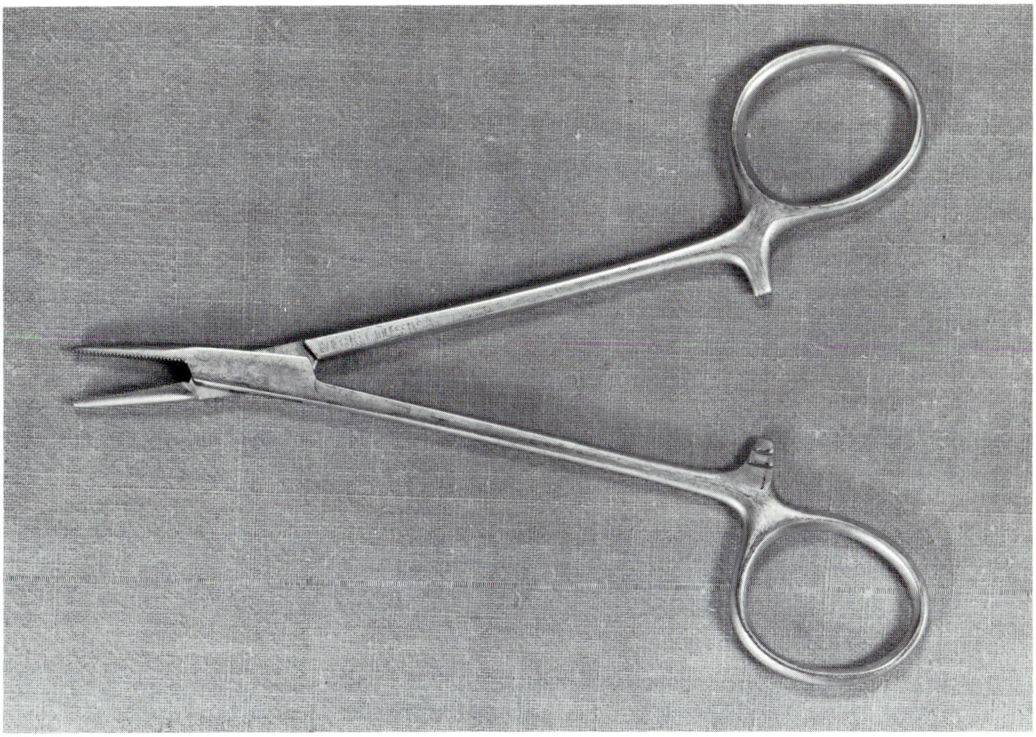

FIGURE 2–35.

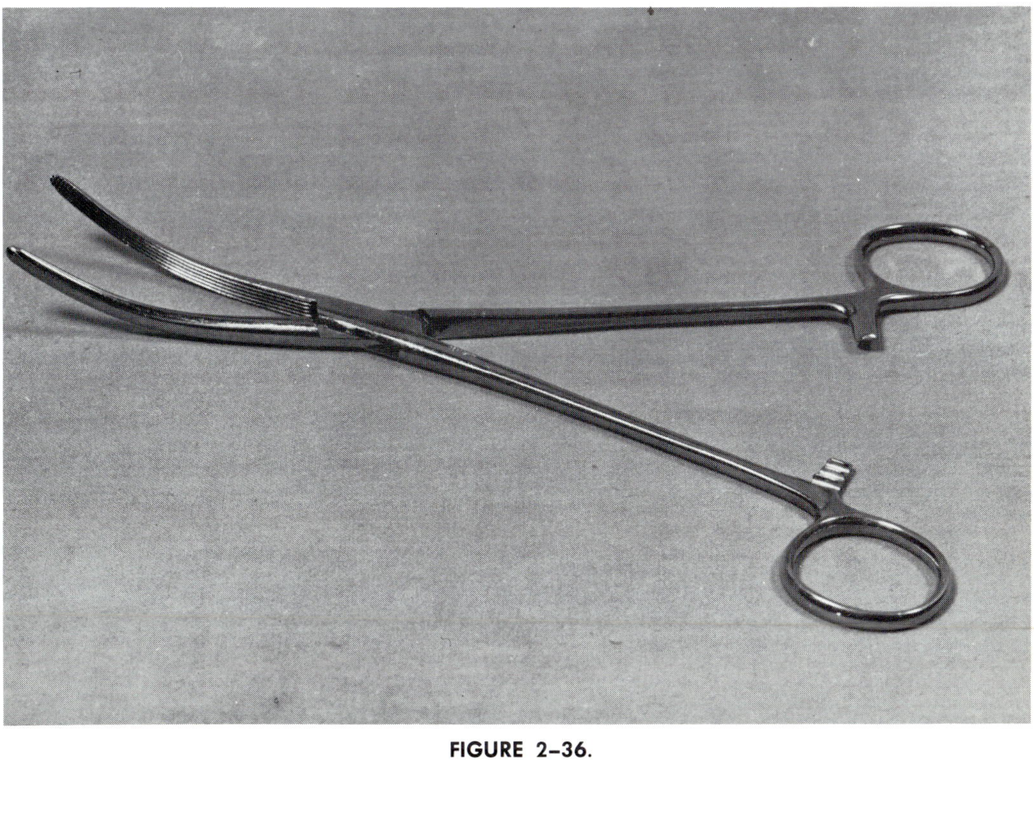

FIGURE 2–36.

FERGUSON ANGIOTRIBE. The angiotribe is used to clamp and crush a large bleeding stump such as the ovarian stump (Fig. 2–37). The jaws are interlocking and have a tongue and groove running the length of the blades. This causes a crimping action on the wide crushed area. Such forceps should be tested before using to make certain that center crushing action does not cut through the tissue. The test is made by clamping the forceps on a piece of grocery twine. If the twine is not cut by the forceps, it is safe to use on tissue.

ALLIS FORCEPS

The Allis forceps comes in a variety of shapes and sizes (Fig. 2–38). Essentially this forceps differs from others in that the tip of the jaw blade is curved inward and flared so that only the tips make contact. The grasping surface is at right angles to the jaw and possesses three to six shallow intermeshing teeth. This forceps is designed for grasping tissue without severely damaging it. It has rather dull teeth and width of purchase. The jaw blades are quite flexible and exert a light, steady pressure.

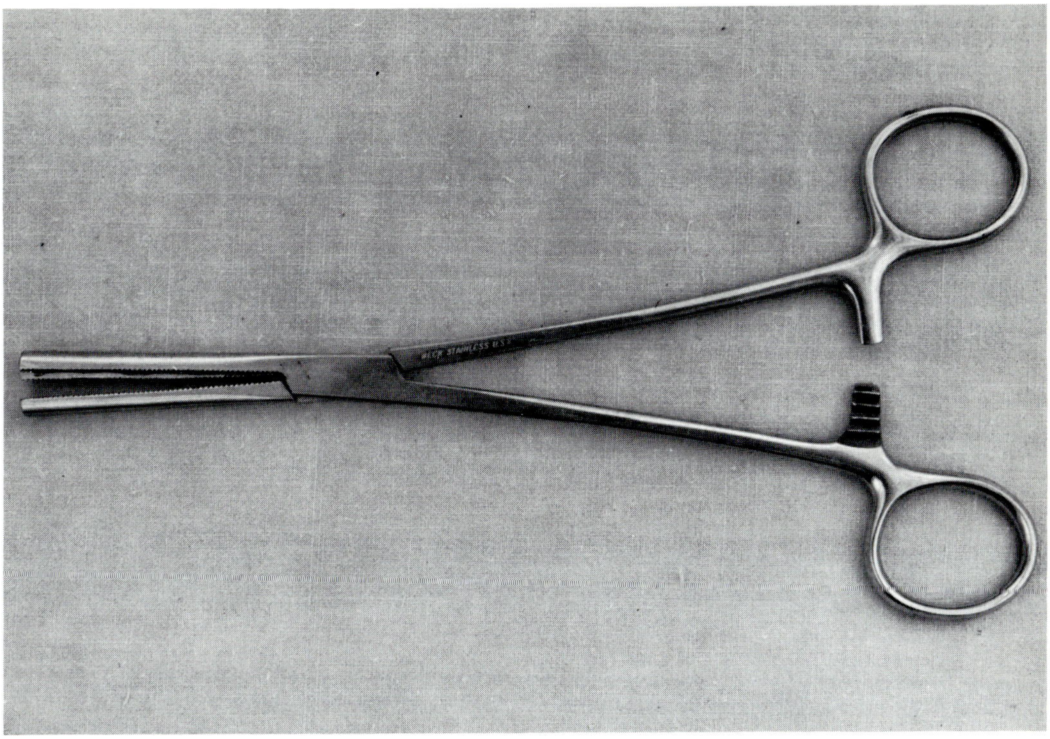

FIGURE 2–37.

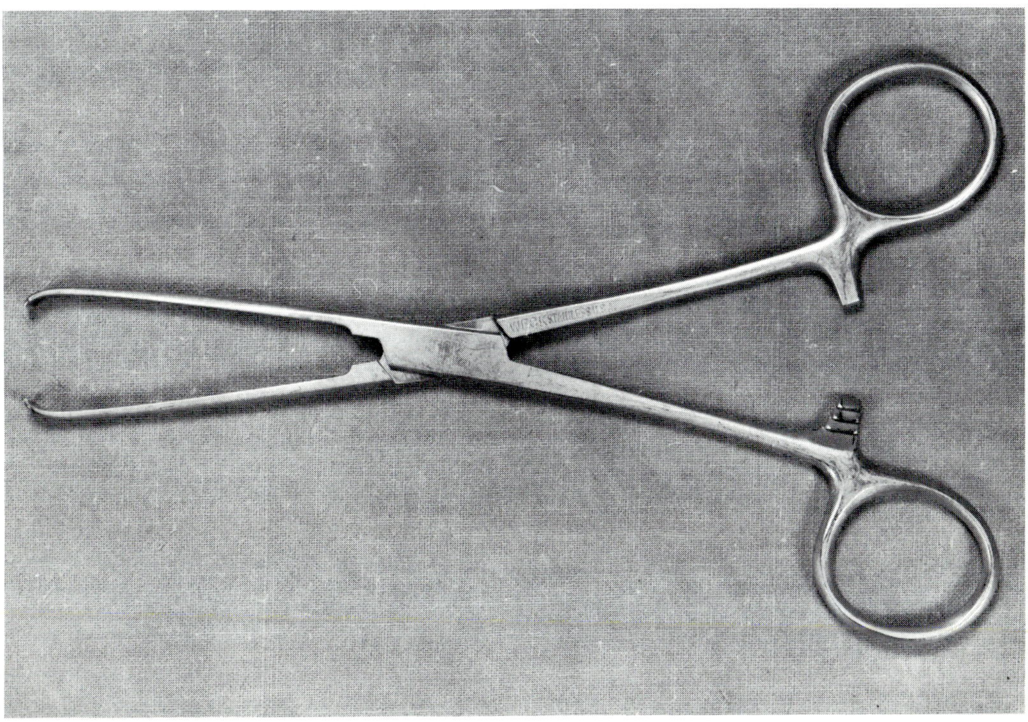

FIGURE 2–38.

SPONGE FORCEPS

Sponge forceps are relatively large with open rings fashioned at the blade tips (Fig. 2–39). The primary use of these forceps is in handling sponges, but they can be used as general utility forceps for handling materials. They are seldom used on tissue except in obstetrics: they make excellent forceps for handling placental membranes.

NEEDLE HOLDER

The selection of a needle holder rests largely with individual preference and to some degree on the type of surgery being performed. There are several choices as to size and shape for each procedure, whether it be abdominal surgery or eye surgery. A good all-purpose needle holder is the Mayo Hegar with narrow jaws (Fig. 2–40). In general, this holder is available in 6, 7, or 8 inch lengths. The ratchet should lock securely, and all sharp edges should be chamfered to prevent snagging of the suture material. Most manufacturers will supply needle holders for either left- or right-handed surgeons.

TOWEL CLAMPS

In canine surgery the towel clamp serves a double purpose: it tacks drapes together to prevent separation, and it anchors the drape to the patient to avoid slipping. Although other types are available, the clamp commonly used has two sharp prongs that grip the skin of the patient. The Backhaus clamp is made like a forceps and can be locked in place by means of a ratchet (Fig. 2–41). This clamp is available in a 3 or 5 inch size.

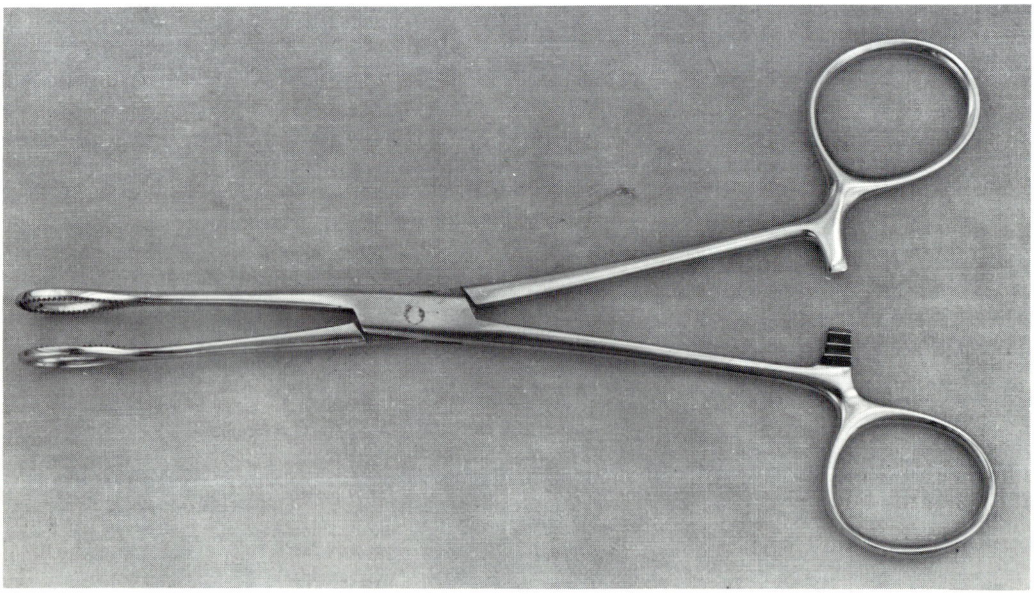

FIGURE 2–39.

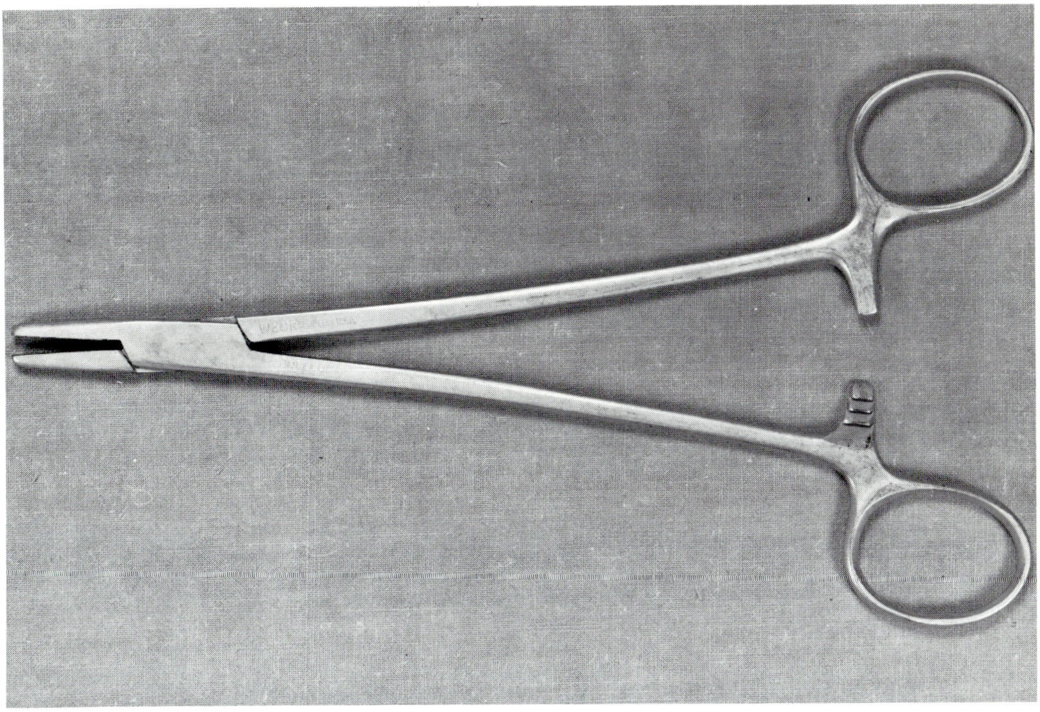

FIGURE 2–40.

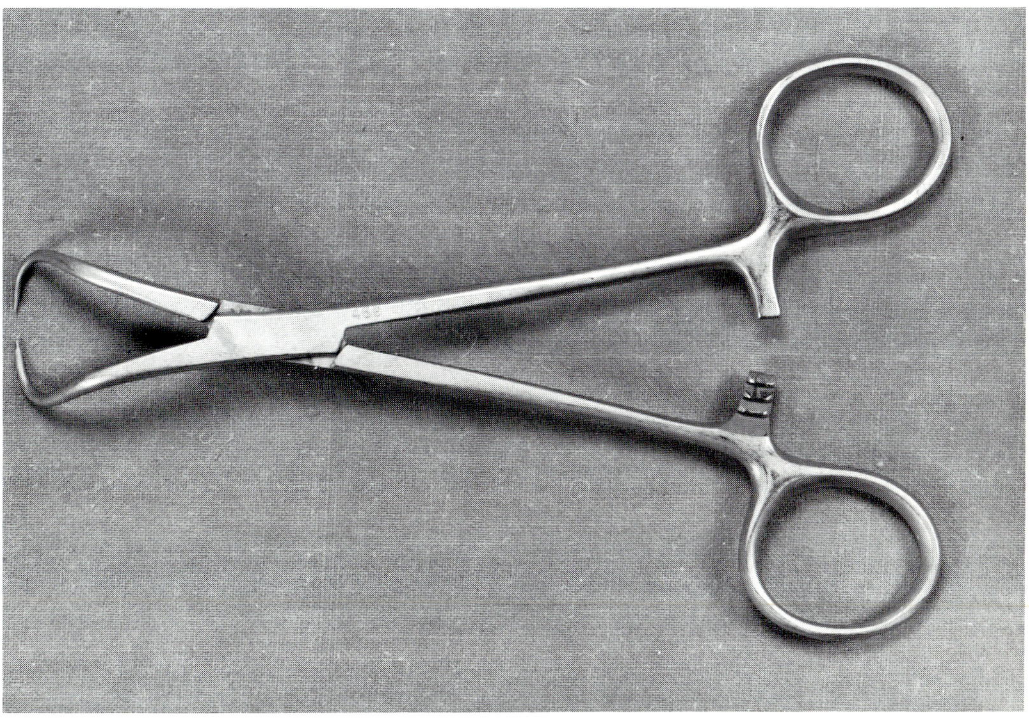

FIGURE 2–41.

PREPARING INSTRUMENTS FOR SURGERY

Good stainless steel instruments are a wise investment. They are easier to clean and keep in repair than chrome instruments because there is less corrosion. They will also last much longer if kept in good repair and handled properly. Most of the deterioration in instruments comes about through improper cleaning and abuse. Surgical instruments should not be used as pliers, screwdrivers, or hammers. Another common abuse is the use of surgical scissors to cut bandages and iris scissors to trim fingernails. Scissors used in this way are often sprung beyond repair.

Cleaning is the first step in preparing instruments for surgery. This step must be thorough. Blood left in the box lock or serrations becomes extremely hardened from the heat of sterilization and thereby interferes with the action and effectiveness of the instrument. Mechanical cleansing is not enough to clear all the debris, and brushing is not recommended because the bristles often become enmeshed in the box lock. If there is delay between surgery and the cleaning process, instruments should be placed in a receptacle of cold water and allowed to soak with all ratchets released and blades open.

The instruments should be washed in cold water to remove the gross soil and then immersed in a good cleaning solution (Figs. 2–42 and 2–43). Immersion in Weck cleaner for 10 minutes is recommended. This solution is made by adding ½ ounce of Weck cleaner to 1 gallon of water. After cleaning, the instruments are thoroughly rinsed in hot running water and placed between two towels so that they can be dried by blotting (Fig. 2–44). They are then sorted, and the basic instruments are placed in a stainless steel or enamel tray ready for packing. Special instruments are wrapped separately. The arrangement in the tray is optional, but it should be orderly and all locking devices should be open. If a tray 8 by 12 inches is used, there will be adequate space for placing a smaller tray within the larger one to hold small instruments such as hemostats and needles. The smaller tray can be used for fluids if necessary during surgery. There will be ample room in the large tray for the remaining basic instruments as well as a good supply of sponges.

When the packing is completed, the tray is placed in the center of a double-thickness muslin wrapper on a diagonal so that the sides face the corners of the wrapper (Fig. 2–45). This wrapper should be 36 by 60 inches unfolded and 36 by 30 inches folded. The use of a large wrapper makes it possible to use the same wrapper as a sterile covering for the instrument stand when the tray is opened for use. The tray is wrapped by folding the wrapper in the same manner as was described for the gown. The wrapper is folded over the short sides of the tray first (Figs. 2–46 to 2–49).

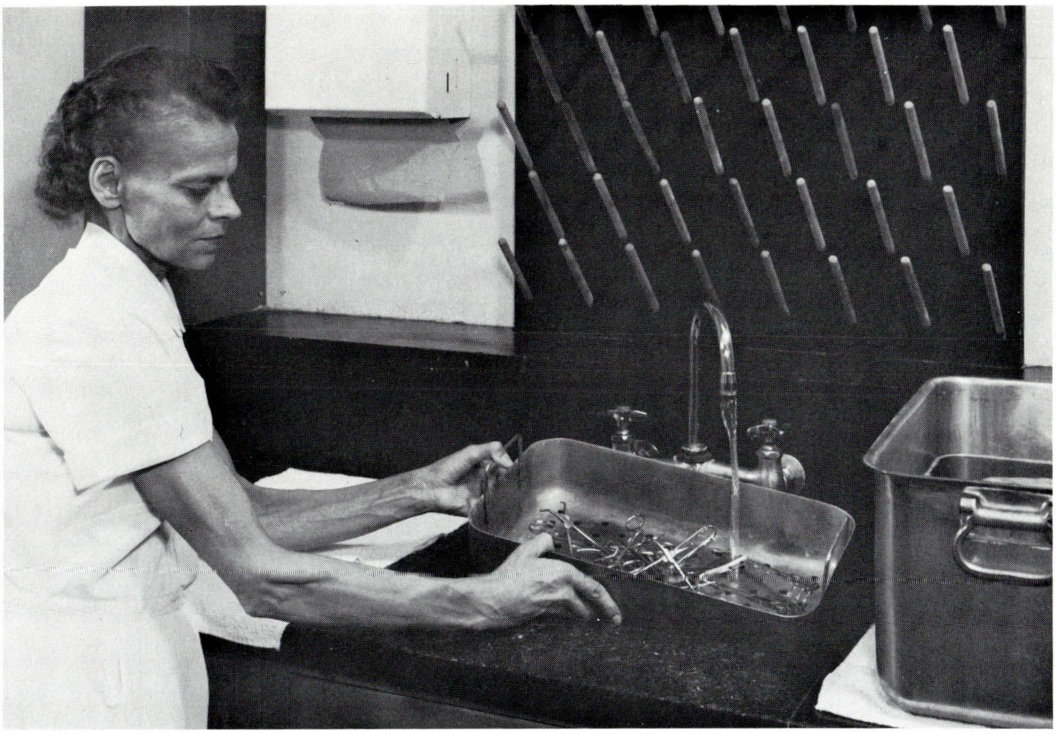

FIGURE 2-42.

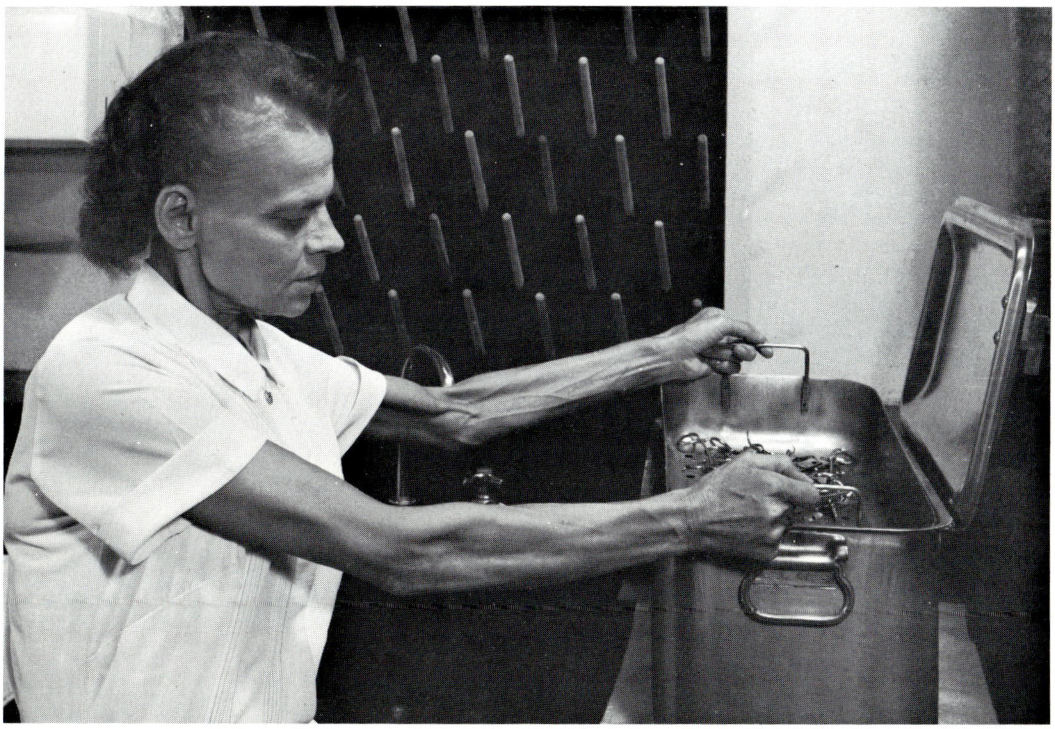

FIGURE 2-43.

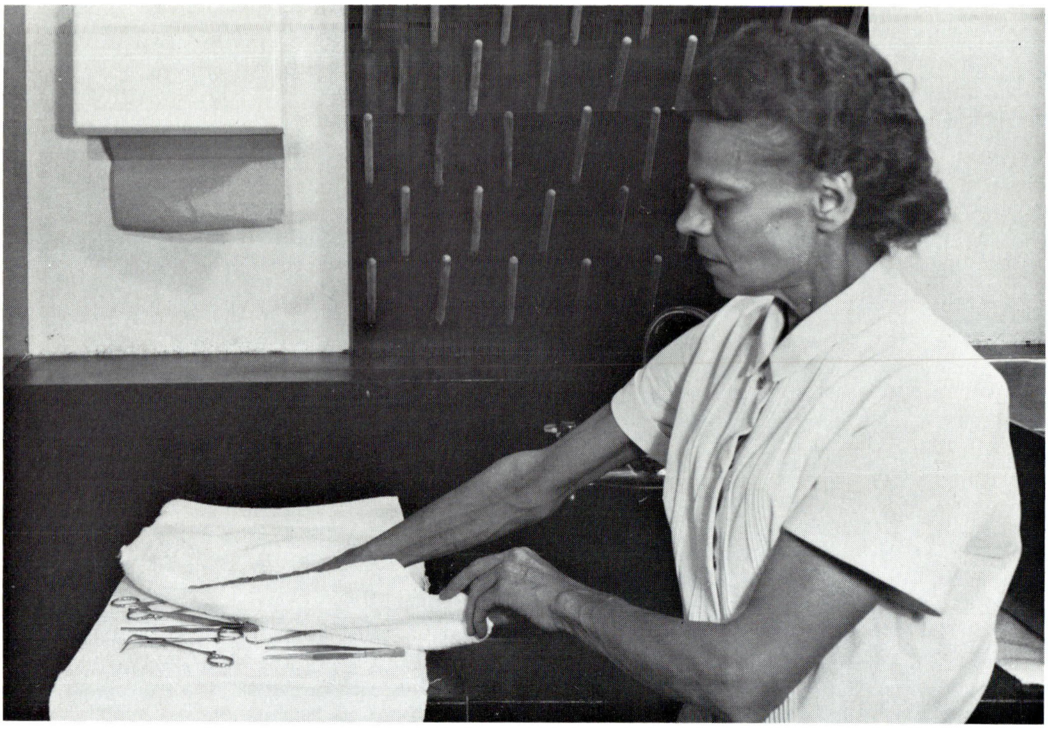

FIGURE 2–44.

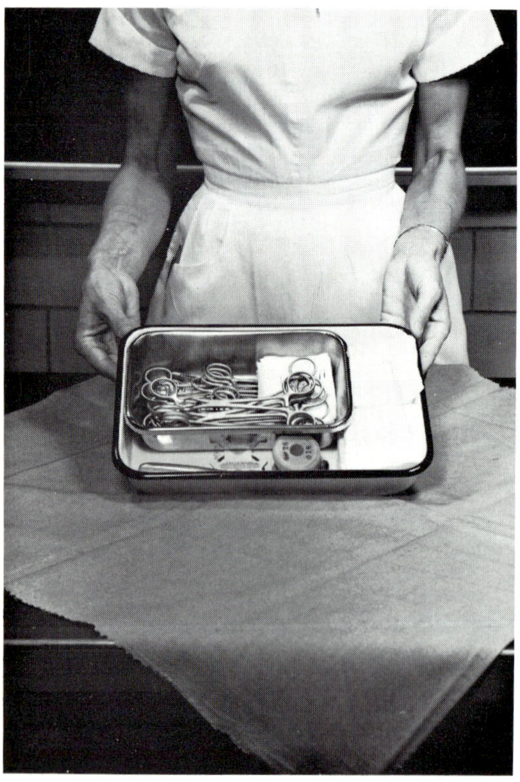

FIGURE 2–45.

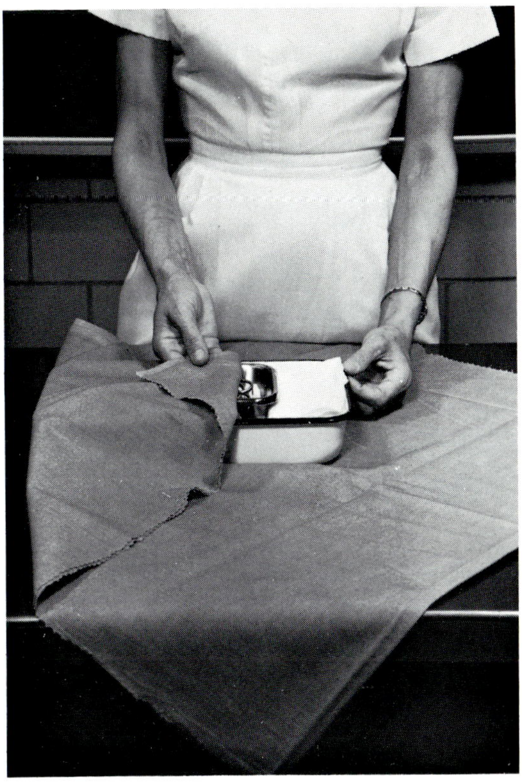

FIGURE 2–46.

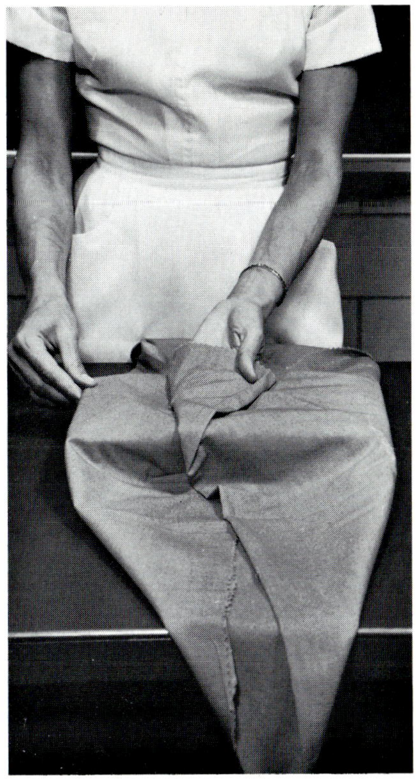

FIGURE 2–47.

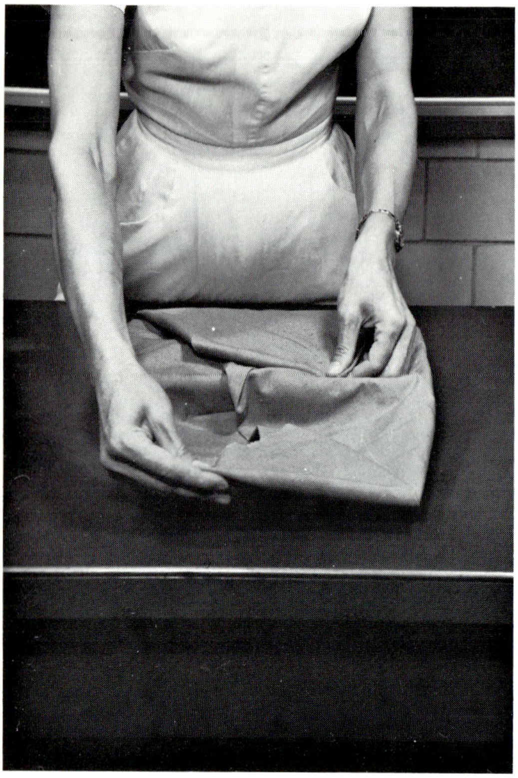

FIGURE 2–48.

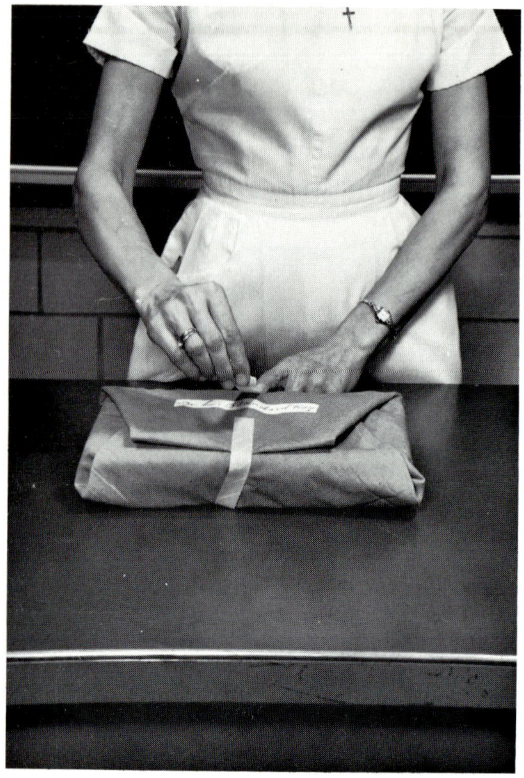

FIGURE 2–49.

Special instruments, syringes, catheters, and small sterilizable equipment should be wrapped separately and labeled for easy identification. Plastic tubing in various diameters is available for easy packaging and identification. After selecting the proper diameter, the tubing is cut at the desired length. The instrument is inserted into the tube and the ends are closed by folding (Fig. 2–50). The fold is held in place by pressure-sensitive indicator tape or a paper clip. Syringes should be packed disassembled with a guard over the needle to prevent puncturing the plastic tubing (Fig. 2–51). They can be assembled inside the pack before it is opened.

Male x-ray catheters should be packed with a tab attached for easy extraction. The end of the tab is folded on the outside of the pack and therefore can only be touched by a nonsterile attendant.

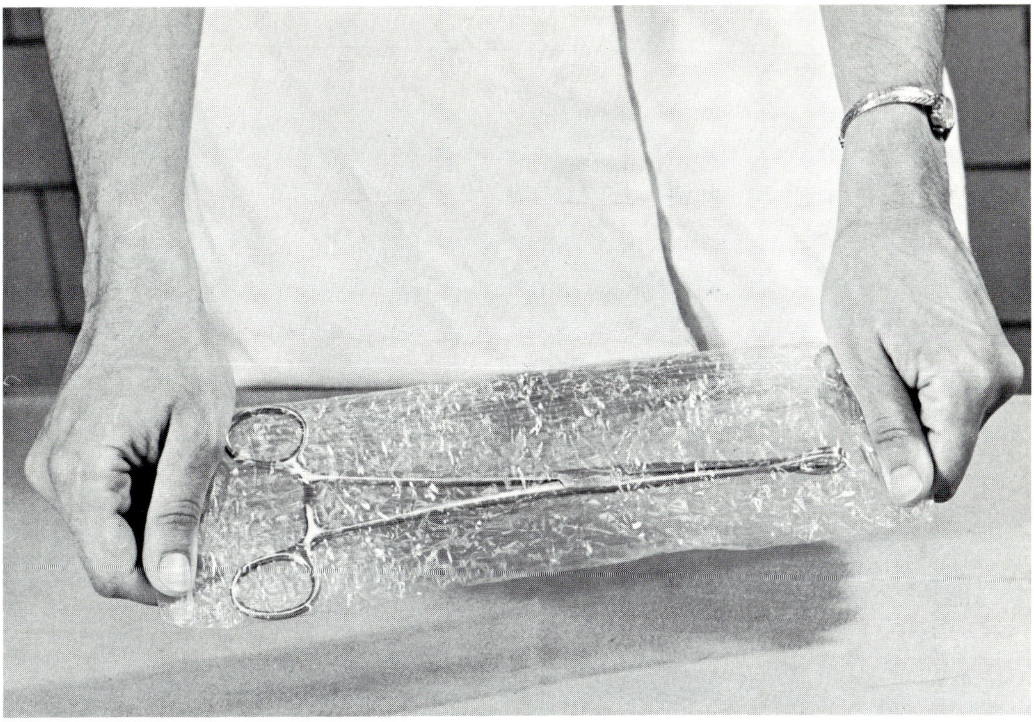

FIGURE 2–50.

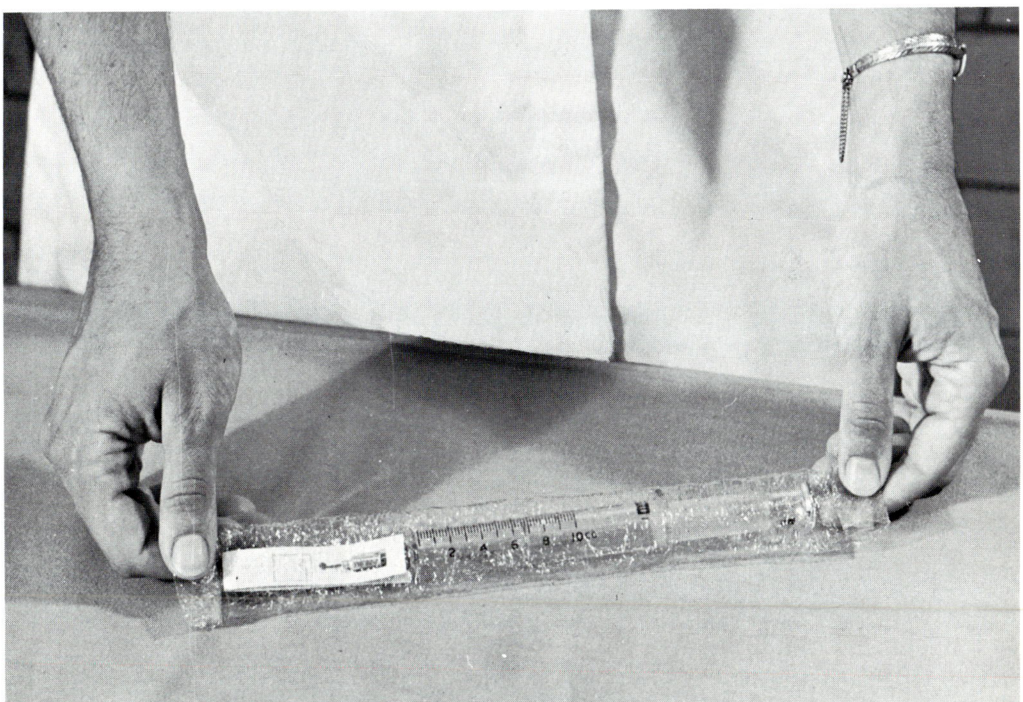

FIGURE 2–51.

SUTURE MATERIALS

A suture has been variously described as a strand, cord, thread, or band of pliable material used to mechanically appose living tissue. By common usage the term "suture" is used as a noun to denote any material used for the purpose of sewing or ligating. When the term is used as a verb, it designates the act of approximating tissue by sewing. Frequently the word "suture" is also used to signify a method of sewing (Cushing suture), but the word "stitch" is preferable (Cushing stitch) because it differentiates the method from the material.

There is a wide variety of materials that can be used for suturing. Some are used externally exclusively; some are used internally, or buried; and some may be used interchangeably. In general, those materials that are used externally are nonabsorbable, whereas those that are buried can be either. Nonabsorbable sutures such as silk, cotton, nylon, polyester fiber, stainless steel, and tantalum are frequently buried in sterile wounds.

EXTERNAL SUTURES

Sutures that hold the skin in apposition and are tied or fastened externally are called external sutures. These sutures usually penetrate only the skin. In some instances, however, they may include the deeper structures, as in the case of the vertical mattress stitch, the vertical figure-of-eight stitch, and the through-and-through stitch. Materials used as external sutures are braided silk, twisted silk, silk specially treated to make it non-capillary, silkworm gut, cotton, nylon, polyester fiber, monofilament or multifilament stainless steel wire, and tantalum. Other materials that could conceivably be classified as external sutures are metal skin clips and plastic skin closure strips.

SILK

Silk is obtainable in either black or white and in sizes from 5 (large diameter) to 7-0 (small diameter). It is processed in a braided form or twisted. Some silk sutures are specially treated with a nonabsorbable coating to reduce capillarity. Usually the fibers in these strands are straight and the surface exceptionally smooth. Silk may be purchased in strands of various lengths or on spools of 25 or 100 yards.

COTTON

Surgical cotton is supplied in sizes from 2 (large diameter) to 5-0 (small diameter) and may be purchased either on 100 yard spools or in precut lengths of 18 to 30 inches. It is made of long staple cotton without filler. The strands are twisted rather than braided. While cotton gains strength when wet, it still does not have the tensile strength of silk.

Ordinary sewing cotton is sometimes used for external suturing; however, it is rougher than surgical cotton and contains fillers which can be irritating. Sizes commonly used are 30 and 60. Mercerized cotton is slightly stronger, but it does not compare in tensile strength with other external suture materials.

NYLON

Nylon, a synthetic nonabsorbable material, is available as a monofilament suture or in a braided form. It is smooth, flexible, and nonirritating in the tissues. It is slightly more resilient than silk or cotton and therefore re-requires extra throws in tying, to prevent loosening of the knot. The monofilament is supplied in sizes 0 to 5-0 and the braided in sizes 5 to 6-0. Usually nylon is dyed a dark color for the purpose of identification.

POLYESTER FIBER

This is a synthetic fiber derived from ethylene glycol and terephthalic acid. The filaments of polyester fiber are braided into sutures of high tensile strength. It is slightly stronger than braided silk or nylon and approximately half again as strong as cotton. It will withstand autoclaving well although, like silk, there is some shrinkage. There is very little tissue reaction to this substance. It may be used either externally or internally. The sizes are 2 to 6-0, and it is marketed under the trade name of Mersilene. Its chief disadvantage is that it requires a bulky knot to prevent slipping.

SILKWORM GUT

Silkworm gut is made from the contents of the silk sack taken from the silkworm. This material, which hardens rapidly, is stretched into strands of about 18 inches and allowed to dry. Three sizes, fine, medium, and coarse, are available and come in lengths of about 12 to 16 inches. Silkworm gut is stiff and must be conditioned by soaking in hot sterile water before use. Its principal use is as a tension suture in the skin.

STAINLESS STEEL

Stainless steel wire has gained wide acceptance as both an external suture and an internal, or buried, suture. Because of the possibility of corrosion in the tissues, only a certain type of stainless steel can be used. It is available as monofilament or multifilament and comes in sizes from 0 (large diameter) to 6-0 (small diameter). Stainless steel monofilament may also be purchased on spools with diameters given in wire gauge. Common sizes in use range from 26 gauge (large) to 40 gauge (small), although wire as large as 18 gauge is available. Wire has good tensile strength and is inert in the tissues; therefore, it can be used either externally or internally.

TANTALUM

Tantalum, like stainless steel, is a metal that is inert in the tissues. The wire in common use is monofilament in sizes from 4 to 6-0. A braided strand is also available. It can be used either externally or internally.

METAL CLIPS

Although metal clips are frequently used in human surgery, their use in small animal surgery is limited. They will hold the skin in apposition over flat surfaces if not disturbed by movement or interference, but dogs and cats are inclined to lick and chew or otherwise dislodge metal clips.

SKIN CLOSURE STRIPS

These adhesive strips are available in sterile packets of 10. They are ¼ inch wide and 4 inches long (6.3 mm. by 102 mm.) and can be placed across an incision to hold the skin edges in apposition. There is very little use for them in small animal surgery, but they can be used to good advantage in human plastic surgery of the face.

OTHER EXTERNAL SUTURE MATERIALS

There are a number of specially prepared suture materials and synthetics that have appeal to veterinarians for one reason or another, but in most cases their disadvantages outweigh their advantages. None holds an overall superiority to those already mentioned.

INTERNAL SUTURES

Sutures that are buried in the tissues or enclosed within the body are referred to as internal sutures. Both absorbable and nonabsorbable materials are used for this purpose. It is desirable, however, to use absorbable sutures wherever possible if the factors of infection, edema, and prolonged stress are not present. Absorbable sutures do not maintain tension for long periods, and their disintegration produces an inflammatory reaction. Nonabsorbable sutures are encapsulated and remain as a foreign body in the tissues. If infection is present, such materials as silk and cotton may harbor organisms and set up a focus of infection and abscess formation. Stainless steel and tantalum are impervious and are therefore safer in the presence of infection.

CATGUT

Catgut is the suture material most commonly used for internal suturing. This material is obtained from the submucosal layer of sheep intestine and is made into catgut by a lengthy processing procedure. It is not, as the name implies, a product procured from the feline family.

The word "catgut" has a very interesting derivation. It has its origin in the word *kitgut*, which was the name given to the strings on the violin used by the ancient Arabians. These strings were made from the intestines of various mammals. The violin was known as a *kit*; hence the word *kitgut*. It is thought that, with the passage of time, *kit* was misinterpreted as referring to a kitten, which accounts for the eventual change from *kit* to "cat."

Catgut is sealed in a foil packet with a small amount of storage fluid. This fluid is composed of isopropyl alcohol, sodium nitrite, diethylethanolamine, and water. Because the catgut is packaged this way, it is nonboilable.

Like any protein, catgut is converted to gelatin in the presence of water and heat. The nature of the storage fluid therefore determines whether the packet can be sterilized by heat on the outside. Heat by boiling would destroy the gut in this storage fluid. It should be kept away from all forms of heat.

The foil packet is sealed in an outer covering, or "pull-apart" package. The packet is then sterilized by irradiation with cobalt–60 or by dry heat and ethylene oxide gas. The outer package can be handled by a nonsterile person who can pull it open and drop the foil packet directly on the instrument tray. If the packet is not used, it must be kept in storage fluid or returned to the manufacturer for repackaging and resterilization.

By tearing the foil packet, the catgut is exposed for use. No attempt should be made to salvage catgut that has been removed from the packet.

Another method of packaging in general use is a double envelope of plastic material.

Catgut can be purchased in a variety of lengths and in sizes from 3 to 6-0. It is an absorbable suture in which the rate of absorption is controlled by chromicizing (tanning) the strands. Tissue enzymes cannot digest chromic catgut as rapidly as plain catgut, and the more heavily the catgut is chromicized the longer it maintains its tensile strength. However, the length of time that any type of catgut remains intact is relative. The kind of tissue, the condition of the patient, the presence of fluids or infection, and many other factors determine the rate of absorption. According to its ability to maintain strength in the tissue, catgut is classified in ascending order as Plain—type A, Mild Chromic—type B, Medium Chromic—type C, and Extra Chromic—type D. The types most commonly used are Plain and Medium Chromic. The various types, sizes, and lengths are available in sterile form.

NONABSORBABLE INTERNAL SUTURE MATERIALS

Many external suture materials can be used internally with good results if there is due respect for the fact that these sutures remain in the tissues as encapsulated foreign bodies. Small sizes of suture should be employed, stitches should be of an interrupted type, and knots should be simple. It has been found that less inflammatory reaction is caused by several rows of small size interrupted stitches than by fewer rows of large size interrupted or continuous stitches. It is important, therefore, to reduce the amount of nonabsorbable suture to the minimum acceptable for good closure.

SILK. Silk has been buried in the tissues by surgeons since the middle of the nineteenth century. The extensive use of silk for internal suturing was advocated by Halsted, and this practice has continued to the present day. Silk can only be used successfully in tissues that are sterile, and even then granulation and cyst formation may occasionally occur as the result of mild irritation. The degree of inflammatory reaction of the tissues to silk is much less than that caused by the digestion and absorption of catgut. It should not be allowed to protrude into the lumen of hollow organs (stomach, intestines, bladder), because it creates a nidus of infection. This may result in the formation of ulcers in the digestive tract and calculi in the urinary tract.

COTTON. Of all the nonmetallic suture materials, cotton produces the least inflammatory reaction. The ends can be cropped closer because of the improved friction of the knot, and there is less likelihood of the strand untwisting. There is less tissue ingrowth and therefore fewer sinuses due to the presence of infection. It does not retain its tensile strength as well as silk or nylon, however.

Because it shrinks when sterilized, it should be removed from the spool and wound on rubber tubing or a folded gauze sponge.

LIGATURES

Any suture material that can be used internally may be used for ligating. Materials such as catgut, cotton, and silk are most commonly used. Metals in the form of clips have been recommended from time to time since Cushing first used them in 1911. The early clips were made of silver, but those in present-day use are of tantalum. The most recent clip made of tantalum is applied with a special forceps which closes the tips of the clip first, thereby preventing extrusion (Fig. 2–52). The clip can be removed if necessary with another special forceps. When closed, the clip measures about 5 mm., which is slightly larger than necessary for some hemostatic work in small animals.

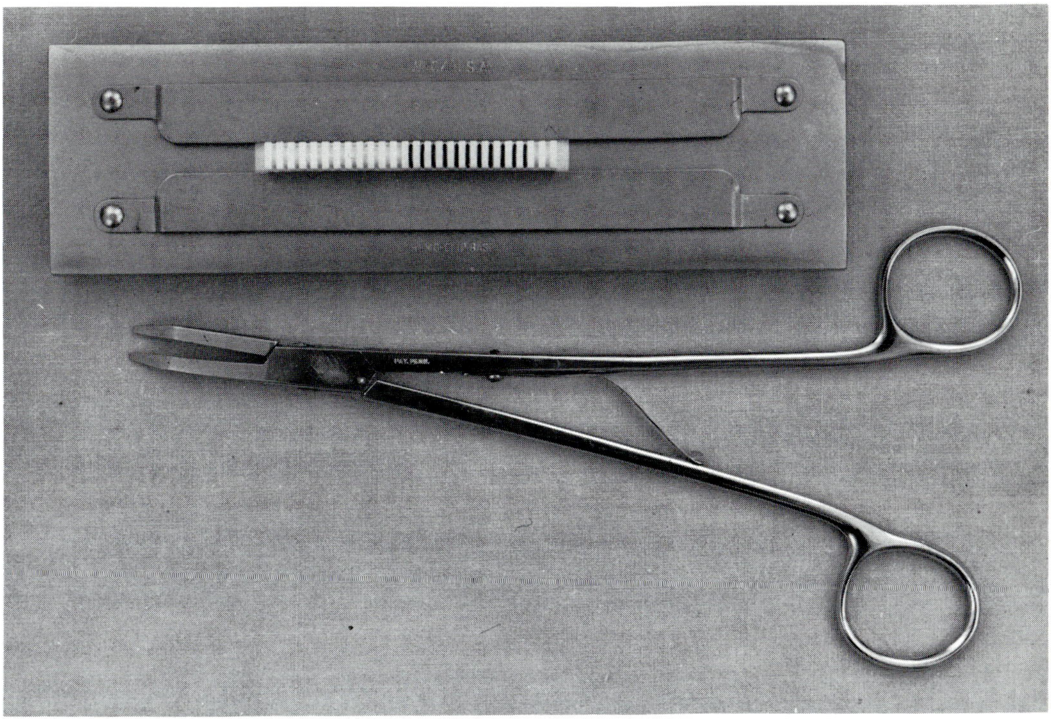

FIGURE 2–52.

REFERENCES

Achsner, A. *J.A.M.A.* 117:2143, 1941.
Artandi, C., and Van Winkle, W., Jr. *Isotopes Rad. Tech.* 2:321–328, 1965.
Cushing, H. *Ann. Surg.* 45:549, 1927.
Ethicon Suture Handbook. 1961.
Guthrie, D. *J.A.M.A.* 117:2143, 1941.
Meade, W. H., and Achsner, A. *Surg.* 7:485–514, 1940.
Meade, W. H., and Long, C. H. *J.A.M.A.* 117:2140–2143, 1941.
Pudenz, R. H. *Surg.* 12:791, 1942.
Samuels, P. B., Roedling, H., Katz, R., and Cincotti, J. J. *Ann. Surg.* 163:427–431, 1966.

Chapter 3

SUTURING AND KNOT TYING

In general it might be said that the principal purpose of suturing and knot tying is to retain tissues in their proper position until they are healed. There are many methods for accomplishing this, only a few of which are adopted by each individual. As long as the basic principles of suturing, ligating, and knot tying are observed, individual preference makes little difference. For example, the continental method of placing a stitch is from near to far, whereas most American surgeons place the stitch from far to near. This reverses the tying procedure, but the basic principles are the same. Each surgeon learns a few procedures well and does not undertake to become proficient in all methods. Experience has shown that well-executed, simple methods are the most effective.

Essentially the fundamental principle involved in suturing, ligating, and knot tying can be stated very simply: Make a firm approximation of all tissues and produce the least amount of trauma possible. In achieving this goal, the tissues must be handled gently, and small size suture material and needles must be used. Each stitch should be placed far enough from the incision so that it does not interfere with healing, but it should not include a large mass of tissue. The stitch should not be tied tightly enough to strangulate the tissue.

Hemostasis must be maintained. Ligatures should not include large masses of tissue and should not be drawn tight enough to cause sloughing of the blood vessel. Fixation of the ligature on large vessels is imperative.

Each tissue layer should be approximated, but not under great tension. Most of the sutures should be placed in the tissues that have the greatest tensile strength, and only enough tension to maintain close approximation should be used. Dead space must be obliterated, even though it requires retention sutures or perhaps a few stitches in tissues of low tensile strength.

Knots should be made simple but secure. The ends should be cropped short. It is well to remember that the body reacts to foreign materials and in some cases encapsulates sutures. For this reason, suture material that is to be left in the tissues should be used in the smallest possible amounts. This can be accomplished by using interrupted stitches of fine material and avoiding bulky knots with long ends. Catgut, because of its tendency to slip, must be cropped slightly longer than silk, cotton, or stainless steel.

MECHANICS OF SUTURING

Accurate apposition of tissues and a smooth closure depends upon accurate mechanical knowledge of the lines of stress in the tissue. It also depends upon the suture material, the needle, and the manner in which they are applied.

SURGICAL NEEDLES

Basically a needle is composed of a point, a shaft, and an eye. Points may be classified as cutting, taper, trocar, triangular, or saber (Fig. 3–1).

Needles are most commonly classified according to the shape of the shaft (Fig. 3–2). They may be five-eighths circle, half circle, or three-eighths circle, depending on the arc formed by the shaft. They may also be half curved, in which case the shaft is partly curved and partly straight, or they may be straight. Some special needles may have shafts that are shaped in other ways (Fig. 3–3). In general, needles with taper and trocar points have round shafts, needles with saber points have oval shafts, and needles with cutting points have triangular shafts. The apex of the triangle forms a cutting edge on the concave surface of the shaft of the curved needle. Needles with the apex of the triangle on the convex surface are known as reverse cutting-edge needles.

Some needles have eyes and others are eyeless. The eyeless needle is known as an atraumatic needle, since it does not require a double strand of suture to follow it through the tissue. The butt end of the needle is hollow, and the suture strand is inserted in it and held in place by pressure. The passageway made by the needle is slightly larger than the suture, and the strand is allowed to pass without further injury to the tissue.

A recent innovation in atraumatic needles is the ribbed needle. This needle has grooves in the shaft which prevent its rotation in the jaws of the needle holder. These grooves are especially helpful in grasping curved needles (Fig. 3–3).

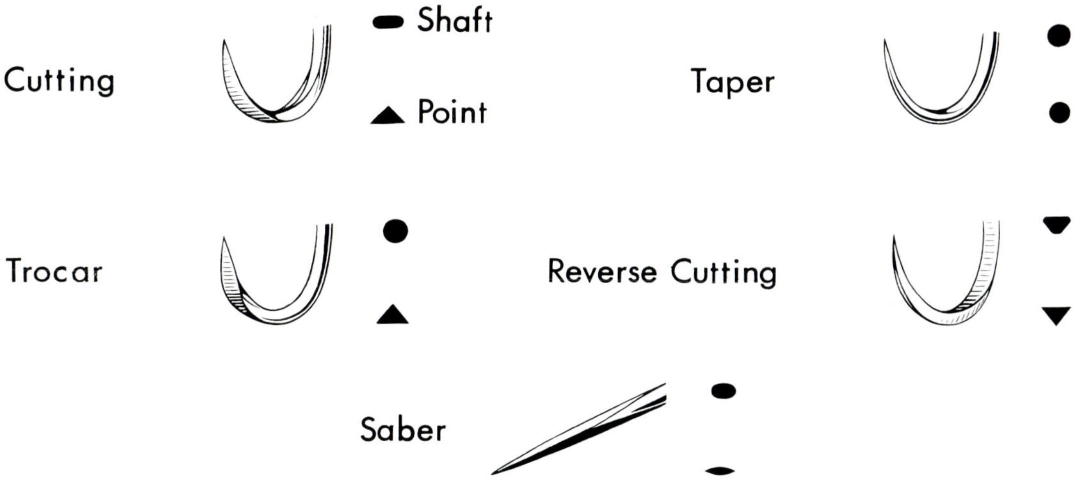

FIGURE 3–1. Needle points.

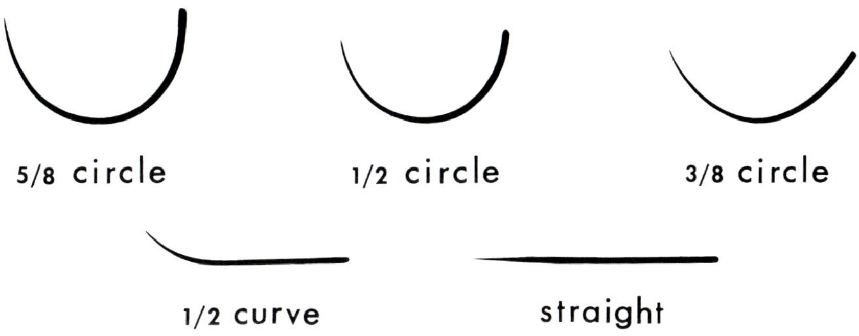

FIGURE 3–2. Needle shafts.

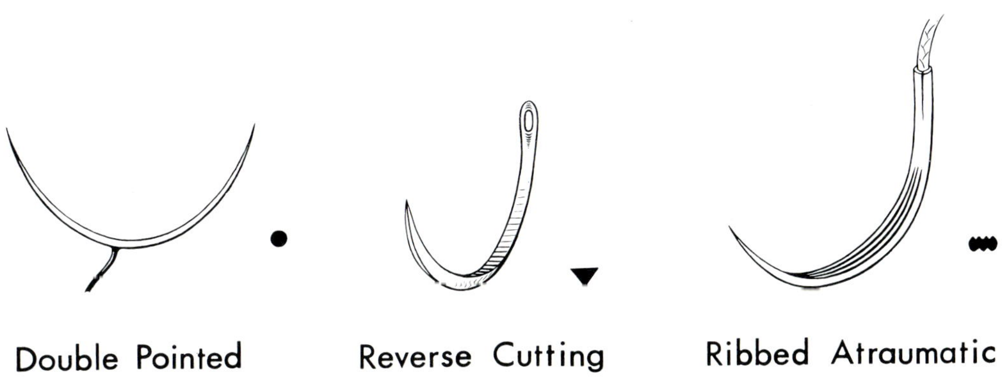

FIGURE 3–3. Special needles.

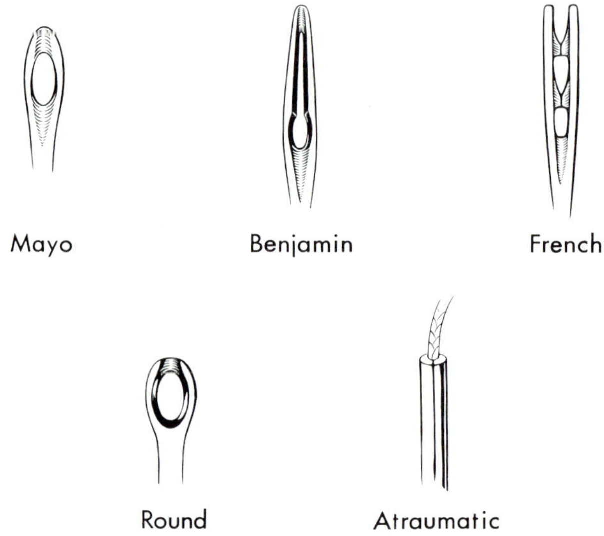

FIGURE 3–4. Needle eyes.

Needle eyes are made in a variety of shapes (Fig. 3–4). Perhaps the most common type of eye is the Mayo. This eye is oblong and grooves extend from the eye to the butt of the needle. The grooves accommodate the doubled strand of suture material after the fashion of a milliner's needle. The Benjamin eye is tapered so that the suture strand will wedge and become self-retaining. The French spring eye is designed for rapid, easy threading. The butt end of the needle is split so that the suture strand can be forced into the eye by stretching it taut across the end of the needle. The round eye, the square eye, and the Hagedorn eye are other types that are occasionally used.

The eyeless or atraumatic needle is gradually replacing the eyed needle. It can be procured in a variety of shapes and sizes that are swaged to accommodate various types of suture material. There are also special needles, such as the double-pointed needle for vascular surgery and the micropoint needle for delicate corneal surgery.

THREADING A NEEDLE

There is no problem involved in threading a needle when the eye is large and the suture small, but when both are approximately the same size, some skill may be required.

Suture material should be cut, not broken, so that the end is smooth. A broken end is frayed and therefore difficult to pass through the eye. One should use suture scissors rather than fine surgical scissors. Occasionally it is necessary to moisten the end of a cotton or silk suture in order to obtain cohesion of the fibre ends. The seamstress accomplishes this by moistening the end with her lips, but the surgeon must moisten it by using sterile saline, or in an emergency he may touch the suture tip to the surgical wound.

The suture is held tightly between the thumb and forefinger, with the end pointing upward at a right angle to the fingers (Fig. 3–5). The tip of the suture should be barely visible. It should be remembered that the suture is not threaded through the eye of the needle, but rather, the needle is placed on the suture. While the suture is held firmly with one hand, the needle eye is forced downward over the suture. Pressure on the suture should be maintained until the needle emerges on the opposite side of the finger and thumb. In the case of curved needles, the concave side should face downward so that the suture will be threaded from inside the curve.

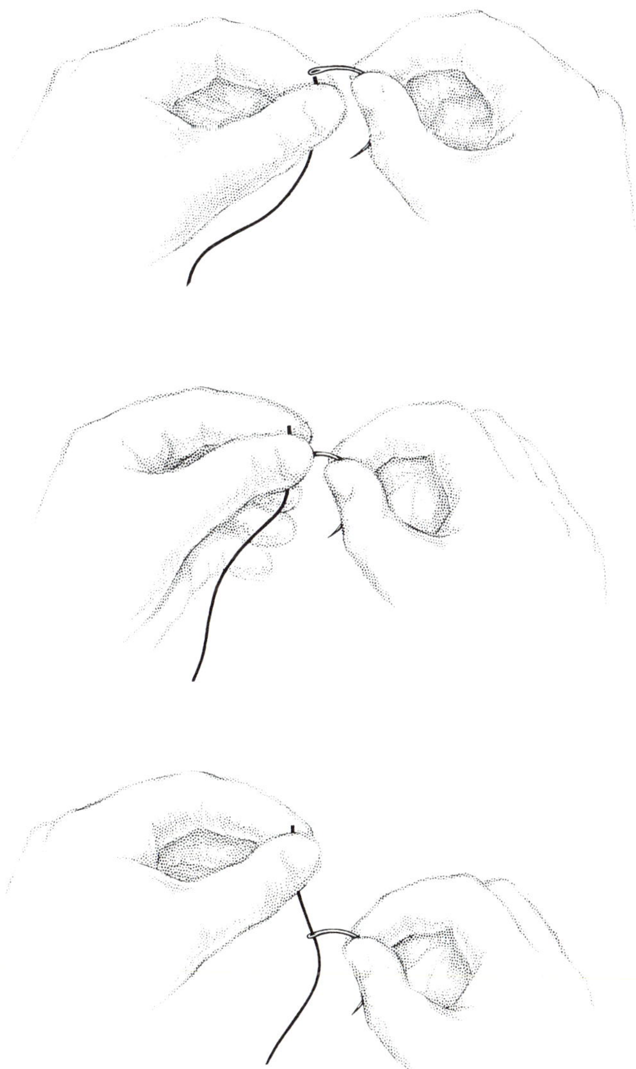

FIGURE 3–5. Threading the needle.

HOLDING THE NEEDLE

Needles should not be hand held in any aseptic surgical procedure, because of the danger of tearing or puncturing the gloves. A suitable needle holder is used to grasp the needle somewhere between the middle of the shaft and a point within one-quarter inch of the eye. Curved needles should be held by the tips of the jaws of the needle holder. Needles should not be clamped near the eye, because of the danger of breaking, nor should they be clamped near or at the point, because of damage to the tip or the cutting edge.

INSERTING THE NEEDLE

Whenever a curved needle is used, the act of inserting the needle into the skin should initiate with a rotation of the wrist so that the movement of the needle is a circular one. If one attempts to insert the needle by applying force in a line which subtends the arc of the needle, the result is a bent or broken needle or at best a difficult insertion.

As stated previously, whether the needle is inserted away from the surgeon or toward him is of little consequence as long as it is properly inserted and as long as all insertions are made in the same direction. Taper-point needles are commonly used in softer tissues such as the hollow organs of chest and abdomen, the blood vessels, the tendons, and the nerves. Cutting needles are required in tissues such as skin and fascia. The reverse cutting-edge needle is particularly advantageous in these tissues. With the cutting edge on the back, this needle does not "cut out" or make openings larger than necessary.

APPROXIMATION OF TISSUES

All other things being equal, the tissues of a surgical wound should be replaced in their normal position. This is not always possible or feasible, but it can be used as a general rule for the closure of most incisions. Healing time can be minimized by the proper approximation of tissues. Special attention should be paid to peritoneum and fascia. The importance of the skin closure has frequently been overemphasized to the detriment of the patient simply because the skin incision is visible following surgery. The condition of the skin closure is often an indication of the type of workmanship that it covers, but if the deep closure is properly done, the skin closure becomes less important. If the deep closure is improperly done, the skin closure is of no importance.

Accurate approximation infers that the suture is not too tight or too loose; that other tissues do not interpose; that tissue layers are not widely separated; and that the wound edges are not unnecessarily traumatized by rough handling, careless clamping, or superfluous suturing. It further infers that only tissues of common histological structure should be sutured and that dead space is to be avoided. Whenever tissue is properly handled and approximated under aseptic conditions, the result will be first intention healing.

The approximation of tissues should be done with gentleness. Unnecessary handling and roughness such as pulling, twisting, tearing, crushing, and rubbing with dry sponges (or even the gloved hand) produces trauma and delay in the healing process.

The interposition of adipose tissue during wound closure can be a detrimental factor in the healing process. In fact, it can and often does lead to wound disruption.

EXTERNAL SUTURING

Sutures that are exposed either on the integument or mucous membrane require slightly different treatment than those that are buried. Since external sutures are removed after the skin or mucous membrane is healed, it is not necessary to be quite so meticulous about the bulk of the knot or the length of the ends. In some cases it may be advantageous to crop the ends comparatively long to facilitate removal.

Exposure to infection can occur either on the body surface or within the skin layers by way of the hair follicles or sebaceous glands. Noncapillary materials, placed only in the skin and less frequently in the mucous membrane, ensure against deep infection from suturing.

TYPES OF STITCHES

There are many types of skin stitches, a few of which will be described. Each surgeon has his favorite way of closing the skin, but for the surgery student the best skin closure is the simple interrupted stitch. A continuous stitch is easily loosened by the disruption of a single bite or by the loss of a single knot.

INTERRUPTED STITCH

The interrupted stitch should be placed in the skin so that it penetrates both the epidermal and corium layers but no more (Fig. 3–6). It should not be placed too near the edge of the incision. An average location would be 5 mm. from the incision, with 5 mm. between stitches. Circumstances can vary these measurements, but these should be considered minimum. The purpose of this stitch is to hold the skin in apposition, but not under tension. If the subcutaneous closure is properly made, there is no need for tension on the skin stitches. The knot should be placed to one side of the incision so that it does not interfere with healing.

CONTINUOUS STITCH

The continuous stitch, sometimes called a running stitch, is started in the same manner as a simple interrupted stitch—that is, by placing the first bite across the incision and tying (Fig. 3–6). The second and subsequent bites may be placed at right angles to the incision or diagnonally to it. In the first case, the exposed suture will run diagonally to the incision, and in the second it will run at right angles. To tie such a stitch, one may hold the free end while the last bite is made, and then tie the loop and the end together. Another method is to take an extra bite parallel to the last bite but in the reverse direction; this leaves a loop to tie to the free end.

MATTRESS STITCH

There are two types of mattress stitch: the horizontal and the vertical (Fig. 3–6). The general rule in making a mattress stitch is to make it as nearly square as possible. The space between bites should be the same as the length of the bite. The horizontal mattress is seldom required in canine surgery and does not give a good cosmetic result, because the edges of the incision are turned outward. This produces oozing during healing and a wide scar afterward. If a mattress suture seems necessary in the skin, the perpendicular mattress can be used to advantage. The deep bite is placed some distance from the incision, and the shallow bite is placed through the corium of the skin so that there is perfect apposition of the skin edges.

RETENTION STITCH

Retention stitches (also called tension stitches, or stay stitches) are frequently referred to and illustrated in surgical texts, but they are seldom used in small animal surgery unless there is a large loss of tissue or undue tension on the suture line for some reason. In most cases the problem can be solved in other ways. This is fortunate, because the skin of the dog will endure very little extra pressure or tension. The retention stitch is placed some distance from the wound and frequently involves some of the deeper tissues. Depending on the tension, it may be padded to distribute pressure.

SPECIAL STITCHES

Probably every surgeon has at least one special stitch that he likes to use under certain circumstances. One example is the figure-of-eight stitch used in an ovariectomy incision in the cat (Fig. 3–6). It is used primarily to facilitate removal. This stitch is placed by inserting the needle diagonally across the incision, crossing the surface to the same side of the incision, and inserting the needle in the opposite diagonal direction. The two ends of the suture are then opposite each other and can be tied. This stitch requires but one snip of the scissors at the spot farthest from the knot to remove it.

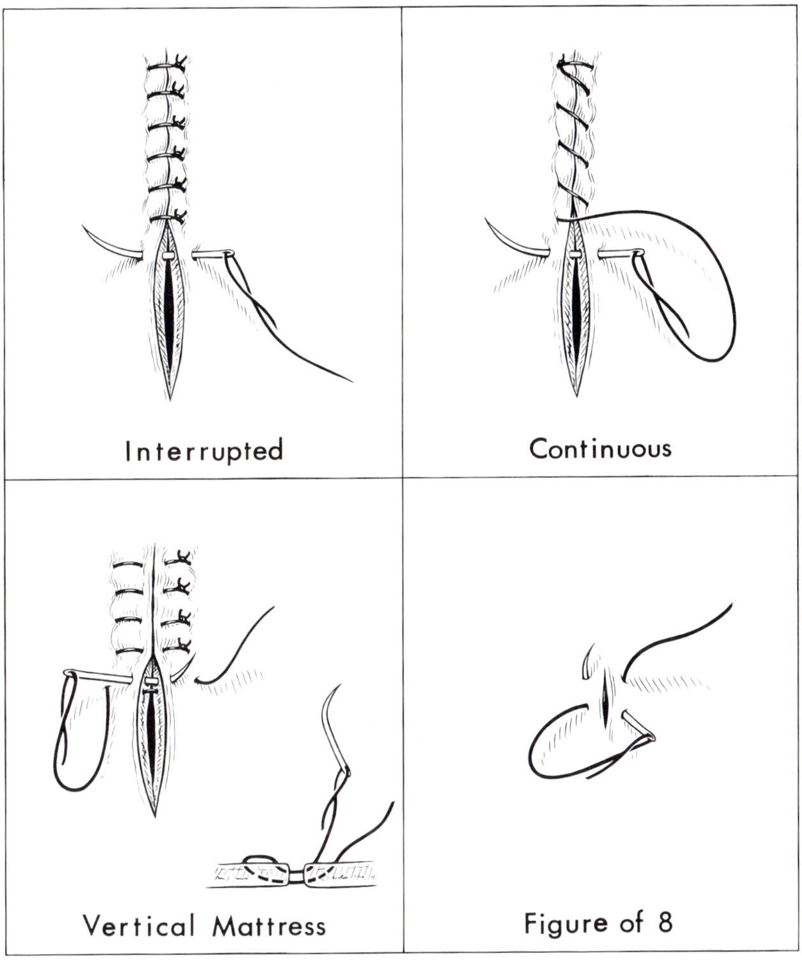

FIGURE 3–6. External stitches.

A special stitch often used for closing the anus and occasionally for other openings is the purse string. In placing this stitch, the bites should be deep enough to give good holding power, and there should be enough bites so that pressure can be evenly distributed. The stitch should be placed about 0.5 cm. from the mucocutaneous border and tied with a bow knot so that it can be released without cutting the suture. This simplifies the problem of replacing the stitch if the need arises.

INTERNAL SUTURING

The principal difference between external suturing and internal suturing is that the suture material is usually removed in the former but seldom removed in the latter. More thought must therefore be given to internal suturing in the way of kinds of material, amounts of material, and types of stitches. The buried suture must be absorbed or encapsulated. If neither occurs the material is extruded. The capillarity of the buried suture is not as important, provided there is no contamination present. The amount of material that is buried depends upon the type of stitch that is made, the bulk of the knot, and the length of the ends. It is therefore important to keep the stitches simple, the knots small, and the ends cropped short.

TYPES OF STITCHES

There are many types of stitches used for internal suturing because there are several types of tissue involved. Some of these tissues heal well when joined end to end and others do not; some hold stitches exceedingly well and some do not; some are exposed to contamination and some are not. Stitches are therefore varied according to the internal conditions.

INTERRUPTED STITCH

The interrupted stitch is the most common internal stitch for the same reason that it is the most common external stitch: It is simple, effective, and safe (Fig. 3–7). Fascia is the tissue most frequently sutured during internal closures, and this tissue lends itself well to the interrupted stitch. These stitches should be small so that they do not include surrounding tissue, and they should be placed close together so that there are no gaps in the suture line or dead space in the incision.

CONTINUOUS STITCH

While seldom used as the principal buried stitch in wound closure, the continuous stitch is commonly used to close the peritoneum (Fig. 3–7). If properly placed, it provides an excellent seal by maintaining uniform pressure along the entire length of the peritoneal opening. Without this seal, wound dehiscence will begin at the peritoneum and spread outward. In old or debilitated animals, the added safeguard of using stainless steel suture for the continuous stitch is well worthwhile. Because of its usefulness in maintaining uniform pressure along an incision, several adaptations have been made for use on hollow organs.

LEMBERT STITCH

The Lembert stitch is used as a continuous as well as an interrupted stitch when it is necessary to appose the serous coats of hollow organs such as

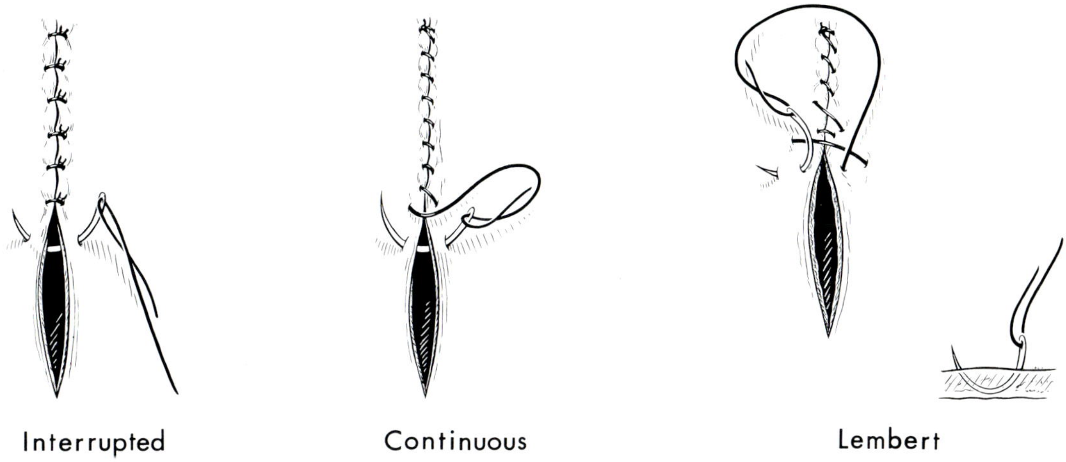

FIGURE 3–7. Internal stitches.

the stomach, intestine, or uterus (Fig. 3–7). The bite is made by inserting the needle through the serous and muscular layers into the submucosal layer. At this point the path of the needle is reversed so that it emerges without penetrating the mucosa. The stitch is then carried across the incision, and the needle is inserted in a like manner on the opposite side. This may be continued for the length of the incision, or it may be separated into individual stitches. The purpose is to roll the external serous surface inward so that the incision will quickly seal when the two serous surfaces are apposed. A taper-point needle should be used to suture hollow organs so that the trauma to tissues will be minimized. This needle also gives a better "feel" for various types of tissue. For example, the needle penetrates the serous and muscular coats very easily but requires more pressure to enter the tougher submucosal layer.

CZERNY STITCH

The Czerny stitch is used to close hollow organs. It is placed in the same direction as the Lembert stitch, i.e., at right angles to the incision. However, the bite is started fairly close to the incision, and when the needle reaches the submucosa, it is directed across the incision into the submucosa on the opposite side. It emerges from the serosa on the opposite side of the incision but in direct line with its entry. Such a stitch can only be used in the first line of a closure. It has the disadvantage of being partly exposed to the contents of the organ during the healing period.

CZERNY-LEMBERT STITCH

Whenever a Czerny stitch is followed by a Lembert stitch the combination is known as a Czerny-Lembert stitch (Fig. 3–7). This combination may be used in organs with a small lumen where two rows of sutures are required.

CUSHING STITCH

The Cushing stitch (Fig. 3–7) is begun in the same manner as the Lembert, but after the first tie is made, the needle is directed parallel to the incision instead of transversely. Bites are made into the submucosa because this is the only tissue of sufficient strength to hold the stitch. Each succeeding bite is begun after crossing the incision to a point opposite the last emergence of the needle. When the stitch is drawn together, the suture should form a straight line.

CONNELL STITCH

The only difference between the Connell (Fig. 3–7) and the Cushing stitch is that the Connell penetrates all layers, including the mucosa. This stitch is sometimes used as a first closure line and followed by a Cushing stitch for a second closure line.

SUBCUTICULAR STITCH

The subcuticular stitch is usually considered an internal stitch, since it is beneath the surface and is not ordinarily removed (Fig. 3–7). It is placed in the corium, or base layer of the skin, and is frequently used in place of external sutures. The stitch is begun by taking bites in the corium on opposite sides of the incision at one end of the incision and tying. Bites are then taken in the corium, parallel to the surface and on alternate sides, until the opposite end of the incision is reached. After pulling the stitch tight, it is ended in the same manner as any continuous stitch, except that the final bite may be placed in the subcutaneous tissue so that the knot will be pulled well below the surface of the skin.

The subcuticular stitch should not be used in areas subject to excessive strain. It does not have strong anchorage and is used mostly where a good cosmetic effect is desired. It should not be confused with the subcutaneous stitch.

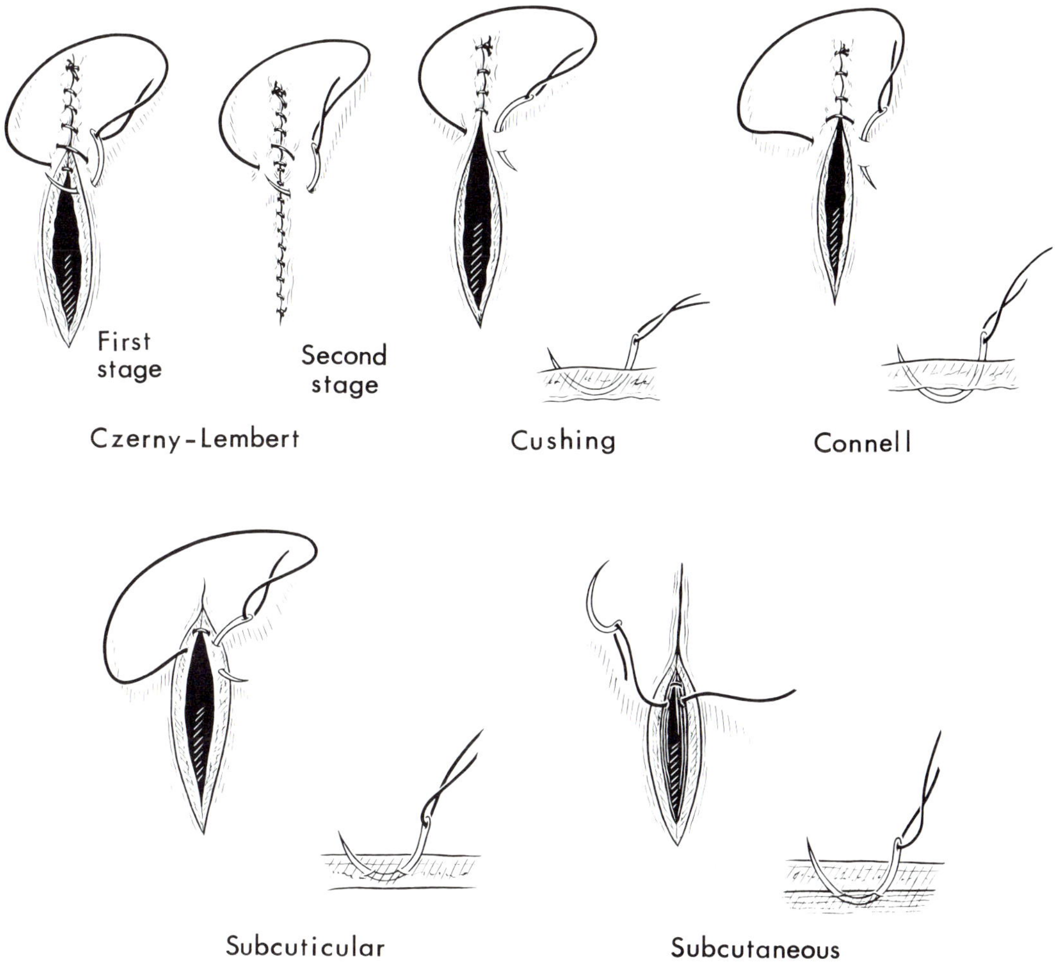

FIGURE 3–7. *Continued.*

SUBCUTANEOUS STITCH

Whenever strong support of the skin incision is needed for proper closure, the subcutaneous stitch is used (Fig. 3–7). This is an interrupted stitch placed in the layer between the corium and the fascia. Situated beneath the skin is a layer of subcutaneous connective tissue composed of oblique elastic fibers, lymphatic and blood vessels, nerves, and fat. When this layer is properly drawn together, there is little or no tension required of the skin sutures.

The subcutaneous stitch is placed by taking a bite on either side of the incision, parallel to the surface, and drawing it together with a square knot. In many instances, when this suture line is completed, the skin will be in apposition.

KNOT TYING

Knot tying is an art that requires considerable practice. This practice, however, should not be devoted to complicated knots and elaborate procedures. One should learn to tie a simple and secure knot. Each "throw"* of the knot should lie flat. To accomplish this, the ends of the second throw must be drawn in the direction opposite that of the first throw. The importance of flat tying is illustrated by the fact that both the square knot and the granny knot are converted to slip knots if they are not tied flat.

The surgeon should be familiar with the square, granny, slip, and surgeon's knots, but he should rely primarily on the square knot in most of his surgery. He should practice this tie until he can accomplish it with ease yet at the same time produce a secure knot. Two-hand ties and instrument ties or a combination of the two produce safer knots because there is less likelihood of producing a slip knot. It is not uncommon to produce a slip knot with the one-hand tie. The combination tie is used whenever the first throw requires tension to keep it in place until the second throw can be completed.

Some suture materials require an extra throw because the surface does not create sufficient friction. Such materials as catgut, nylon, and other synthetics require more than a simple square knot. An extra throw adds much to the safety of the tie.

The following illustrations portray simple methods of tying for both the right-handed and the left-handed operator. It should be borne in mind that the incision line is left to right and that the suture has been inserted toward the operator. The black part of the suture would therefore represent the short end, or trailing end.

SQUARE KNOT

The square knot is the common surgical knot and the most widely accepted. It consists of one throw superimposed upon another, with the second throw in the reverse direction to the first. This knot is also known as the true knot, the reef knot, and the flat knot.

RIGHT-HANDED OPERATOR—TWO HANDS (FIG. 3–8)

STEP 1. The short strand (black) is grasped in the right hand.

STEP 2. It is crossed over the long strand (white).

STEP 3. The two ends are grasped at the crossing point by the thumb and index finger of the left hand.

STEP 4. The left thumb and index finger are rotated to force the short end through the loop that has been formed.

STEP 5. The short end is picked up by the right hand.

STEP 6. The loop is drawn tight by pulling the long strand away from the operator with the left hand and the short strand toward the operator with the right hand.

---

*Variously referred to as a simple knot, a half-hitch, and a loop.

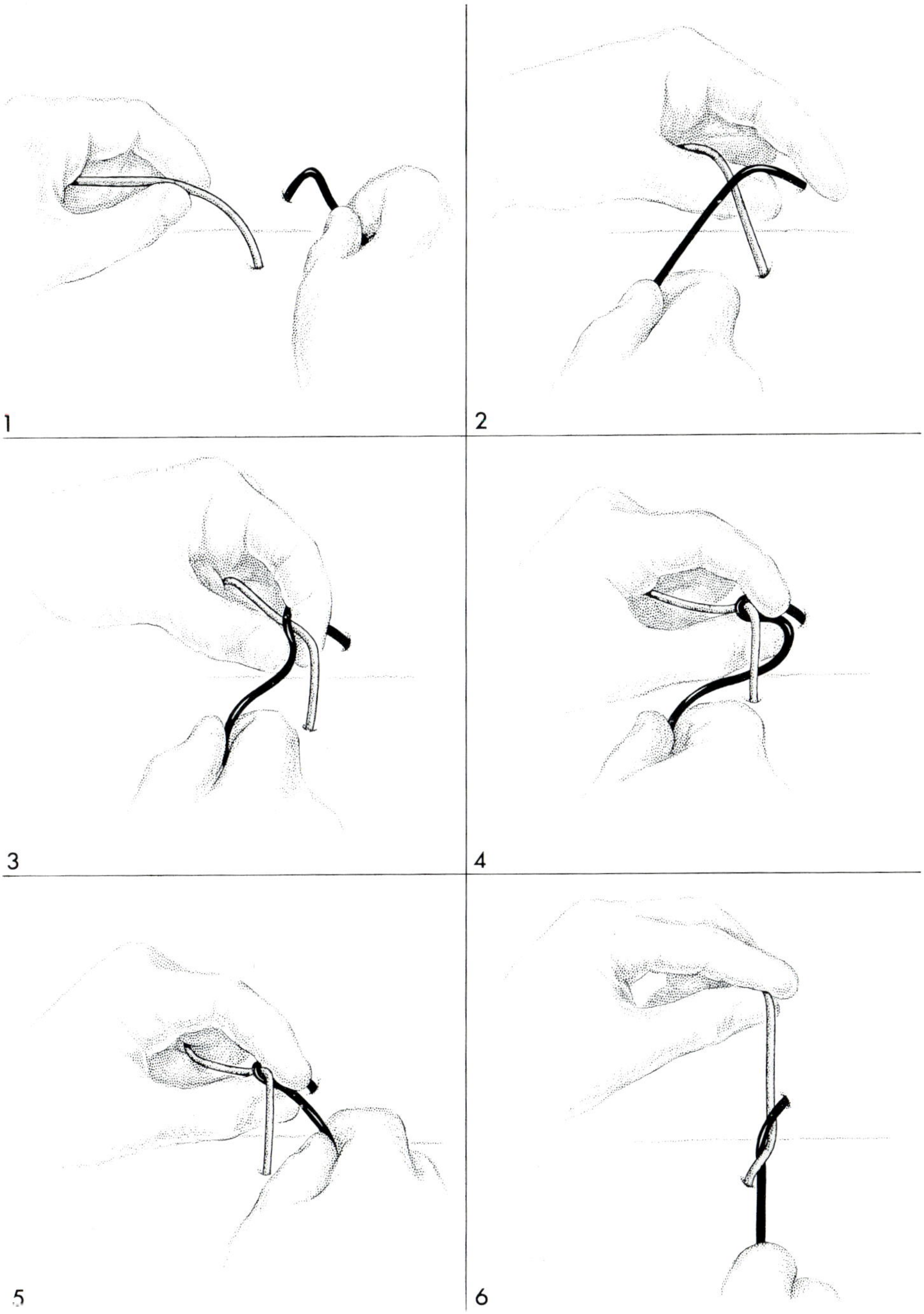

FIGURE 3–8. Square knot. Two-hand tie for right-handed operator.

RIGHT-HANDED OPERATOR—TWO HANDS (FIG. 3–8) *Continued*

STEP 7. The short strand is looped over the left thumb, and the long strand is lifted with the left forefinger.

STEP 8. The long strand is allowed to drop across the left thumb. At the same time, the short strand crosses the long.

STEP 9. The strands are grasped at the point of intersection by the left thumb and forefinger.

STEP 10. The left index finger rotates the short strand downward through the loop.

STEP 11. The short end is grasped by the right hand.

STEP 12. Traction on the short end is away from the operator and on the long end toward the operator.

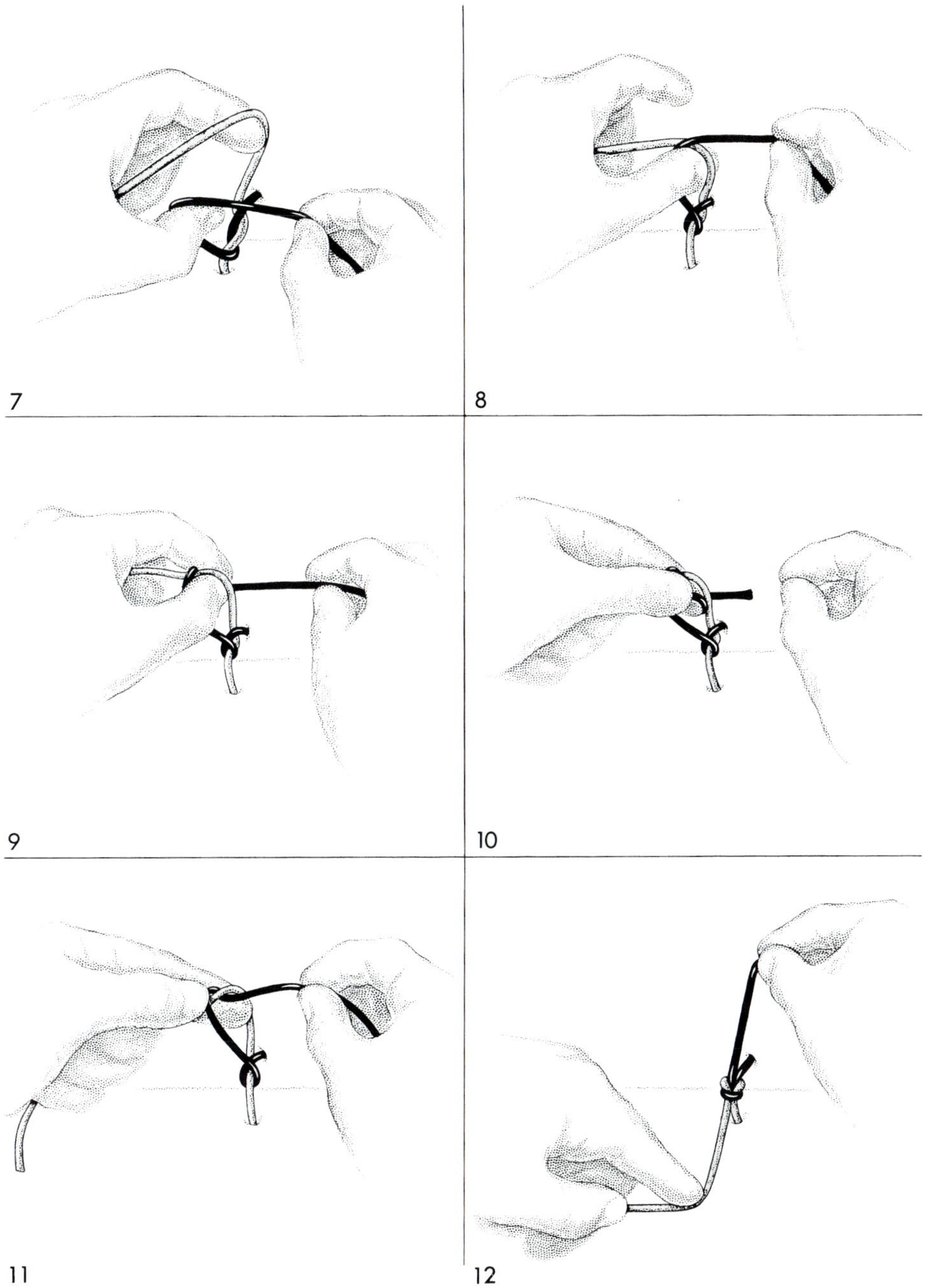

FIGURE 3–8. *Continued.*

RIGHT-HANDED OPERATOR—ONE HAND METHOD I (FIG. 3–9)

STEP 1. The long strand, with needle attached, is held perpendicular or slightly away from the operator by the right hand. The short strand is held between the thumb and middle finger of the left hand, and the index finger is extended.

STEP 2. The fingers of the left hand are brought together around the long strand so that the grasp on the short strand is temporarily transferred to the thumb and index finger.

STEP 3. The middle finger is moved to the far side of the long strand so that the short strand is grasped between the middle and index fingers.

STEP 4. The short end is drawn through the loop that has been made.

STEP 5. Traction directed away from the operator is applied to the long strand by the right hand, and traction directed toward the operator is applied to the short strand by the left hand. This completes the first throw.

STEP 6. The left wrist is rotated so that the thumb is under the short strand.

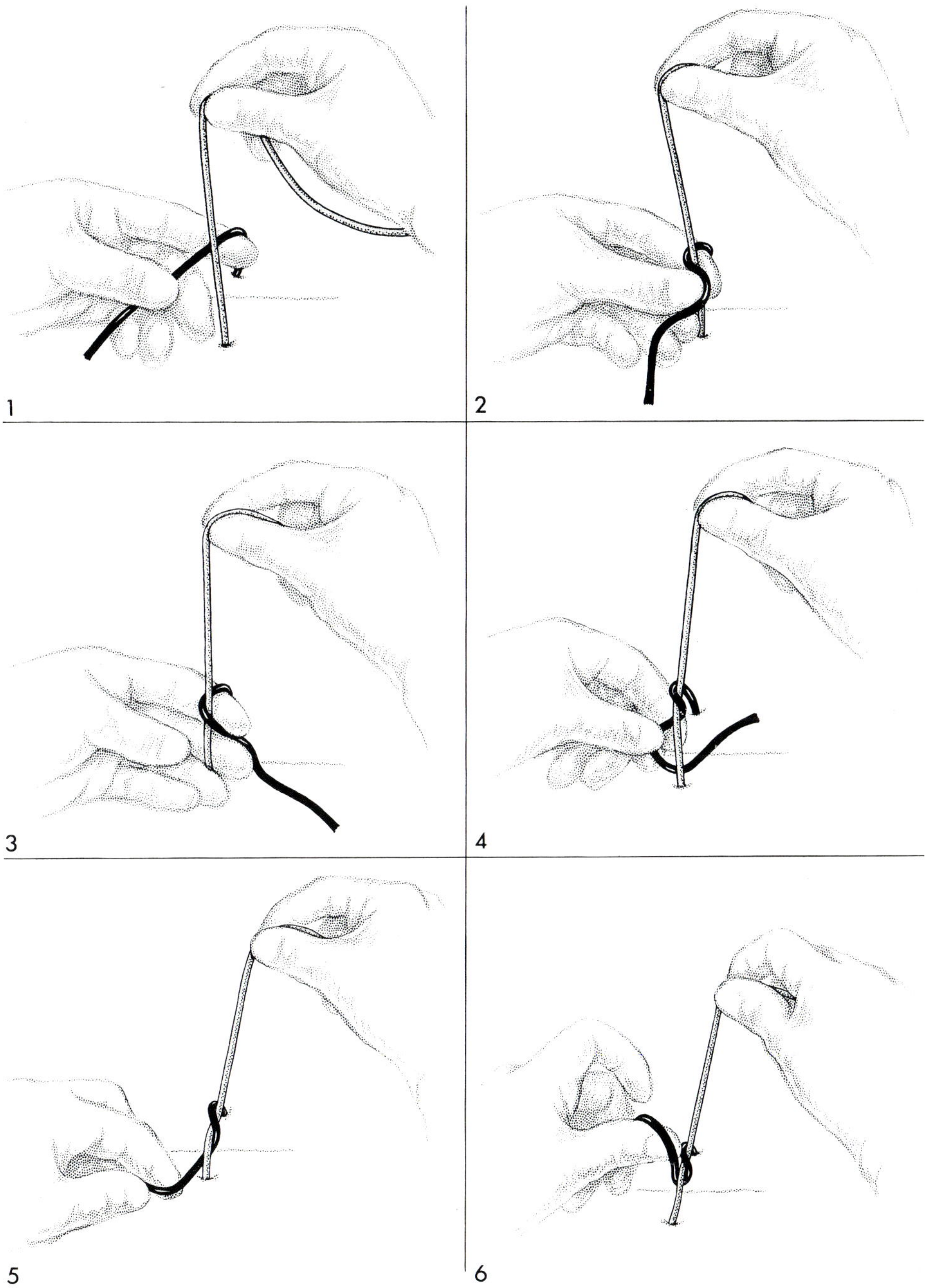

FIGURE 3–9. Square knot. One-hand tie for right-handed operator using Method I.

RIGHT-HANDED OPERATOR—ONE HAND METHOD I (FIG. 3–9) *Continued*

STEP 7. The strands are crossed, with the short strand leading away from the operator.

STEP 8. The middle finger of the left hand pushes the end of the short strand around the long strand in a counterclockwise direction.

STEP 9. The end of the short strand is pushed through the loop by the index finger.

STEP 10. The end of the short strand is grasped between the thumb and middle finger. At this point the long strand is brought toward the operator.

STEP 11. The short strand is directed away from the operator who makes sure that both throws are lying flat.

STEP 12. The knot is tightened to the proper degree.

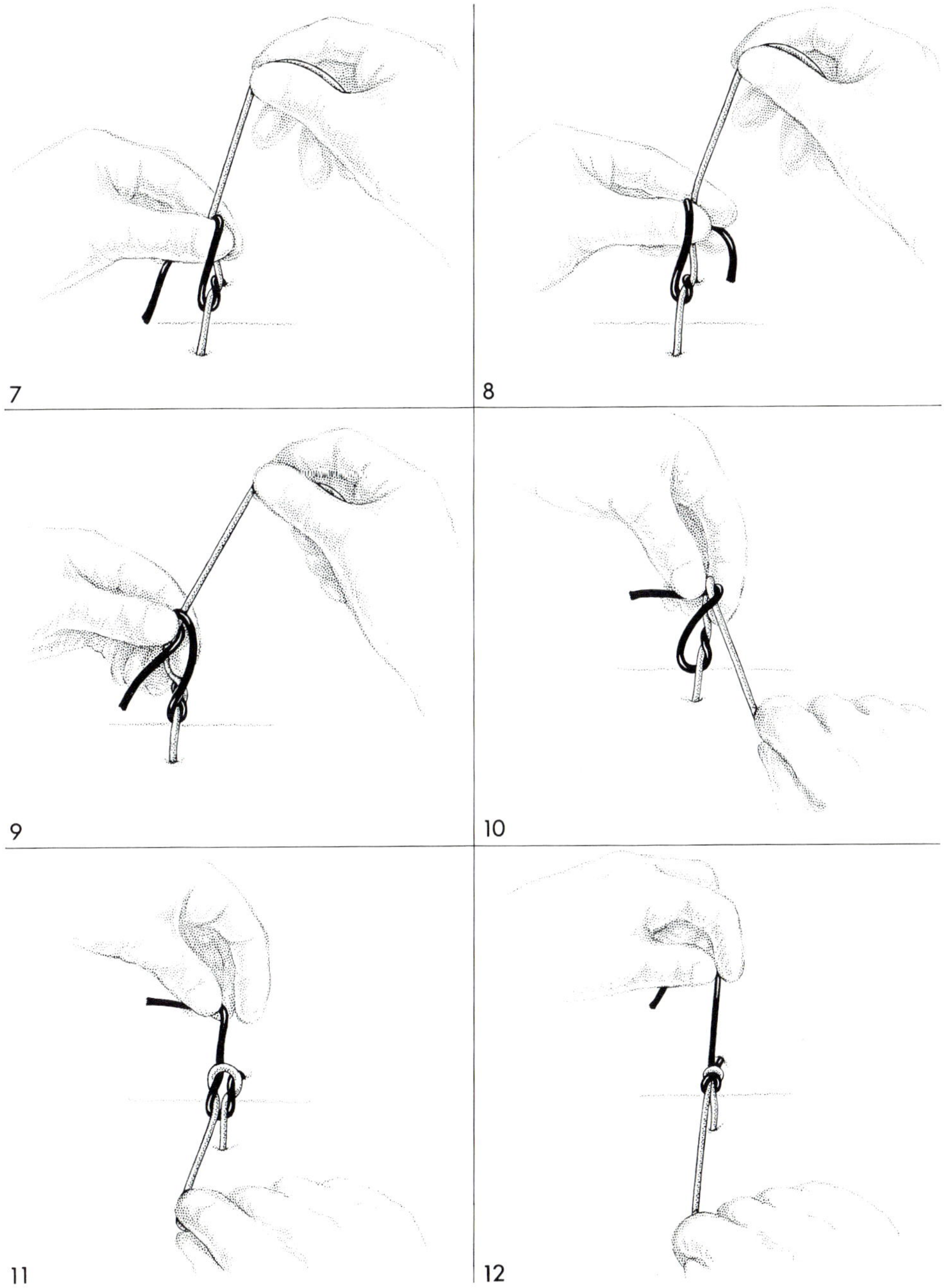

FIGURE 3–9. *Continued.*

METHOD II (FIG. 3–10)

STEP 1. The long strand, with needle attached, is held perpendicular or slightly away from the operator with the right hand. The short strand is looped over the left index finger and held between the middle finger and the ring finger. The thumb presses an arc in the center of the strand.

STEP 2. The short strand is pressed against the long strand. The pressure of the thumb forms a loop behind the long strand.

STEP 3. The left index finger is passed through this loop.

STEPS 4 AND 5. By flicking the left index finger backward, the short strand is drawn through.

STEP 6. The first throw is drawn tight by applying traction to the long strand, which is directed away from the operator by the right hand, and to the short strand, which is directed toward the operator by the left hand.

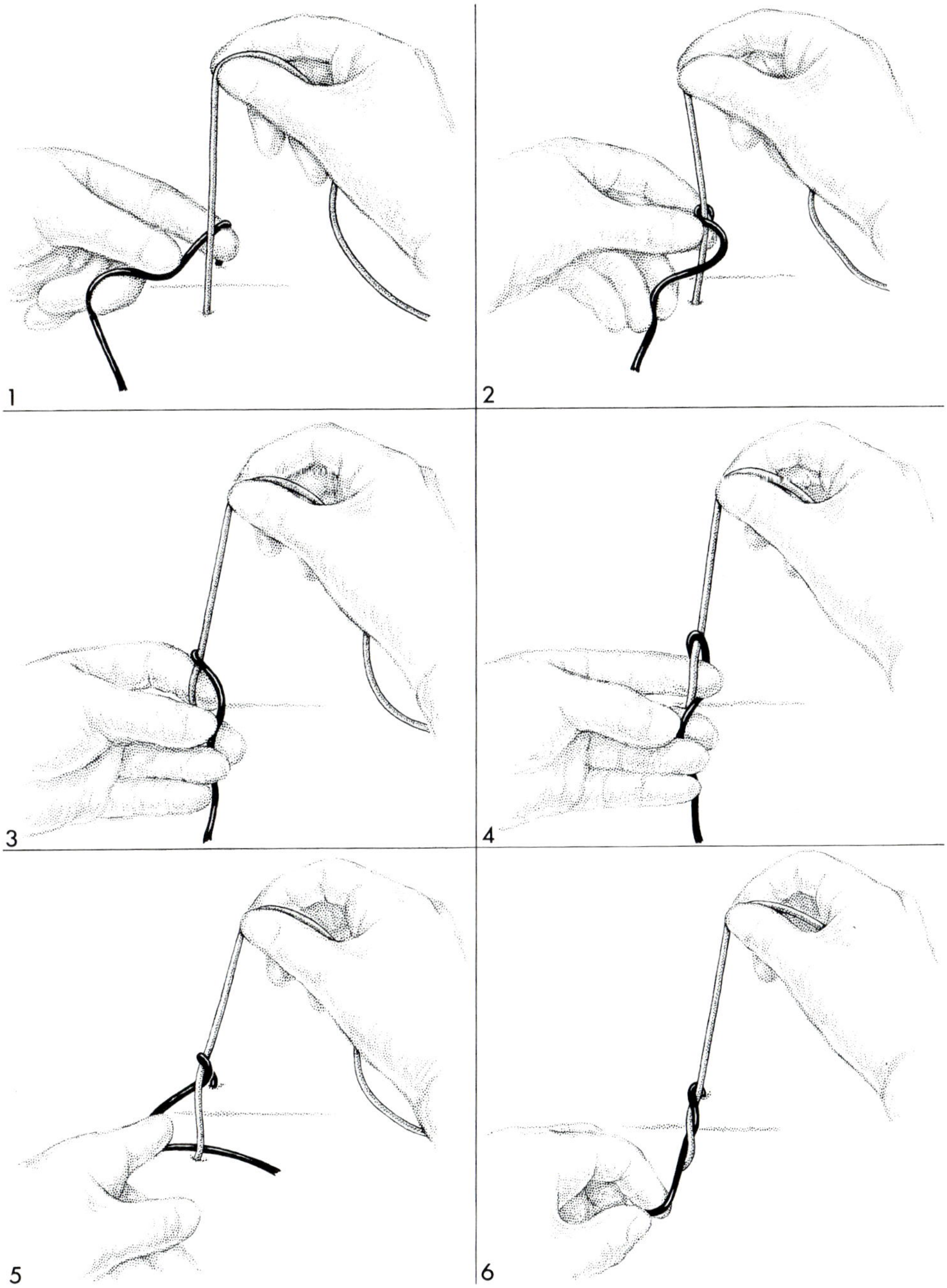

FIGURE 3–10. Square knot. One-hand tie for right-handed operator using Method II.

METHOD II (FIG. 3–10) *Continued*

STEP 7. The second throw is started by holding the long strand in the same position as in Step 1. The short strand is passed across the palmar surface of the fingers of the left hand and is held by the thumb and forefinger.

STEP 8. The long strand is passed over the dorsal surface of the last three fingers of the left hand and is then turned down over the palmar surface of these fingers.

STEP 9. The two strands are now lying side by side. By flexing, the middle finger of the left hand can be placed between the two strands so that the short strand can be made to cross the long strand.

STEPS 10 AND 11. The left thumb and forefinger release the short strand, and the middle finger and ring finger bring the strand through the loop.

STEP 12. The knot is tightened after making certain that each throw is lying flat.

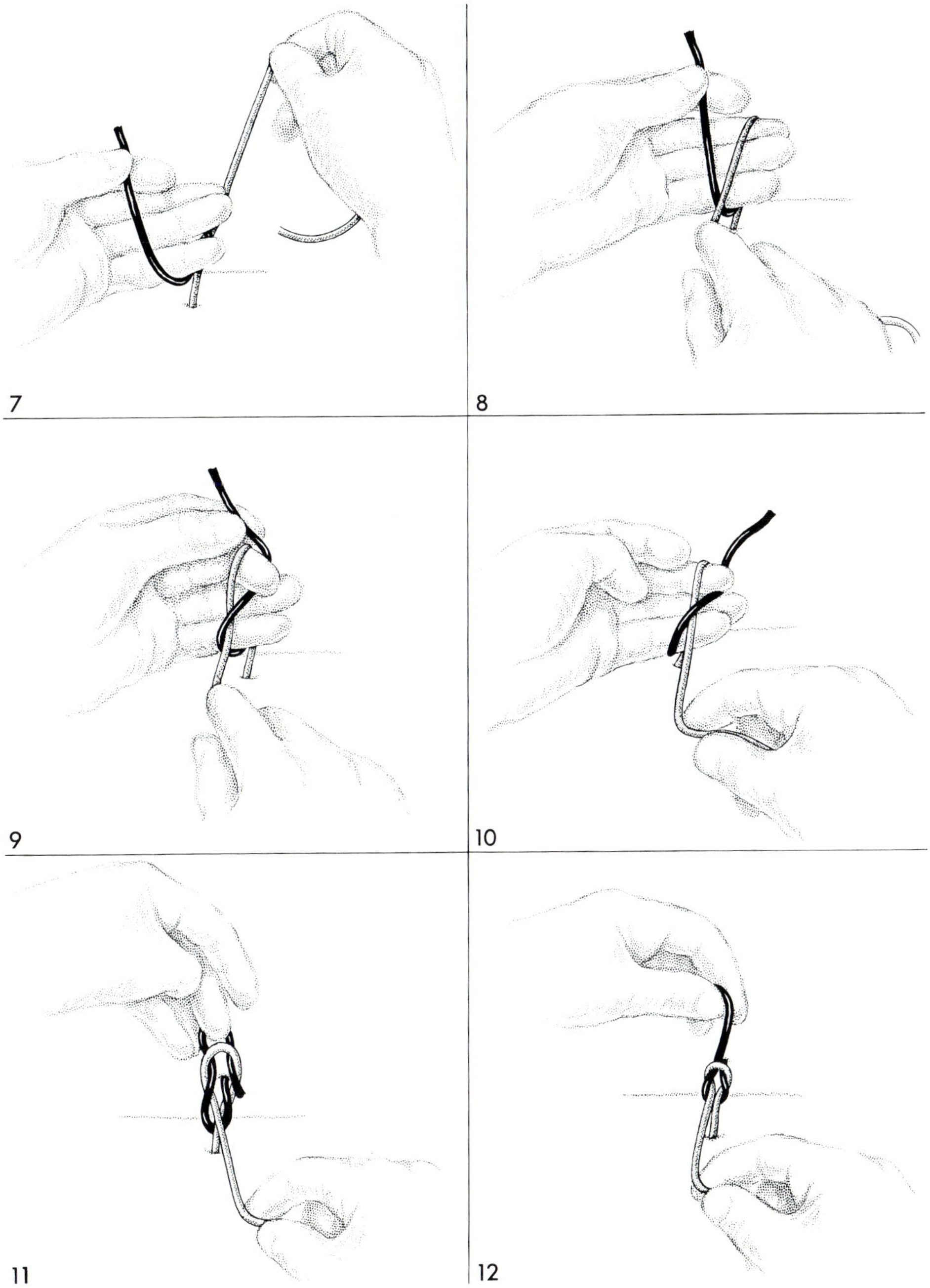

FIGURE 3–10. *Continued.*

LEFT-HANDED OPERATOR—TWO HANDS (FIG. 3-11)

STEP 1. The short strand is grasped in the left hand.

STEP 2. It is crossed over the long strand.

STEP 3. The two strands are grasped at the crossing point by the right thumb and forefinger.

STEP 4. The right thumb and forefinger are rotated to force the short strand through the loop that has been formed.

STEP 5. The short strand is picked up by the left hand.

STEP 6. The loop is drawn tight by pulling the long strand away from the operator with the right hand and the short strand toward the operator with the left hand.

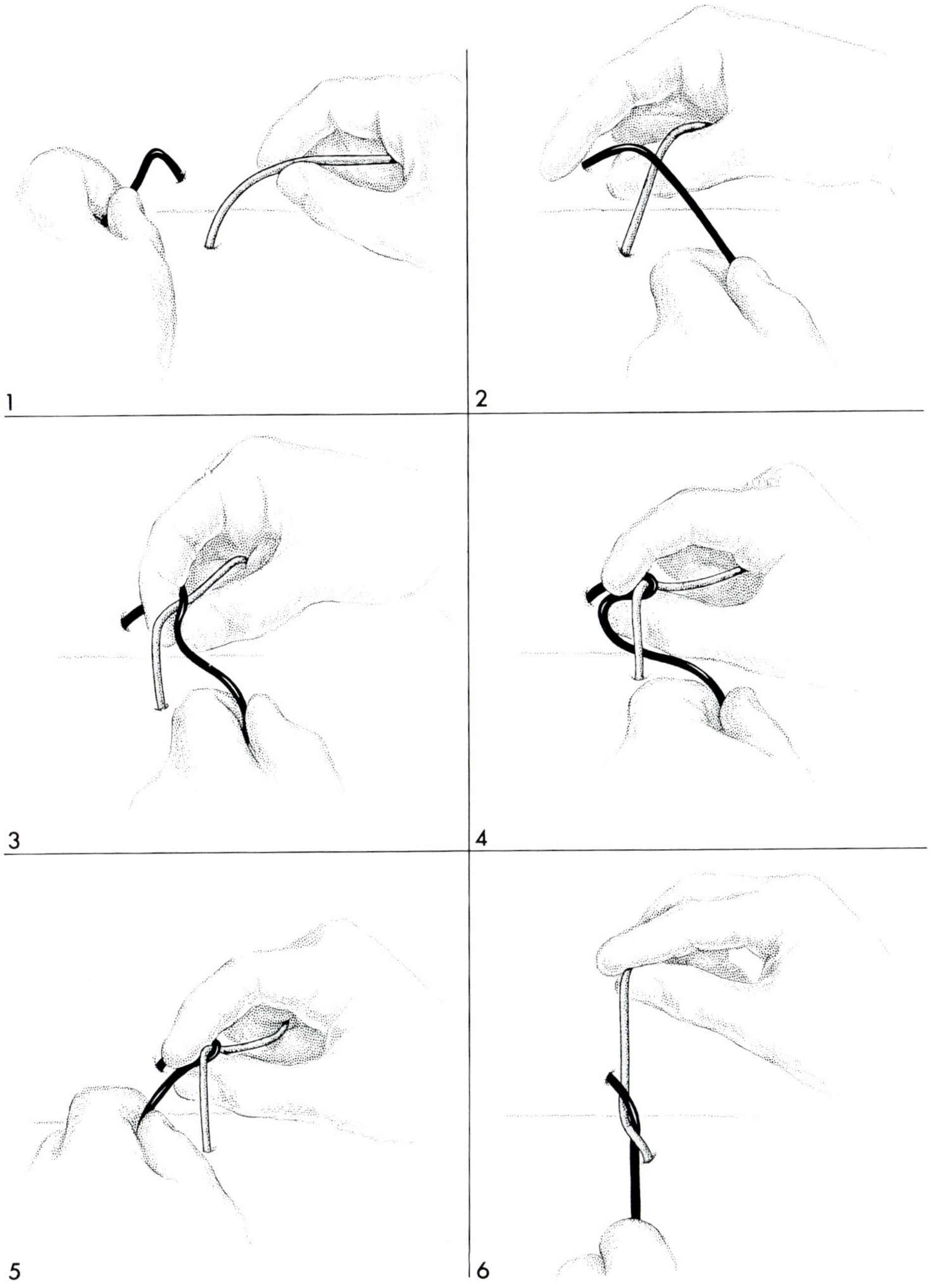

FIGURE 3–11. Square knot. Two-hand tie for left-handed operator.

LEFT-HANDED OPERATOR—TWO HANDS (FIG. 3-11) *Continued*

STEP 7. The short strand is looped over the right thumb, and the long strand is lifted by the right index finger.

STEP 8. The long strand is allowed to drop across the right thumb. At the same time, the short strand crosses the long.

STEP 9. The strands are grasped by the right thumb and forefinger at the point of intersection.

STEP 10. The right forefinger rotates the short strand downward through the loop.

STEP 11. The short end is grasped in the left hand.

STEP 12. Traction on the short end is away from the operator and on the long end toward the operator.

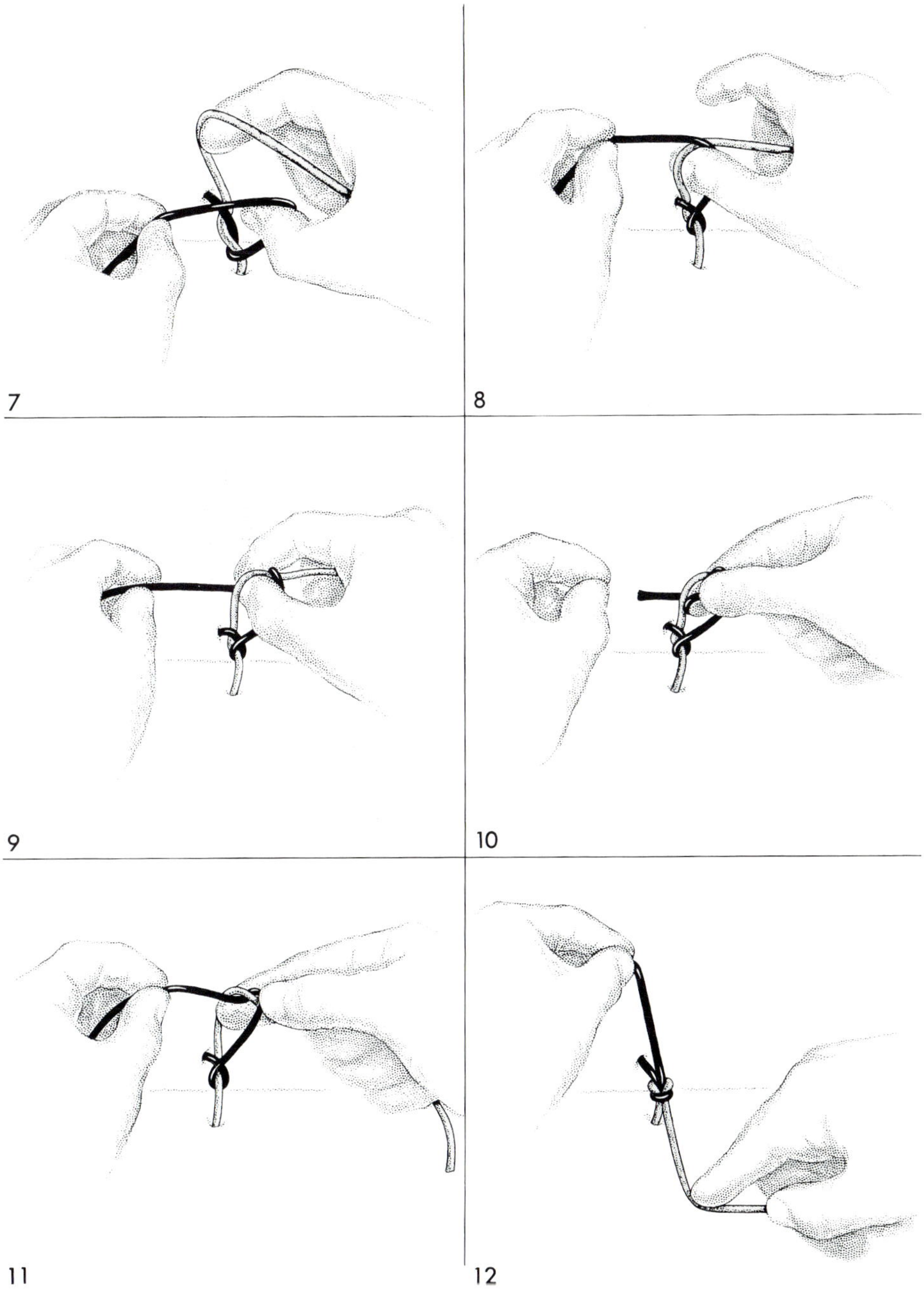

FIGURE 3–11. *Continued.*

LEFT-HANDED OPERATOR—ONE HAND METHOD I (FIG. 3–12)

STEP 1. The long strand, with needle attached, is held perpendicular or slightly away from the operator in the left hand. The short strand is held between the thumb and middle finger of the right hand, and the index finger is extended.

STEP 2. The fingers of the right hand are brought together around the long strand so that the grasp on the short strand is temporarily transferred to the thumb and index finger.

STEP 3. The middle finger is moved to the far side of the long strand so that the short strand is grasped between the middle and index fingers.

STEP 4. The short end is drawn through the loop that has been made.

STEP 5. Traction directed away from the operator is applied to the long strand by the left hand, and traction directed toward the operator is applied to the short strand by the right hand. This completes the first throw.

STEP 6. The right wrist is rotated so that the thumb is under the short strand.

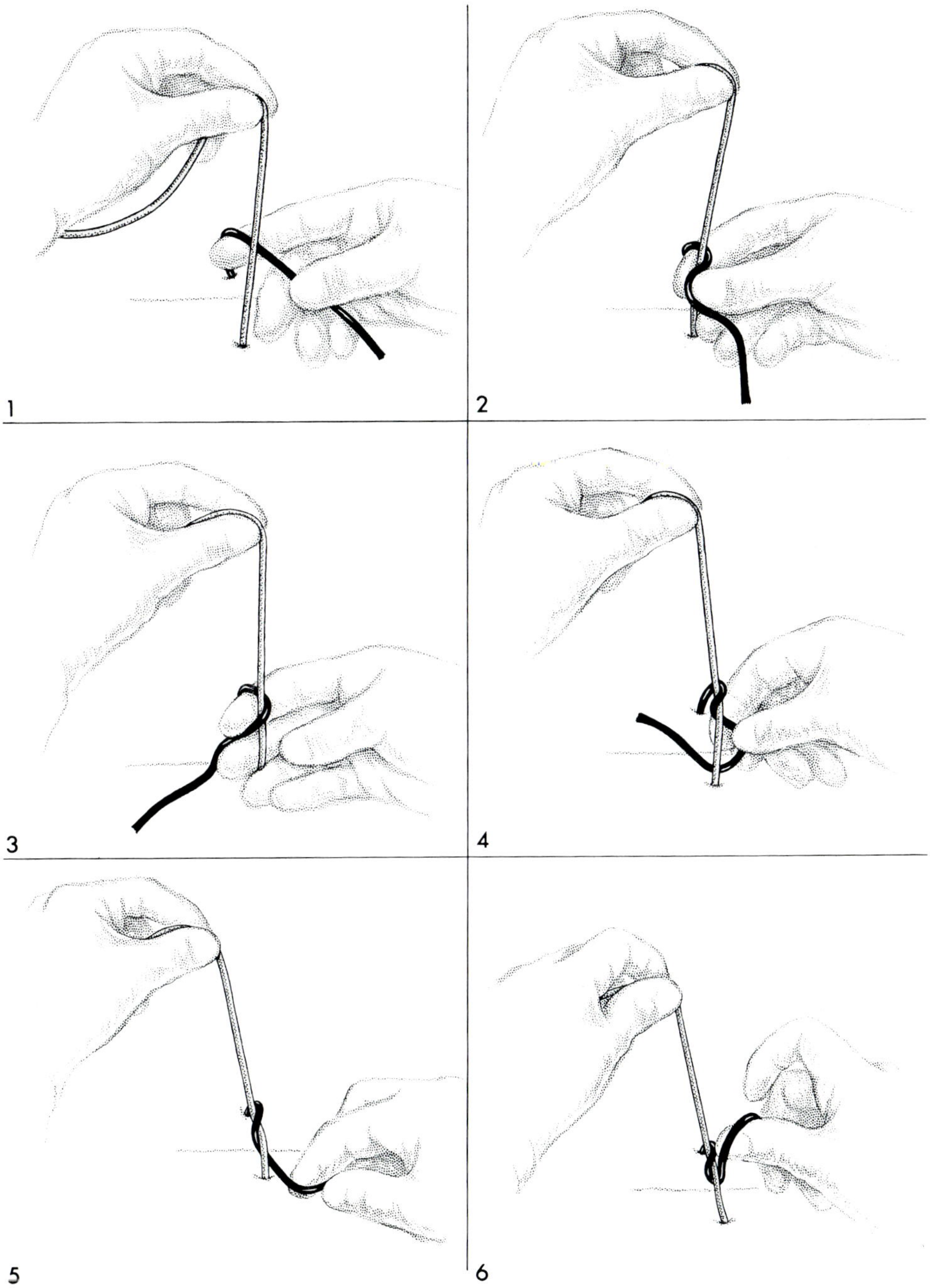

FIGURE 3–12. Square knot. One-hand tie for left-handed operator using Method I.

LEFT-HANDED OPERATOR—ONE HAND
METHOD I (FIG. 3–12) *Continued*

STEP 7. The strands are crossed. The short strand is leading away from the operator.

STEP 8. The middle finger of the right hand pushes the end of the short strand around the long strand in a counterclockwise direction.

STEP 9. The end of the short strand is pushed through the loop by the index finger.

STEP 10. The end of the short strand is grasped between the thumb and middle finger, and the long strand is brought toward the operator.

STEP 11. The short strand is directed away from the operator, who makes sure that both throws are lying flat.

STEP 12. The knot is tightened to the proper degree.

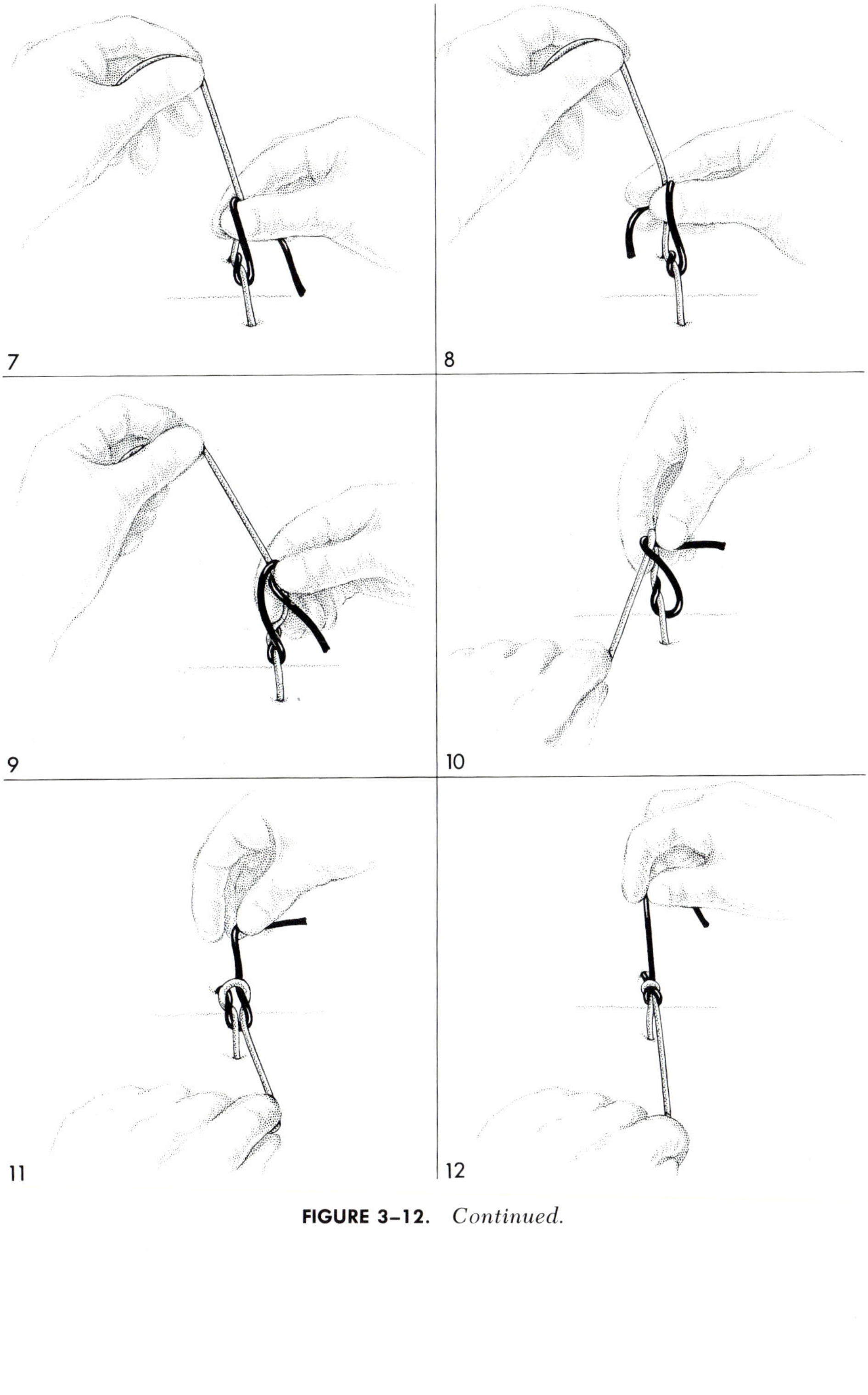

7 8 9 10 11 12

FIGURE 3–12. *Continued.*

METHOD II (FIG. 3–13)

STEP 1. The long strand, with needle attached, is held perpendicular or slightly away from the operator in the left hand. The short strand is looped over the right index finger and held between the middle finger and the ring finger. The thumb is pressing an arc in the center of the strand.

STEP 2. The short strand is pressed against the long strand. The pressure of the thumb forms a loop behind the long strand.

STEP 3. The right index finger is passed through this loop.

STEPS 4 AND 5. By flicking the right index finger backward, the short strand is drawn through.

STEP 6. The first throw is drawn tight by applying traction to the long strand, which is directed by the left hand, and to the short strand, which is directed toward the operator by the right hand.

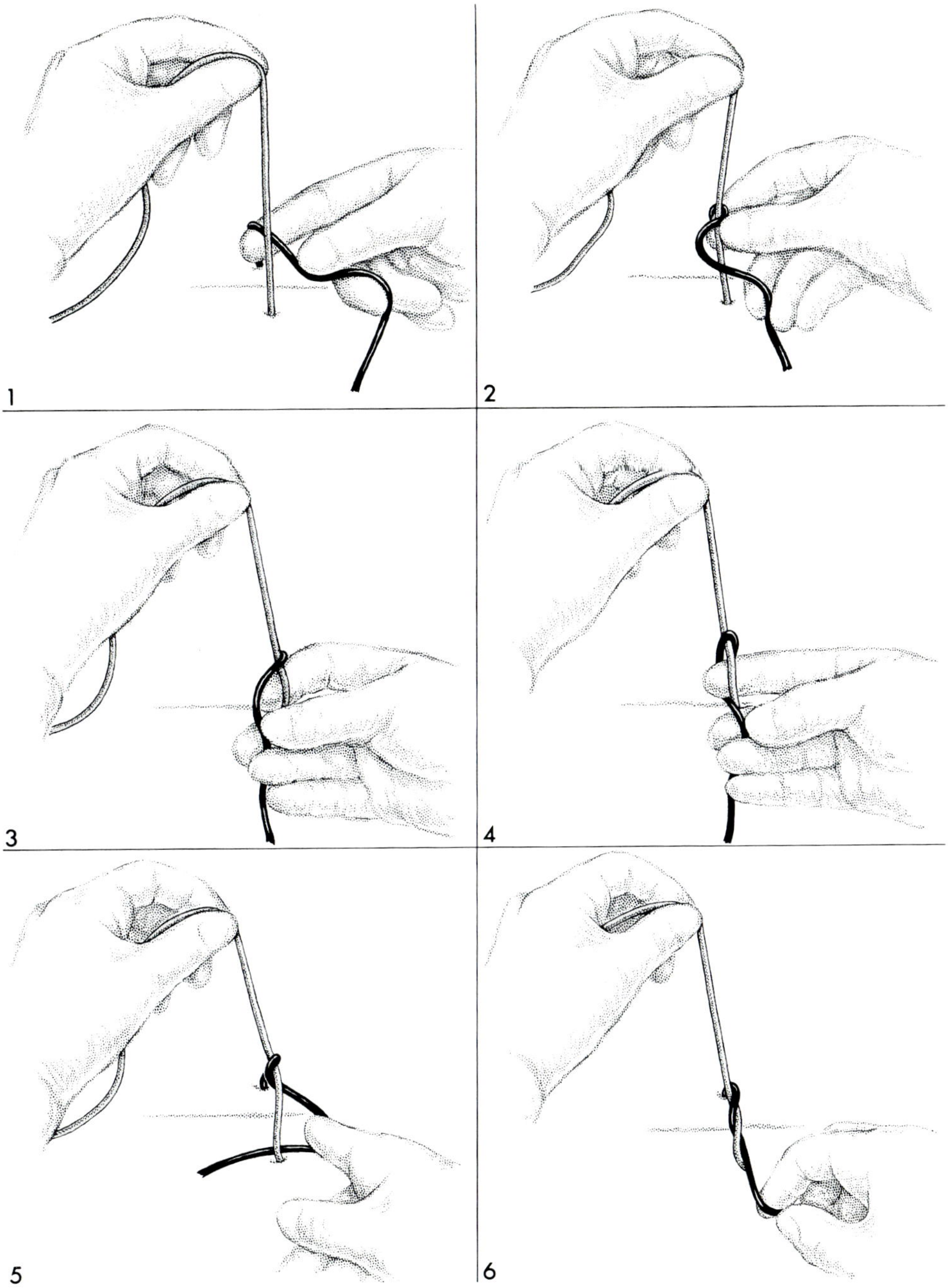

FIGURE 3–13. Square knot. One-hand tie for left-handed operator using Method II.

METHOD II (FIG. 3–13) *Continued*

STEP 7. The second throw is started by holding the long strand in the same position as in Step I. The short strand is passed across the palmar surface of the fingers of the right hand and is held by the thumb and forefinger.

STEP 8. The long strand is passed over the dorsal surface of the last three fingers of the right hand and then turned downward over the palmar surface of these fingers.

STEP 9. The two strands are now lying side by side. By flexing, the middle finger of the right hand can be placed between the two strands so that the short strand can be made to cross the long strand.

STEPS 10 AND 11. The right thumb and forefinger release the short strand, and the middle finger and ring finger bring the strand through the loop.

STEP 12. The knot is tightened after making certain that each throw is lying flat.

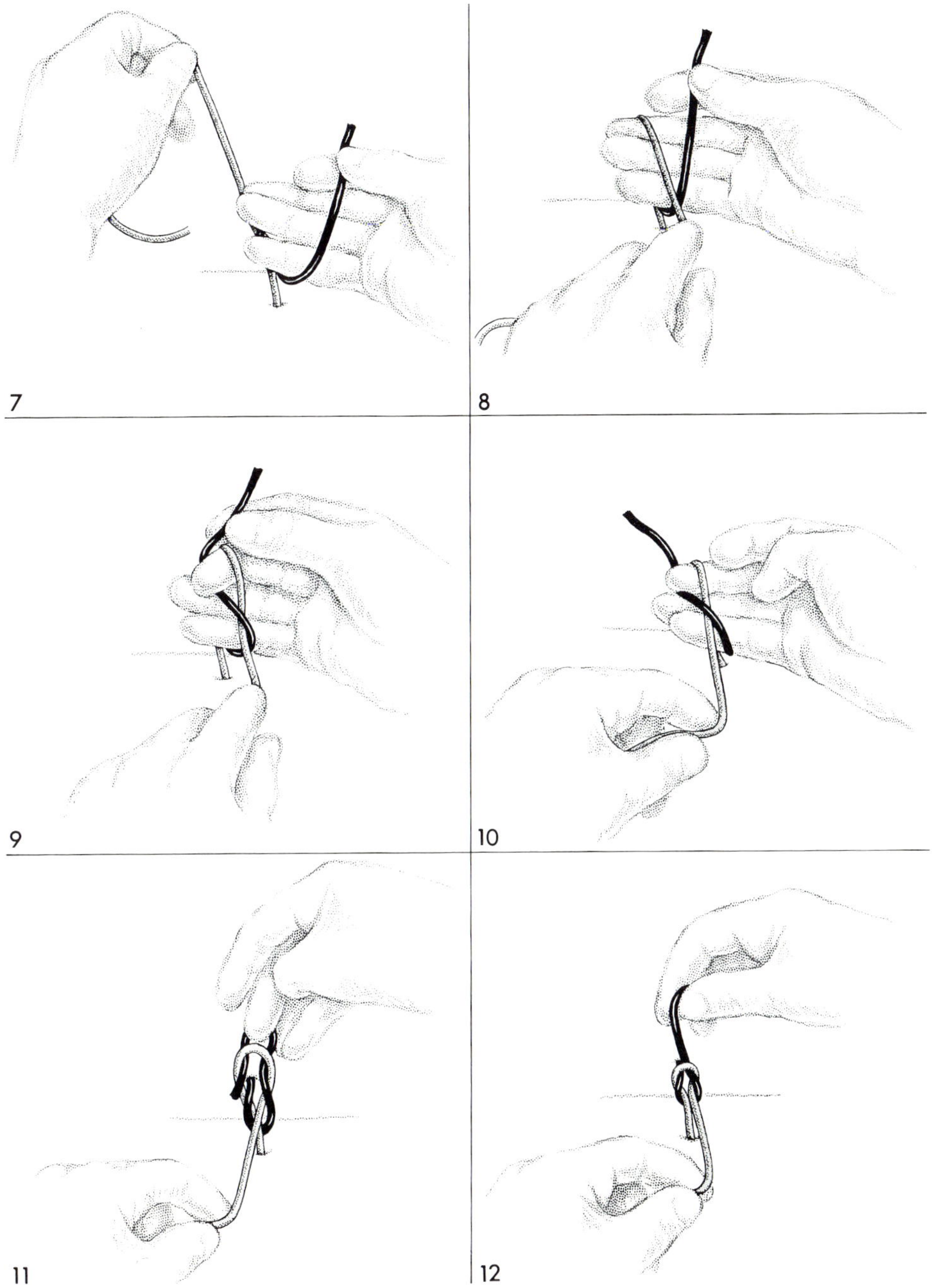

FIGURE 3–13. *Continued.*

RIGHT-HANDED OPERATOR—INSTRUMENT (FIG. 3–14A)

STEP 1. The long strand is passed over the forceps in a loop, and the short strand is grasped by the forceps and pulled through the loop toward the operator. This constitutes the first throw.

STEP 2. The long strand is passed under the forceps in a loop.

STEPS 3, 4, AND 5. The short strand is grasped by the forceps and pulled through the loop in the direction away from the operator.

STEP 6. The knot is tightened if the throws are flat.

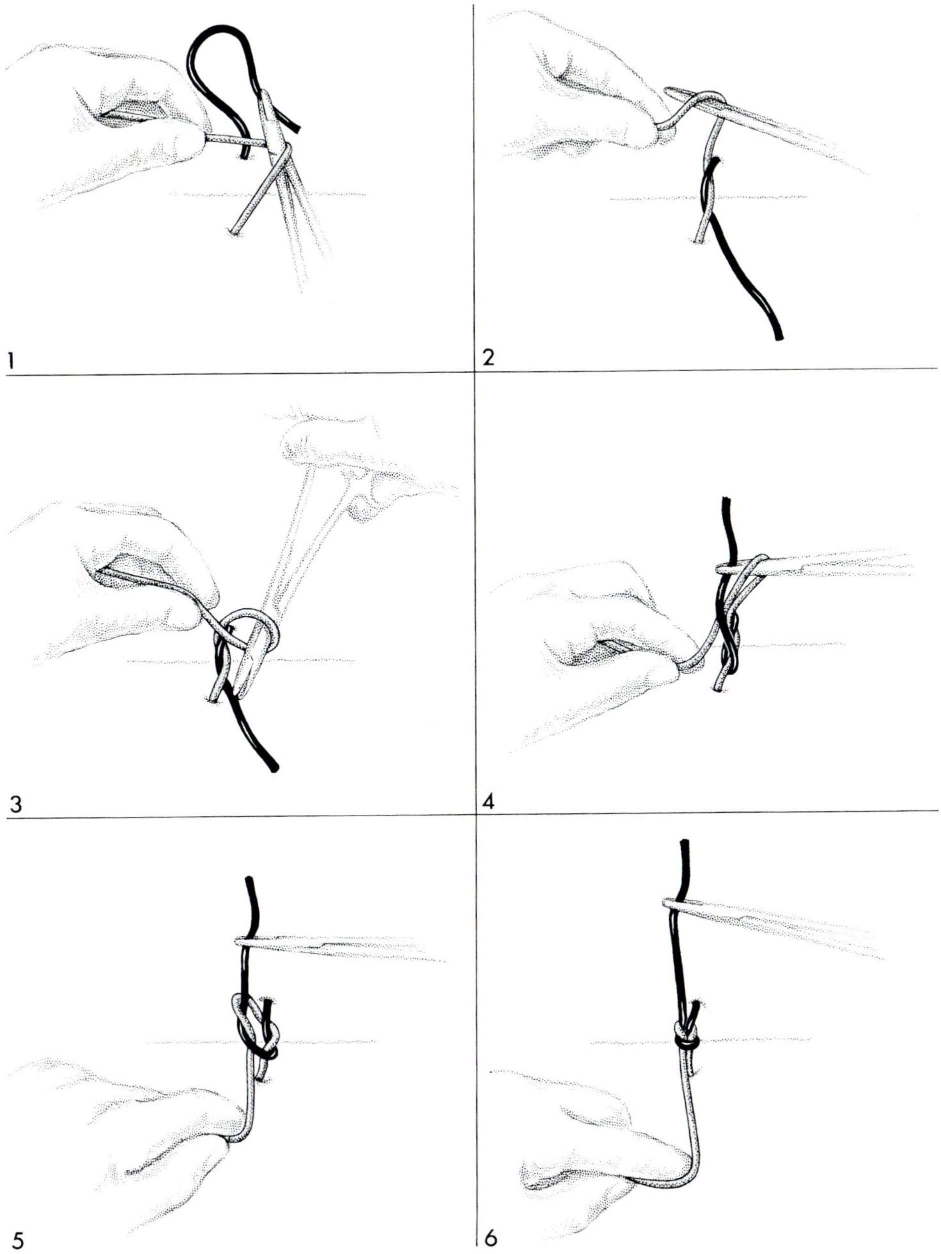

FIGURE 3–14A. Square knot. Instrument tie for right-handed operator.

LEFT-HANDED OPERATOR—INSTRUMENT (FIG. 3–14B)

STEP 1. The long strand is passed over the forceps in a loop, and the short strand is grasped by the forceps and pulled through the loop toward the operator. This constitutes the first throw.

STEP 2. The long strand is passed under the forceps in a loop.

STEPS 3, 4, AND 5. The short strand is grasped by the forceps and pulled through the loop in the direction away from the operator.

STEP 6. The knot is tightened if the throws are flat.

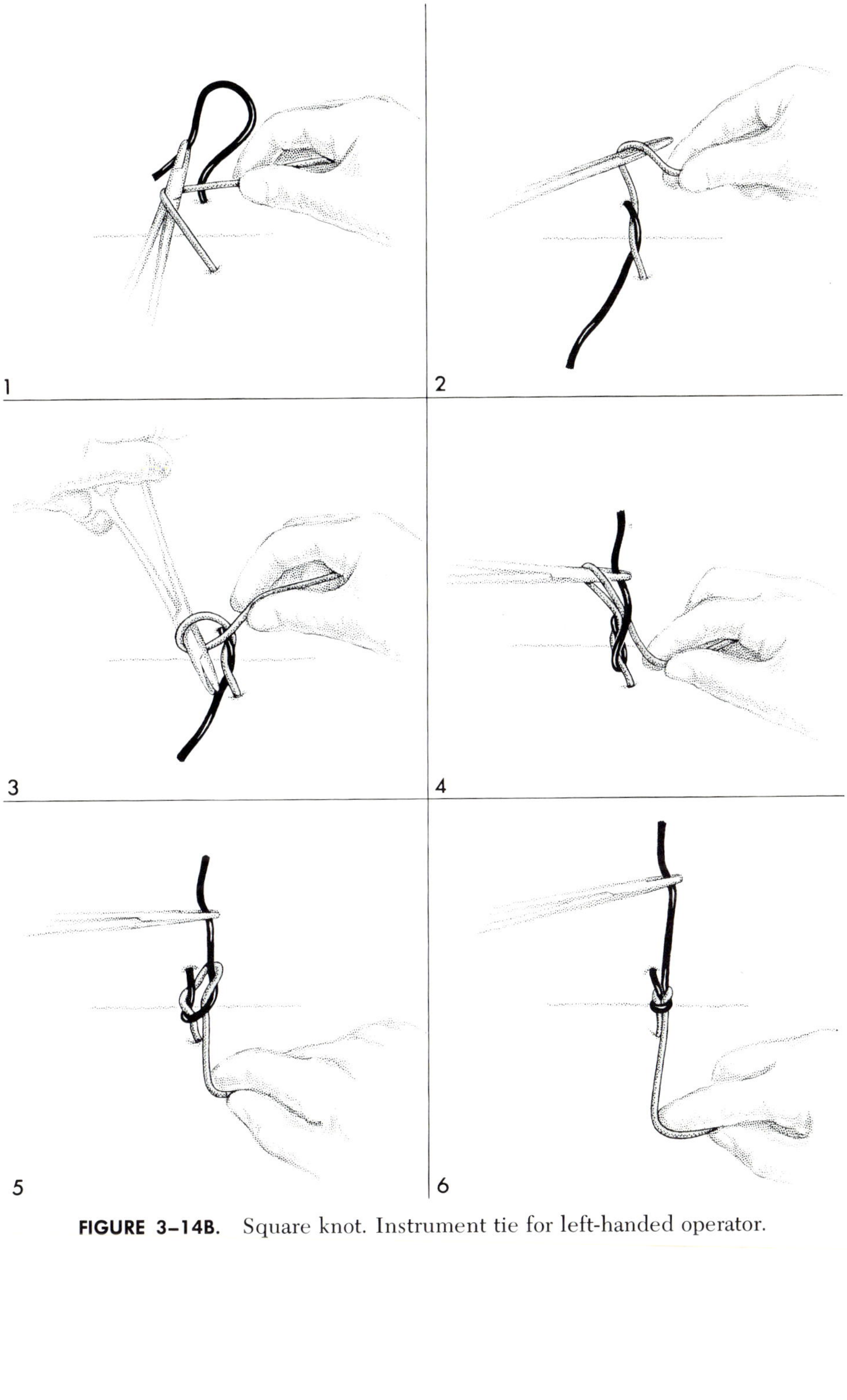

FIGURE 3–14B. Square knot. Instrument tie for left-handed operator.

RIGHT-HANDED OPERATOR—COMBINATION (FIG. 3–15A)

STEP 1. The first throw is made in the same manner as the regular instrument tie.

STEP 2. The simple knot is held snug by crossing the ends and holding them between the thumb and forefinger.

STEP 3. The short end is thrust through the loop by the forefinger and grasped with the forceps.

STEP 4. The ends are pulled tight by carrying the short strand away from the operator and the long strand toward the operator.

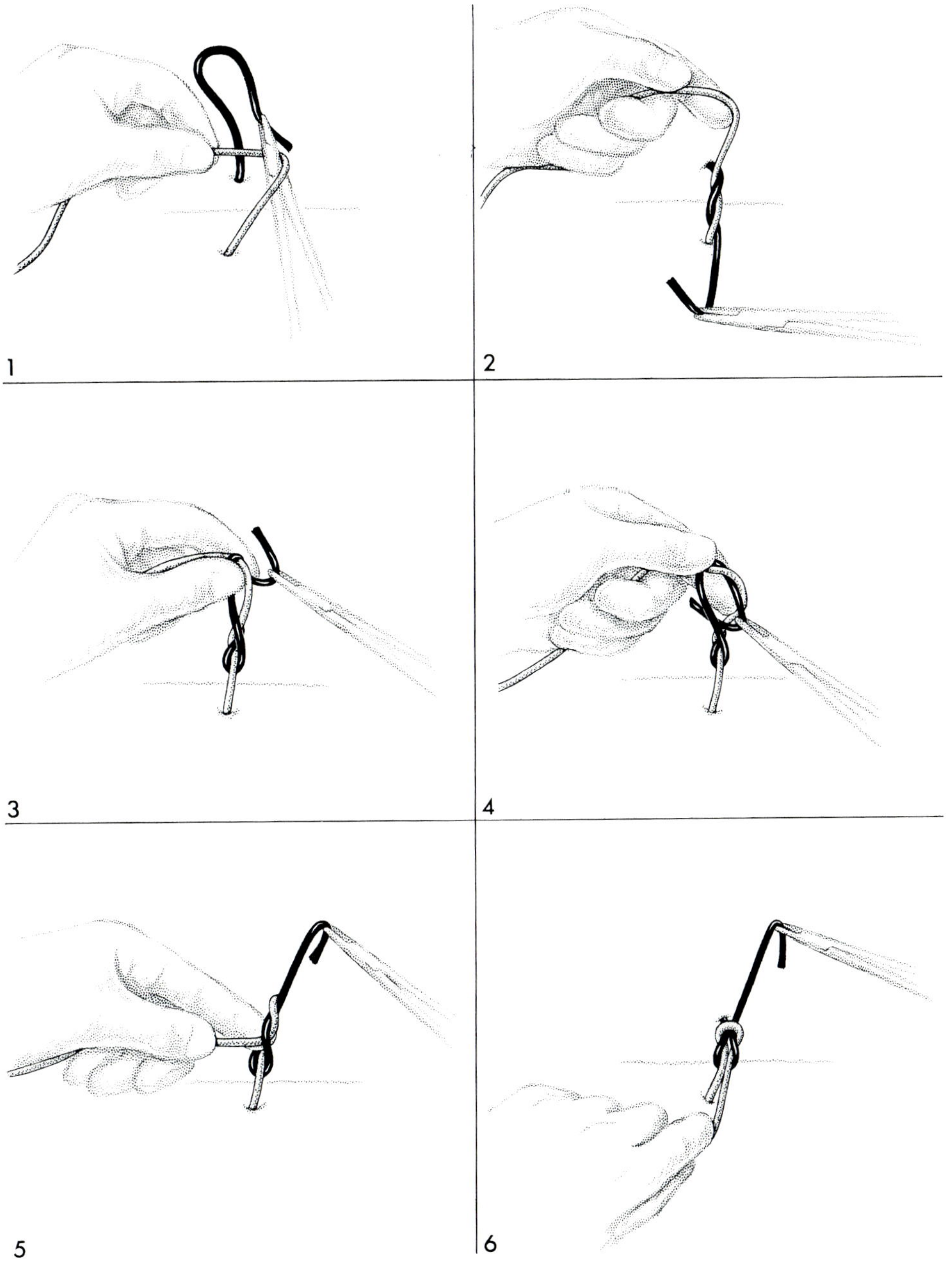

FIGURE 3–15A. Square knot. Combination instrument and hand tie for right-handed operator.

LEFT-HANDED OPERATOR—COMBINATION (FIG. 3–15B)

STEP 1. The first throw is made in the same manner as the regular instrument tie.

STEP 2. The simple knot is held snug by crossing the ends and holding them between the thumb and forefinger.

STEP 3. The short end is thrust through the loop by the forefinger and grasped with the forceps.

STEP 4. The ends are pulled tight by carrying the short strand away from the operator and the long strand toward the operator.

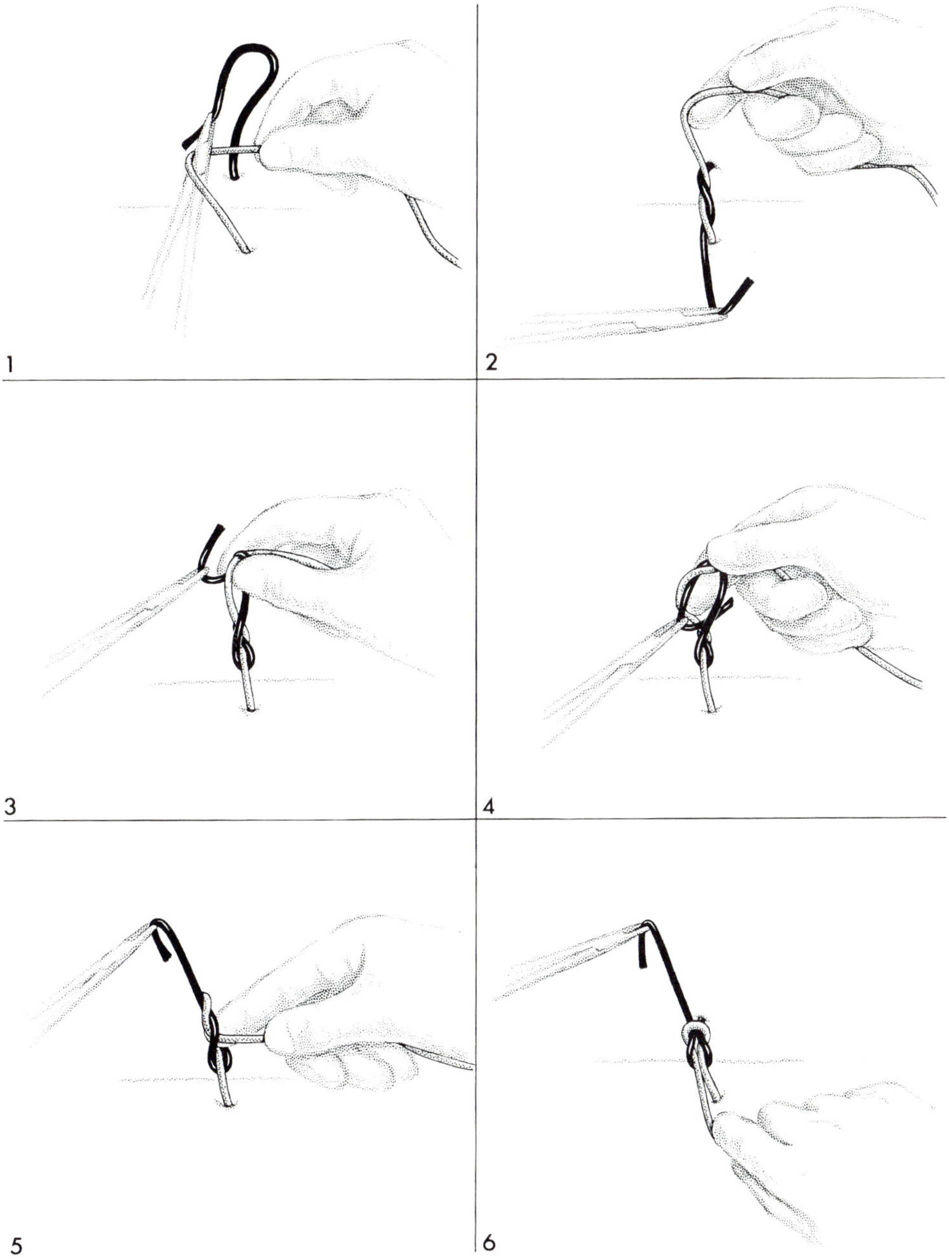

FIGURE 3–15B. Square knot. Combination instrument and hand tie for left-handed operator.

GRANNY KNOT

The granny knot consists of two throws—one superimposed upon the other—the second of which is not reversed (Fig. 3–16). This knot will slip unless it is fortified by a third throw. While this knot is used by some surgeons, it is not as trustworthy as the square knot and therefore cannot be recommended to the student in beginning surgery. It is especially untrustworthy when not tied tightly or when the suture material is smooth and slippery.

SURGEON'S KNOT

Many surgeons use the surgeon's knot to retain the first throw under tension while the second throw is being made (Fig. 3–16). The knot is made by making two wraps instead of one on the first throw. The disadvantage is that the knot is wider at the base, or first throw, than at the second throw. This results in a knot that cannot be tied tightly without danger of breaking the suture and a knot that is too bulky. Where tension is required on the first throw, a combination tie can be used, or an assistant can place his finger on the first throw until the second throw is completed. There is some danger to the suture material when hemostats are used to retain the tension.

SLIP KNOT

The slip knot is mentioned here because it so frequently results from careless tying and is a very dangerous knot to use. One can go through the

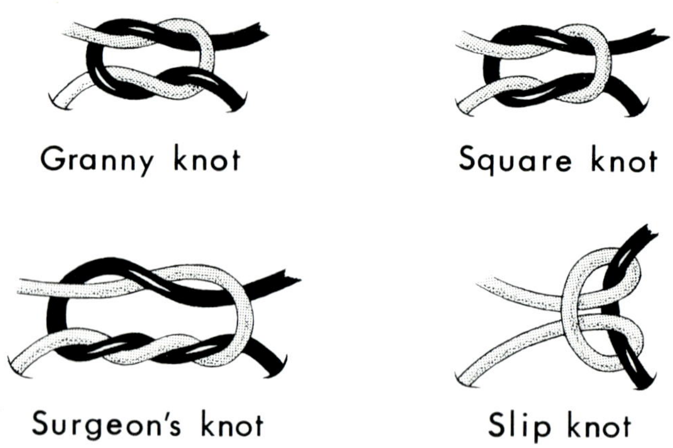

FIGURE 3–16. Knots used in surgery.

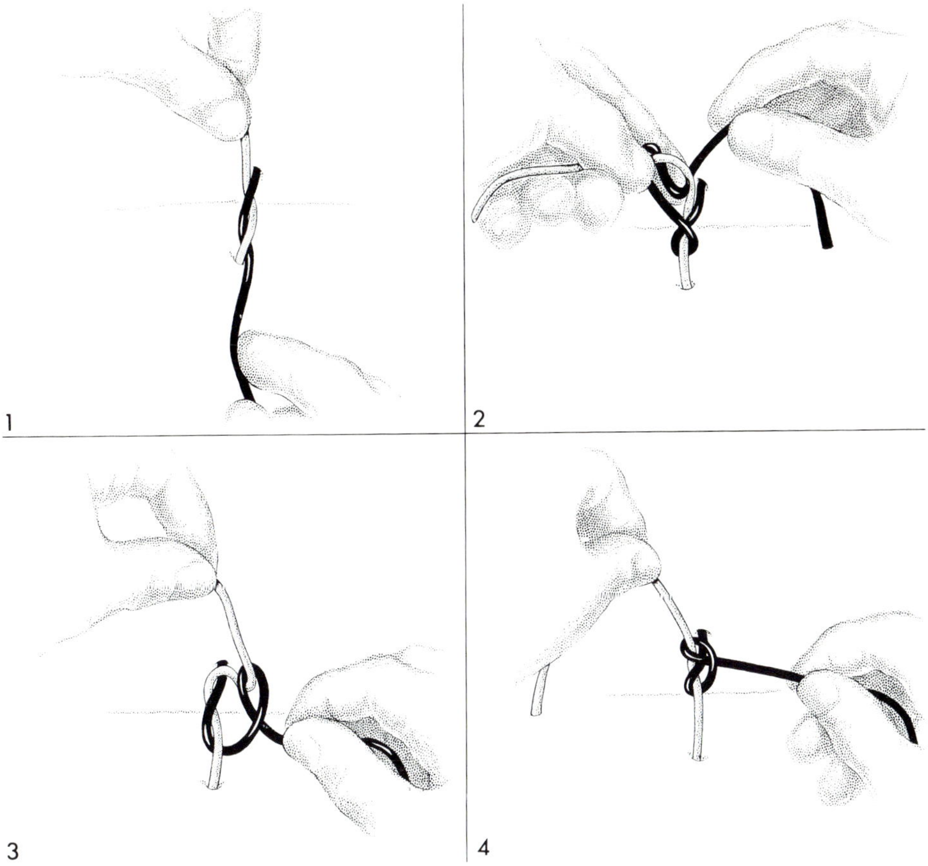

FIGURE 3–17. A slip knot resulting from improperly tied square knot.

motions of tying a square knot and, by failing to lay the throws flat, produce a slip knot unconsciously. The mere movement of the hand in the opposite direction does not ensure a square knot. It is imperative that each throw lie flat (Fig. 3–17).

LIGATION

Knot tying, which is part of ligation, has already been discussed, but the placement of the ligature is equally important. Whenever feasible, blood vessels should be ligated before they are cut. It is often possible to pass a small hemostat under or around a blood vessel and thereby draw a ligature through. This is less hazardous than the use of a needle, but it is not always possible except when dealing with the softer tissues.

Simple ligation of small vessels is usually sufficient, but larger vessels should have a ligature that is transfixed to prevent rolling or slipping. The needle is passed through the vessel and a simple knot is tied. The ligature is then passed around the entire vessel, proximal to the first knot,

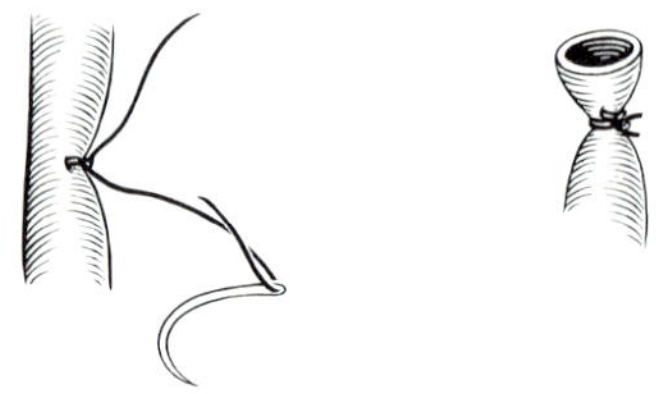

Transfixed ligature on large vessel

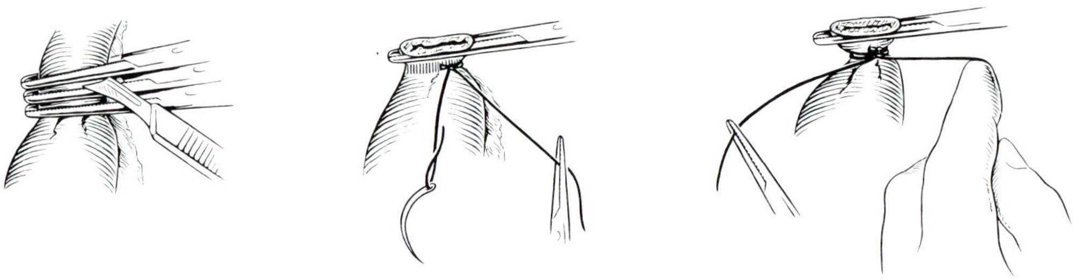

Ligation of pedicle, three forceps method

FIGURE 3–18.

and tied securely with a square knot. In certain instances it is possible to fix the ligature to a satellite structure (the vas deferens in the case of the spermatic vessels), but this should only be done when there is no danger of countertraction on the ligature.

Ligation of a pedicle is best accomplished by the three-forceps method. After the stump is separated between the first two forceps, the third forceps is removed, and a transfixation ligature is placed in the groove left by the third forceps. The second forceps can then be gradually released, and the stump can be tested for bleeding (Fig. 3–18).

Chapter 4

SURGICAL PREPARATION

STERILIZING PROCEDURES

Everything that has any connection with sterile surgery must be prepared for that event in a most meticulous fashion. The sterilizing procedures must produce sterile drapes, gowns, and instruments. Any breakdown in the system may be very hazardous. It is therefore important that whoever is entrusted with this part of the preparation be capable of understanding the various ramifications involved.

PREPARATION OF DRY GOODS

The folding and bundling of drapes and gowns is fully discussed in Chapter 2. These bundles should be as small as possible, since large bundles are often difficult to penetrate thoroughly with steam. The wrappers should be of muslin or some other type of cloth so that the air can be quickly evacuated from the bundle. Paper wrappers do not allow the air to escape rapidly.

Caps and masks are usually laundered and folded in neat piles, but they are not necessarily sterilized. These two pieces of apparel serve the useful purpose of restraining outside contaminants, but they are themselves contaminated when they are put on the head and face.

All rubber goods should be powdered and packaged in such a way as to avoid one rubber surface contacting another under pressure. Paper or cloth placed between layers or folds of rubber is helpful. In the case of rubber gloves, excessive pressure must be avoided.

Catheters, syringes, needles, and all manner of small ancillary equipment may be packaged individually in sterilizing tubing as long as they are not placed in a large bundle. Scrub brushes should have nylon bristles and may be sterilized individually or in a metal rack.

PREPARATION OF INSTRUMENTS

If good stainless steel instruments are used, they should be given good care. This means that they should receive immediate attention following surgery. Perhaps it should be stated that good care of instruments starts with the surgeon. He can help to preserve his instruments by wiping them with a dry sponge after each use. Blood is very corrosive to steel and will spot it if left in contact for any length of time.

At the conclusion of surgery, the instruments should be rinsed in cold water and placed in an instrument cleaning solution. There are several good cleaners available. The author has found Weck cleaning powder to be excellent. One tablespoonful of this powder is added to 1 gallon of water. The instruments are allowed to stand in this solution for 10 to 15 minutes. They are then removed and rinsed in very hot water. Drying is done by spreading the instruments on a towel and blotting them with another towel spread over them (see Figs. 2–42, 2–43, and 2–44).

Instruments with box locks should not be scrubbed with a brush, because bristles become lodged in the lock and spoil the instrument. Clean instruments should be placed in an orderly fashion in a tray or receptacle with their rachets open. Occasionally a drop of oil on a lock is required, but excessive oil should not be used.

Each surgeon has his own way of organizing his instrument tray. The tray should be packed in an orderly fashion, and the instruments should always be placed in the same order so that the surgeon will have no difficulty in finding an instrument when he needs it. After the tray is packed, it is wrapped by placing it diagonally on an extra-large, double-thickness wrapper and folding the portion of the wrapper along the short sides of the tray first, with the corners of the wrapper out, and then the portion along the long sides of the tray, with the corners inward. A strip of pressure-sensitive tape is then placed around the bundle. When this is opened on the instrument stand, the wrapper will act as a sterile drape over the tray.

AUTOCLAVE

All dry goods and most instruments, except cutting instruments, are ordinarily sterilized by steam autoclave. With certain modifications, a pressure cooker may also be used for this purpose. Sterilization requires 30 minutes at 20 pounds pressure and 250° F. or 121° C. Gloves are only subjected to 15 pounds pressure for 15 minutes because of the fragility of the rubber.

Air must be evacuated from the autoclave as well as the bundles so that steam can circulate freely throughout the chamber. It is therefore important not to overload the chamber or pack it too tightly. Shelves of expanded metal are helpful in keeping the load dispersed. Trays of instruments should be placed on their sides so that stream will penetrate to the bottom. When laid flat they may trap air and prevent steam from reaching the deeper instruments (Fig. 4–1).

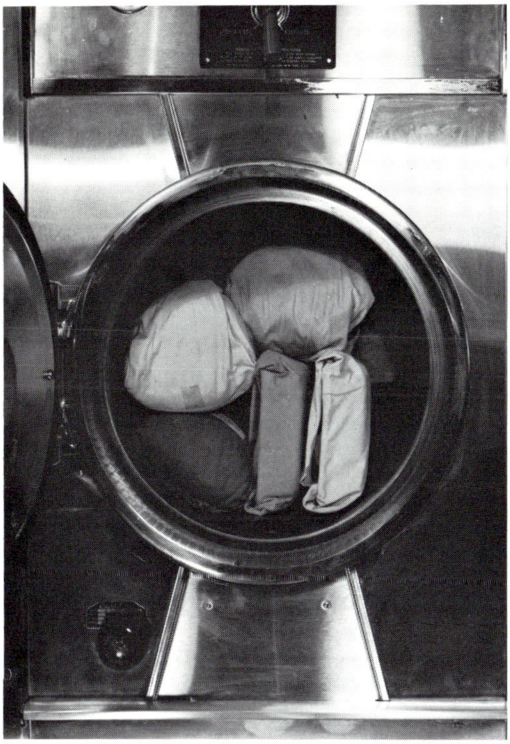

FIGURE 4–1.

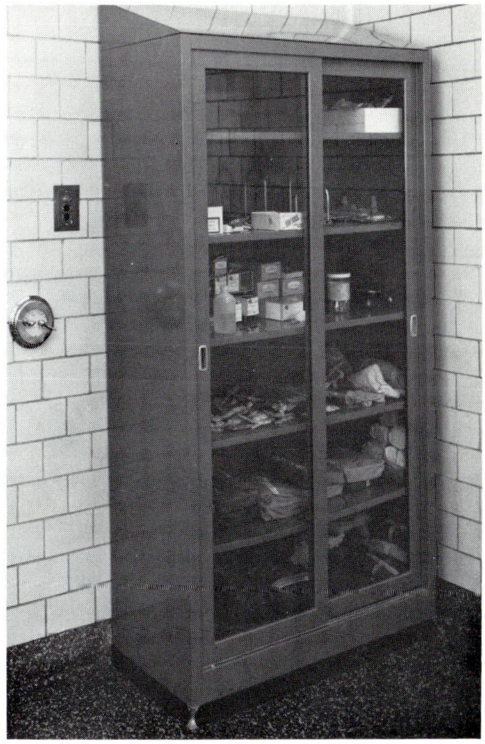

FIGURE 4–2.

The sterilizing period should begin when the pressure gauge shows the proper pressure and not when the door of the sterilizer is closed. At the end of the period, the chamber pressure is released, but the jacket pressure is maintained. The sterilizer door is left ajar so that moist air can escape while the heat from the jacket dries the bundles. The procedure is completed by storing the sterile bundles in dustproof cabinets (Fig. 4–2).

In recent years two other methods of sterilization within a sealed chamber have been used successfully. One method is known as gas sterilization. The advantage with gas is that it can be used for the sterilization of plastics, rubber goods, electric cords, catheters, and other materials which do not withstand repeated steam treatments.

The sterilizing is done under vacuum with a measured amount of humidity. The gas is composed of a mixture of ethylene oxide and carbon dioxide or Freon. This method does not reduce sterilizing time, but it is convenient, since it requires no steam or water connections. An exhaust vent and an electrical outlet are all that is necessary.

The second method is high-vacuum steam sterilization. With this method the temperatures can be elevated to 275° F., and the sterilizing time can be reduced to 3 minutes for dry goods. This reduces deterioration of materials and accelerates the sterilizing time. Because of the forced vacuum, full steam penetration is immediate to all parts of the load. It permits heavier loads and quicker drying time.

BOILING

Boiling water at 212° F. or 100° C. for 30 minutes at altitudes less than 900 feet will sterilize surgical instruments. Longer periods of time are required at higher altitudes. The sterilization time can be shortened by lowering the hydrogen ion concentration. A simple method for achieving this is to add enough sodium carbonate (sal soda) to the water to make a 2 per cent solution.

Instruments are cleaned in the usual manner, eliminating all oil and grease, and then placed in the sterilizer with rachets open. Boiled instruments must be transferred directly to the sterile instrument tray. This limits the amount of preparation that can be done beforehand.

Boilding tends to dull cutting instruments and shortens the life of all instruments. Its use in recent years has been confined mostly to emergency situations.

CHEMICAL STERILIZATION

This form of sterilization depends largely on adsorption. It is therefore imperative that the surface of the instrument be absolutely clean. Raising the temperature of the solution and rubbing the surface helps, but none of the commonly used solutions will kill germs that are embedded in a film of grease or dirt.

Cutting instruments are often sterilized by chemical means. One of the problems with chemical sterilization has been the corrosive action of solutions containing alcohol or formalin. One product which does not have a corrosive effect and yet is an effective disinfectant is Pentacresol (Upjohn).

It should be borne in mind that most chemical disinfectants have no effect on spores. If the presence of spore-forming organisms is suspected, disinfection should take the form of boiling or autoclaving. Fortunately, infections in dogs from spore formers are unusual. These organisms are frequently present in the gut, but they seldom become pathogenic.

THE SURGEON

The preparation of the surgeon for surgery begins with his clothing. A change from street clothing to clean, preferably white attire kept especially for the purpose is desirable. It is equally important to keep footwear spotlessly clean, either by close inspection before surgery or by reserving a pair of shoes for surgery only.

Once the surgeon is properly attired, and before beginning the scrub, a clean cap is placed on the head so that the hair is well covered. This prevents contamination from loose hair and scalp debris (Fig. 4–3). The nose and mouth are then covered by a mask. The mask helps control droplet contamination caused by sneezing, coughing, and talking (Fig. 4–4). Efficiency of the mask is gradually lost during protracted surgery, but its effectiveness can be prolonged by keeping conversation at a minimum. Both the nostrils and the mouth should be covered by the mask, with one tie going over the head and one behind the neck. Persons wearing glasses sometimes encounter the problem of fogging from exhaled air. This can be remedied by fitting the metal nose piece of the mask snugly to the nose (Fig. 4–5) or by rubbing the glasses with hard milled soap and then polishing them (Fig. 4–6).

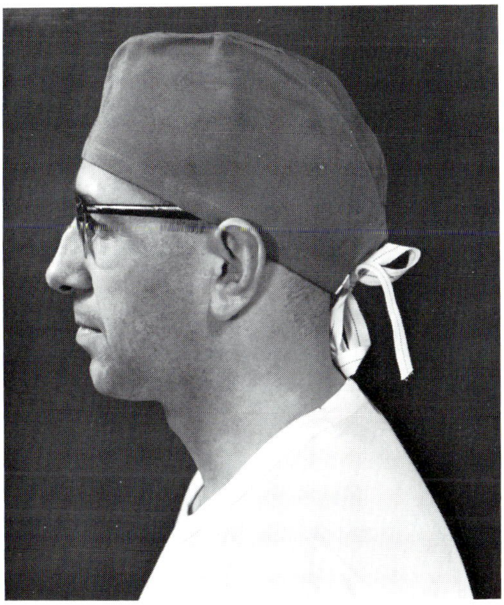

FIGURE 4–3.

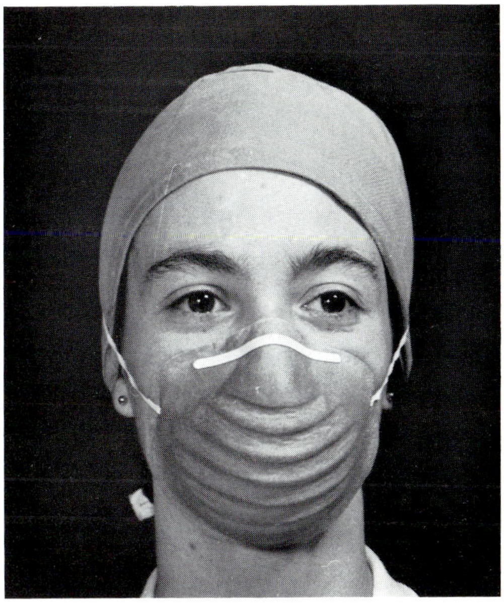

FIGURE 4–4.

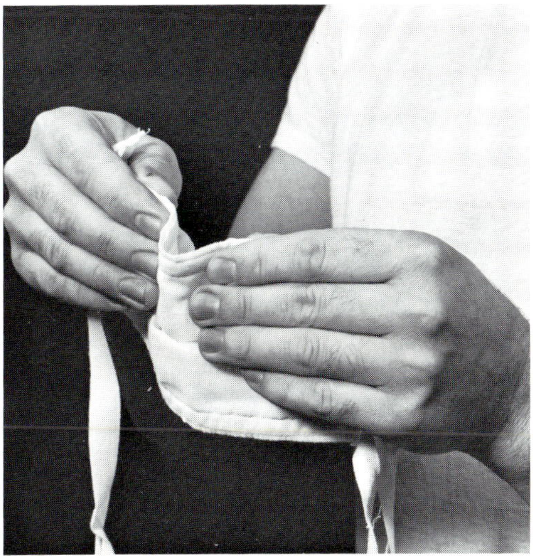

FIGURE 4–5.

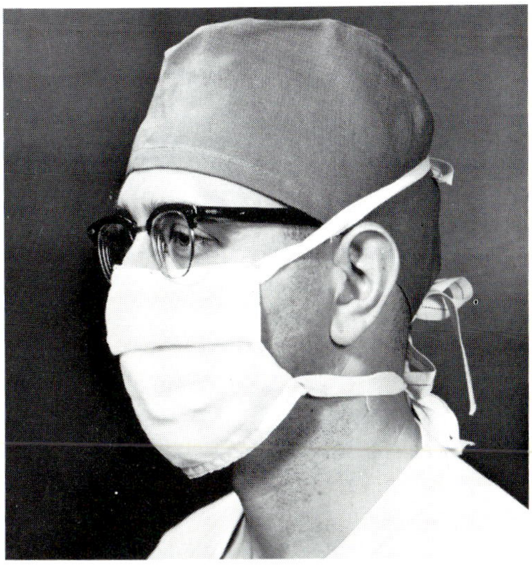

FIGURE 4–6.

SCRUBBING

Preparation of the hands and arms should be done with utmost care. This is no ordinary bathing procedure. Meticulous cleansing of the skin adds an extra safeguard in case the sterile protection (gloves and gown) is penetrated unknowingly during the progress of surgery.

Because there is less likelihood of contamination when foot controls at the scrub sink are used, they are preferred. With this type of control, one can adjust the flow of water with the foot or knee. By the same means, the water temperature can be adjusted and the liquid-soap dispenser operated. The hands and arms are thereby free of contact with anything above the sink level. Scrubbing is begun by a preliminary washing of the hands and arms with soap or detergent and water. Moisten the hands and arms, make a good lather with either bar soap or liquid soap, and wash the hands and arms to a point above the elbows with sufficient briskness to remove all extraneous debris. The fingernails are cleaned next with an orange stick or nail file.

At this point the surgical scrub is started by using a sterile brush to vigorously scrub each of the four surfaces of each finger (Fig. 4–7). If bar soap is used, it should be held in the hand along with the brush until it is no longer needed (Fig. 4–8). It should not be laid down until there is no further need for soap, because the fingers become contaminated in retrieving it. The use of liquid soap and a foot operated dispenser eliminates this minor problem. At least 10 strokes should be given to each surface (Fig. 4–9). The number of strokes and the vigor of the scrub is far more important than the time spent in scrubbing. In all, there should be at least 40 strokes on each finger and 20 strokes each on the nails, the palm of the hand, and the back of the hand. The scrubbing should be done systematically. The surgeon should start with the thumb and then move on to the fingers, the nails, the palm, and finally the dorsum of the hand (Fig. 4–10).

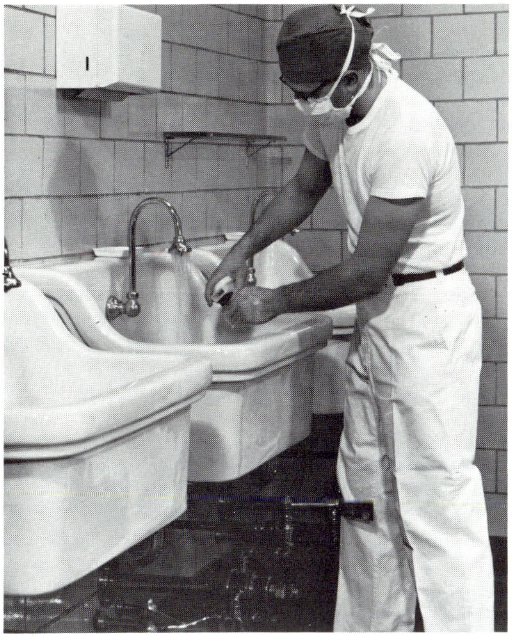

FIGURE 4–7.

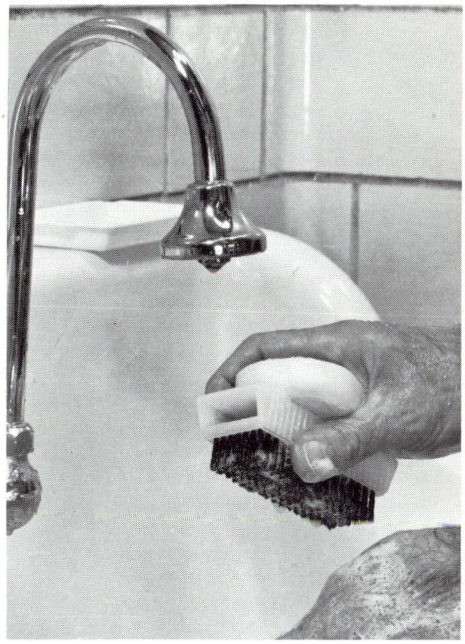

FIGURE 4–8.

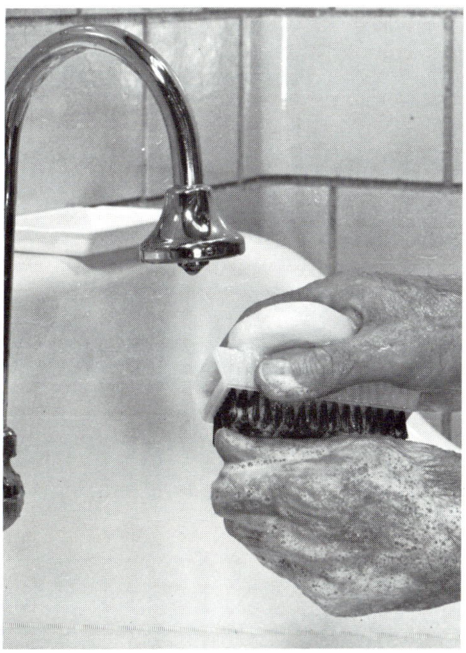

FIGURE 4–9.

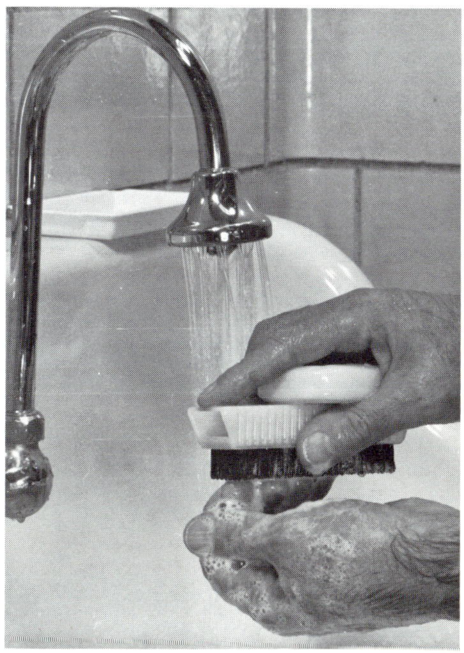

FIGURE 4–10.

Start scrubbing the arm at the wrists and gradually work up tho arm to a point above the elbow (Fig. 4–11). Once scrubbing of the arm is begun, do not bring the brush back to the hands (Fig. 4–12).

Rinsing is done with warm water (Fig. 4–13). Allow it to flow from the hands to the elbow, and always keep the hands above elbow level. Allow sufficient time for water to drip from the elbows before entering the arm-immersion solution. This avoids excessive dilution and prolongs the usefulness of the solution.

The immersion basin should be filled with sufficient solution so that it reaches the elbows when the hands and arms are immersed. This solution may be either 1 : 1000 aqueous Roccal, 70 per cent ethyl alcohol, or 50 per cent isopropyl alcohol. The Roccal solution is frequently used following a scrub with hexachlorophene. It should not be used following a soap scrub, because the soap neutralizes its action. The alcohol solutions remove the hexachlorophene film but are highly effective antiseptics in themselves. Immersion in alcohol for 1 minute will produce the same germicidal effect as scrubbing for 10 minutes. Rubbing of the hands and arms while immersed greatly increases the germicidal action (Fig. 4–14).

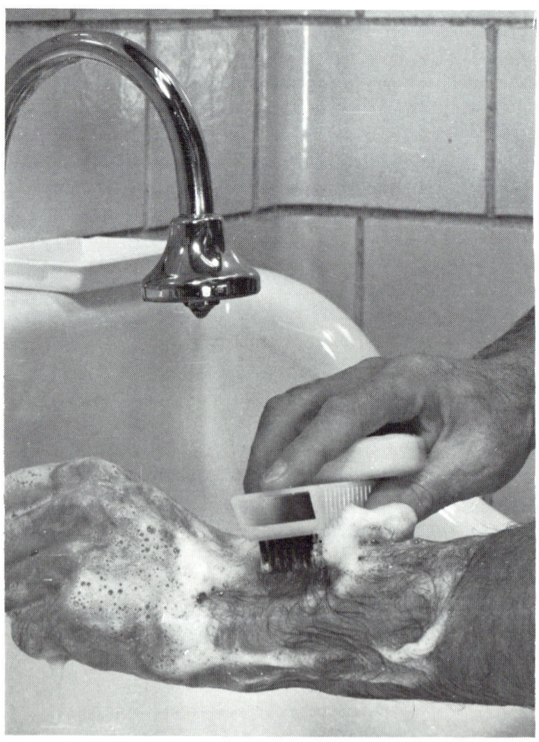

FIGURE 4–11.

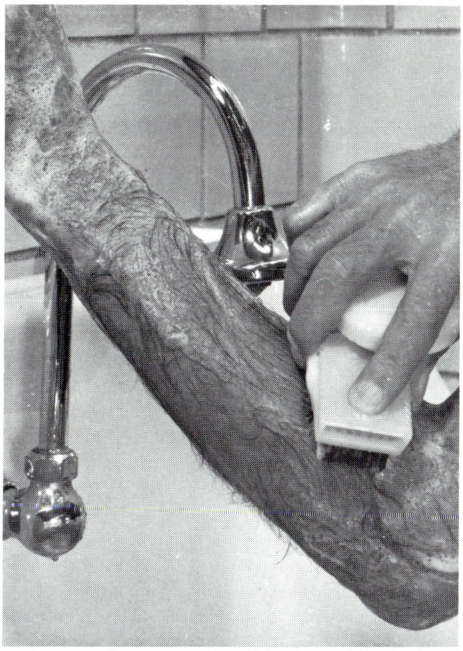

FIGURE 4–12.

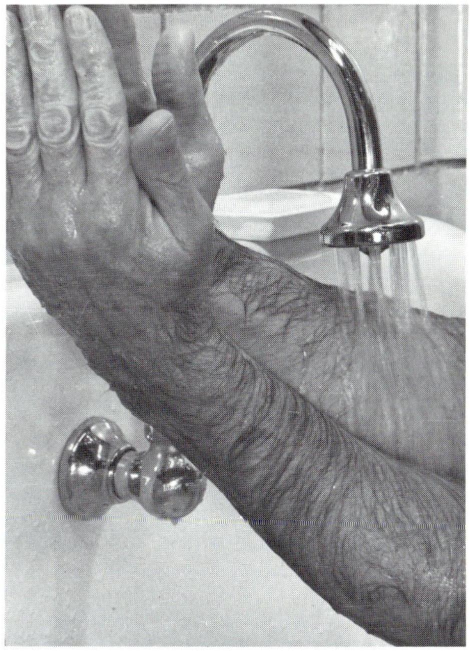

FIGURE 4–13.

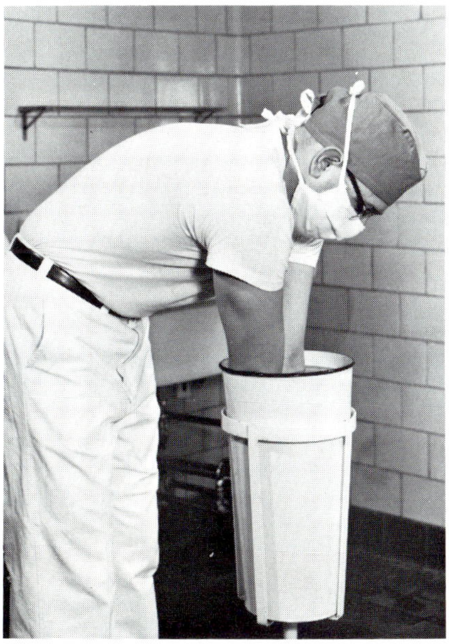

FIGURE 4–14.

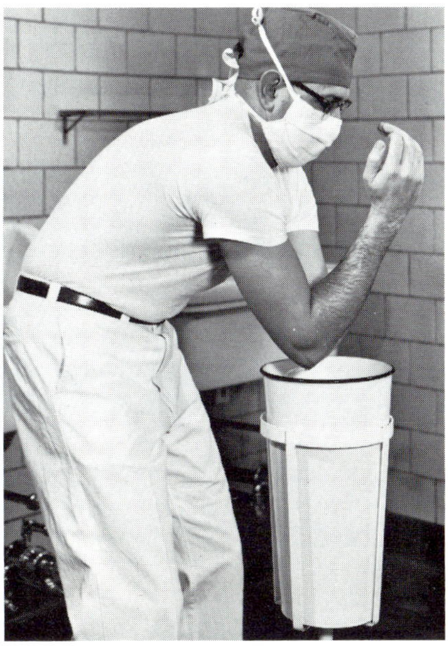

FIGURE 4–15.

When the hands and arms are withdrawn from the immersing fluid, the excess should be allowed to drip from the elbows (Fig. 4–15) before drying with a sterile towel (Fig. 4–16). Unfold the towel and dry the hands first by blotting (Fig. 4–17). Then with short, upward, stroking motions, dry one arm by beginning at the wrist and working upward (Fig. 4–18). Then transfer the towel to the opposite hand, making certain that it is grasped in the same spot (Fig. 4–19), and dry the other arm with a fresh part of the towel after the manner of the first arm (Fig. 4–20). It is important that the interchange between hands be done without the hands contacting that portion of the towel that has touched the arm.

Great care should be taken to avoid any contamination of the hands following the scrub and during the gowning and gloving procedure. Naturally, the principal source of trouble comes from contact with nonsterile parts of the body or with wearing apparel. The face and neck are particularly vulnerable spots. Any of the clothing worn during the scrub or any parts of the sterile operating gown that have contacted nonsterile areas must be carefully avoided by the clean hands. Even the slightest contact breaks the asepsis. To avoid unnecessary exposure, the hands are held in front and the elbows are slightly flexed. It is arbitrarily assumed that nothing below the belt is sterile, even after donning the gown. Therefore, the arms should never be held at the sides or placed in any position below the belt line. Extreme caution should be exercised at all times.

If a wet technique is desired, the sterile gloves can be deposited in the arm-immersion basin. It is then possible to go directly to the donning of the gloves without any intervening drying procedure.

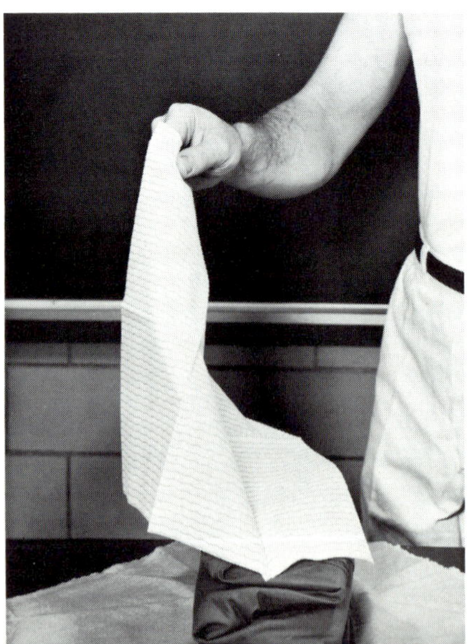

FIGURE 4–16.

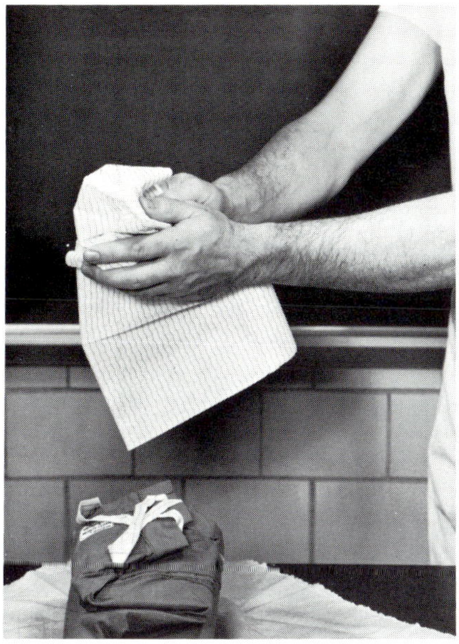

FIGURE 4–17.

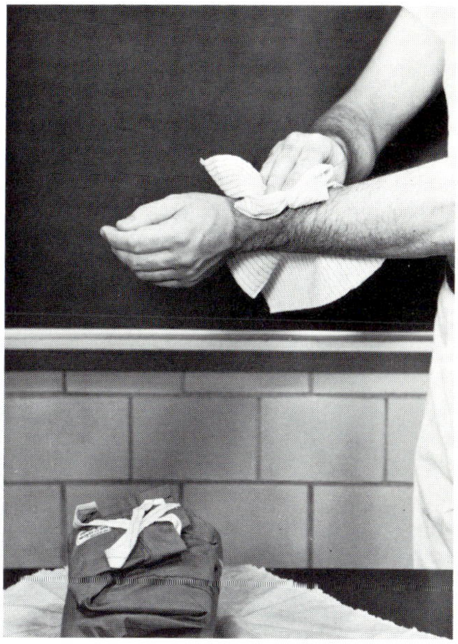

FIGURE 4–18.

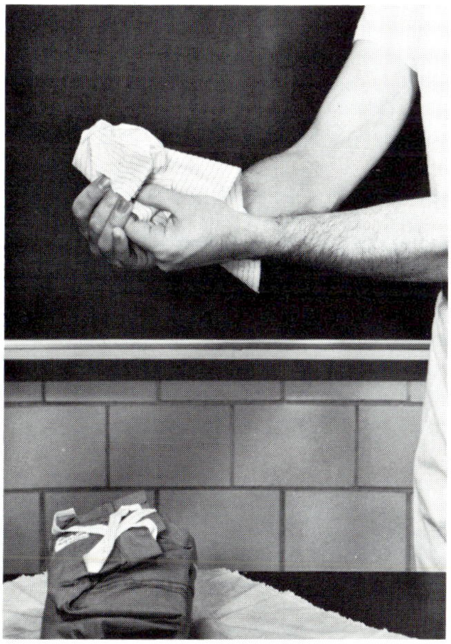

FIGURE 4–19.

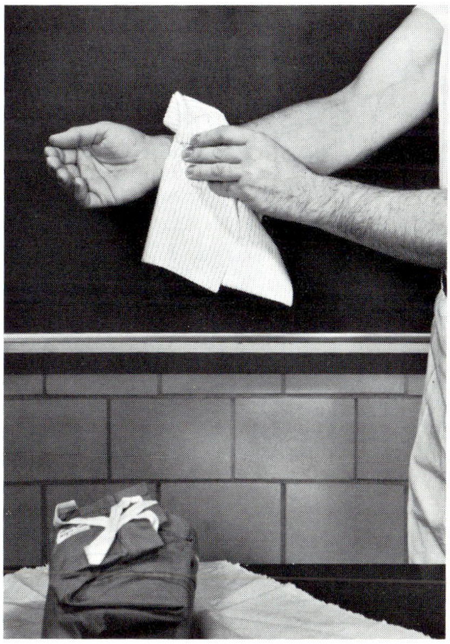

FIGURE 4–20.

GOWNING

The gown may be put on either by the surgeon alone or with the help of an operating room assistant. Since many veterinarians are obliged to perform many services by themselves, it is well to learn to don the gown unaided.

STEP 1. The gown is grasped by the neck ties and lifted from the pack with care so that it does not drag across the tabletop (Fig. 4–21). As the gown is lifted, it unfolds to its full length. For this reason the neck ties should be held as high as possible until the gown clears the table. Hold it at arm's length and turn it so that the inside is toward the operator; at the same time make certain that there is ample room for donning without touching surrounding objects. Shake the gown to free the sleeves and any remaining folds. Toss the gown into the air and catch it by thrusting the hands into the arm holes.

STEP 2. It is important to keep the gown thus suspended on the outstretched forearms until the hands have been thrust through the cuffs (Fig. 4–22). The inside of the gown should not touch the body of the operator until the foresleeves have been adjusted. The sleeve is pulled over the left hand by grasping it with the right hand, which is still covered by the right sleeve (Fig. 4–23). The right sleeve is pulled into place by flexing the left arm, which reaches inside the gown without touching the body or the right arm, and grasps the sleeve through the front of the gown (Fig. 4–24).

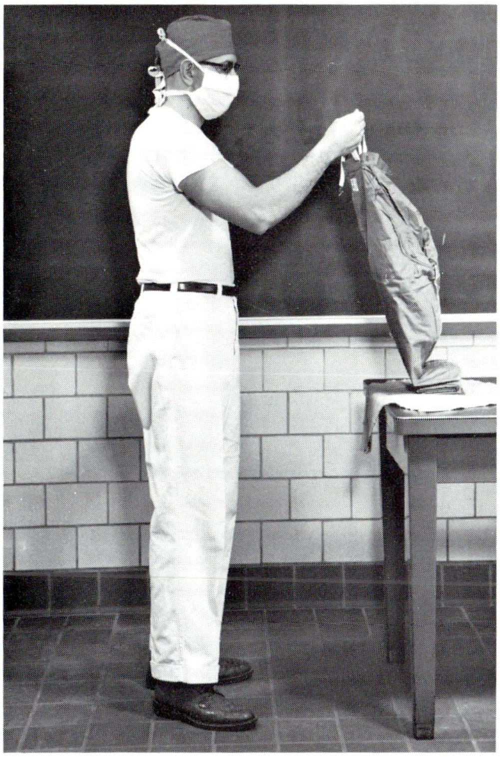

FIGURE 4–21.

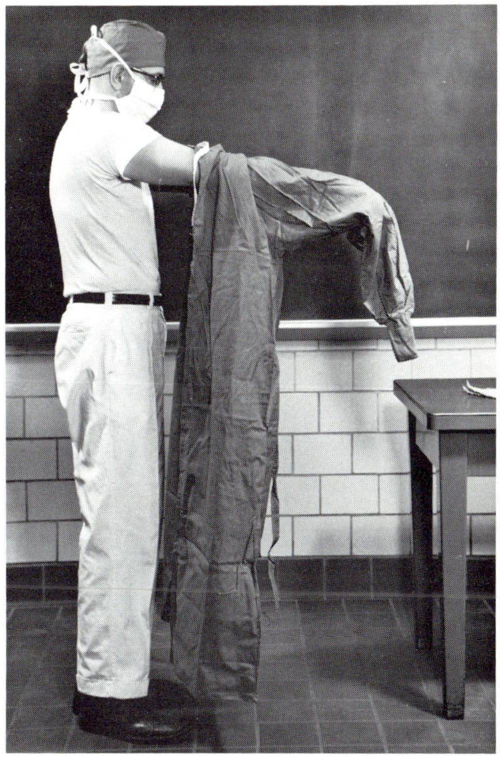

FIGURE 4–22.

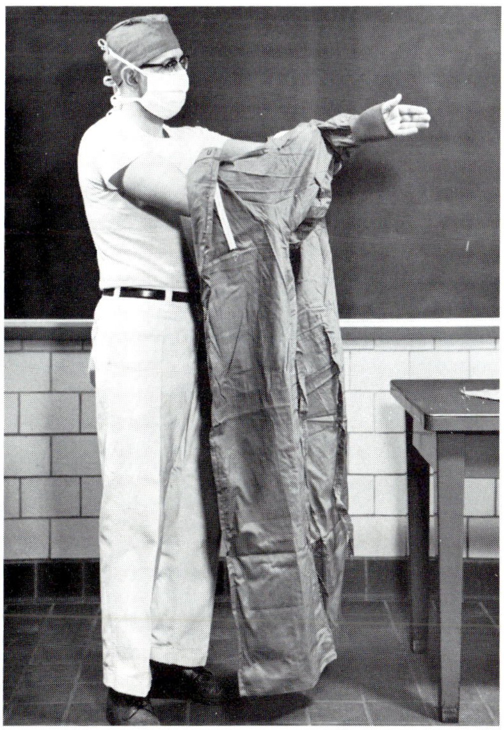

FIGURE 4–23.

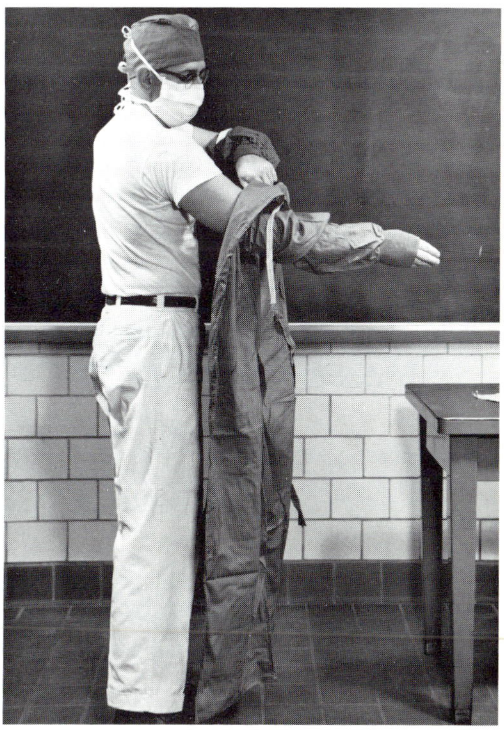

FIGURE 4–24.

STEP 3. When the sleeves are in place on the forearms, the neck ties are again grasped by crossing the hands and reaching over the neckband to the opposite side (Fig. 4–25). After retrieving the neck ties, the hands are reversed so that the right hand holds the right tie and the left hand holds the left tie. The ties are then carried behind the neck, and care is taken that no contact is made with the body. The sleeves can be pulled into place by grasping the ties in one hand and extending the opposite arm (Fig. 4–26). Care must be taken not to touch the back of the head or neck while tying the neck band (Fig. 4–27).

STEP 4. The belt is tied by first leaning forward so that the ties swing free of the gown (Fig. 4–28). They are grasped near the end and are carried in a wide arc to the back. Tying should be done without contact of the hands to any part of the gown or body (Fig. 4–29).

If an assistant is used for gowning, Steps 2, 3, and 4 may be omitted by the operator. At the end of Step 1, the assistant, standing behind the operator, grasps the neck ties and pulls the sleeves into place. After the collar is tied, the operator bends forward and grasps the belt ties near the middle of the free ends and carries them laterally until the assistant can grasp the ends and tie them. No contact should be made between the hands of the operator and the assistant.

Once the surgeon is gowned, he must be especially careful not to brush against objects or personnel in the area. This caution must be practiced until it becomes habitual.

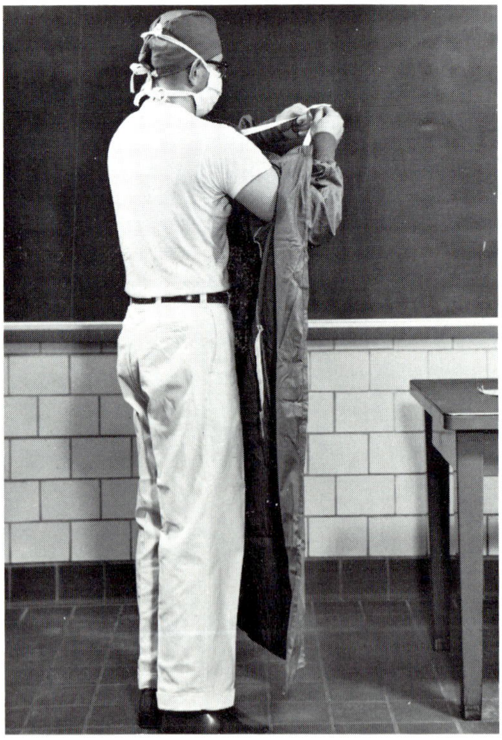

FIGURE 4–25.

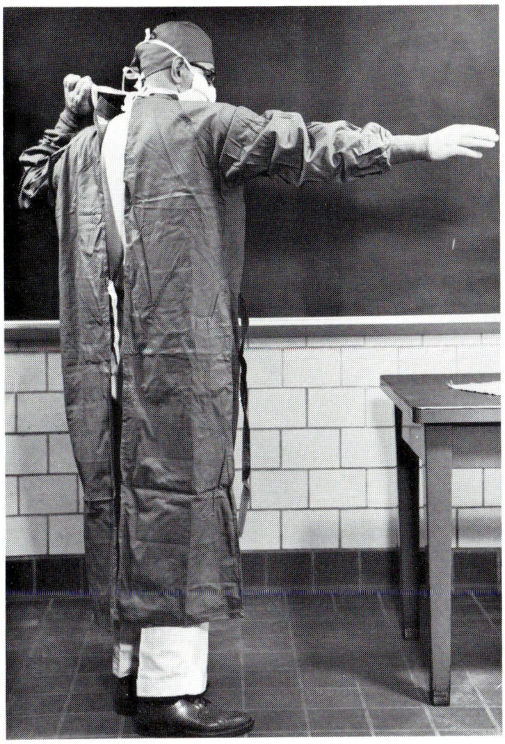

FIGURE 4–26.

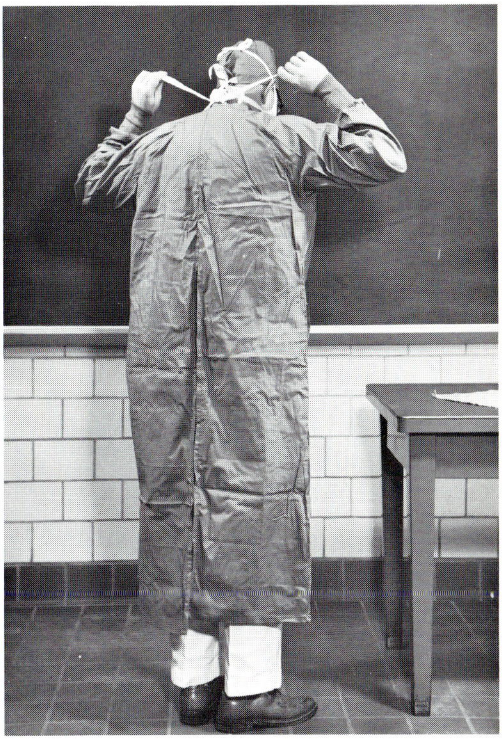

FIGURE 4–27.

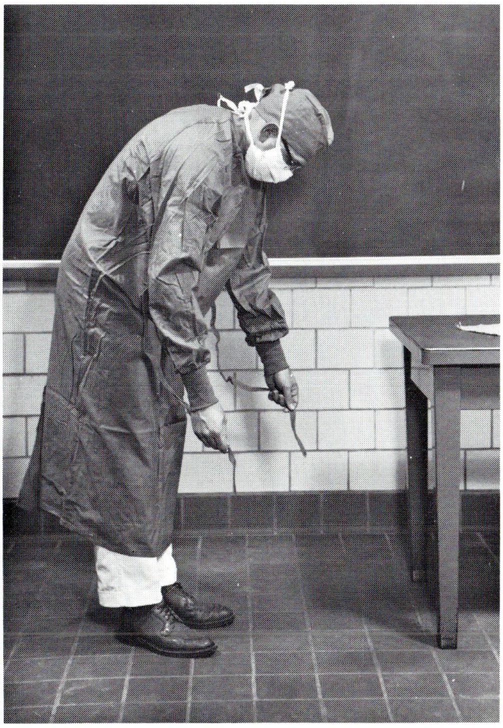

FIGURE 4–28.

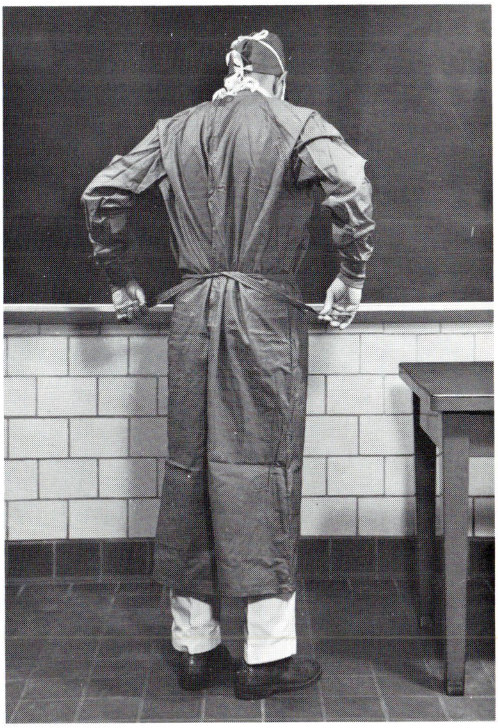

FIGURE 4–29.

GLOVING

The selection of the proper glove size is an important contributing factor toward the comfort and dexterity of the surgeon. Most beginners select sizes that are too large. The glove should fit neatly but not tightly. It should be free of wrinkles and snug enough so that it does not slide on the fingers as the hands are manipulated. Operators with short fingers should wear "cadet" sizes. These gloves are normal in size in all respects except that they have shorter fingers. In the beginning, a properly fitting glove usually feels tight, but as the operator becomes accustomed to the feel of a well fitted glove, this sensation passes. Once the adjustment is made, the sense of touch and the ability to handle fine instruments and sutures equals the acuteness of the bare hand.

Before donning the gloves, the hands should be powdered. This is a form of lubrication which facilitates the insertion of the hand into the glove. The powder ordinarily used is a specially treated cornstarch derivative (Biosorb) (Fig. 4–30). It is applied to the hands over a receptacle with care so that a minimum of dust is created. Spilling on the floor or clouding the air can create a hazard from contamination. A cream (Biosorb cream) may be used in place of the powder (Fig. 4–31). This cream rapidly evaporates and leaves a film of powder on the hands, thereby excluding the danger from dust in the air or on the floor. The cream is actually preferable.

As the gloves are picked up, it is well to remember that only the inside of the glove should be touched. A good way to recall this rule is to repeat the formula "rubber to rubber and skin to skin," meaning that the rubber side of the glove, or the outside, should only be touched by the outside of the other glove, and the skin side, or inside, should only be touched by the bare hand.

The left glove is picked up by the right hand (Fig. 4–32). It is held on the palm side of the everted cuff. The left hand is inserted into the glove while steady traction is applied by the right hand (Fig. 4–33). The fingers should be spread slightly and worked into the glove with minute flexing and extending movements. As soon as the fingers of the left hand are in place, the glove is released, leaving the cuff still everted.

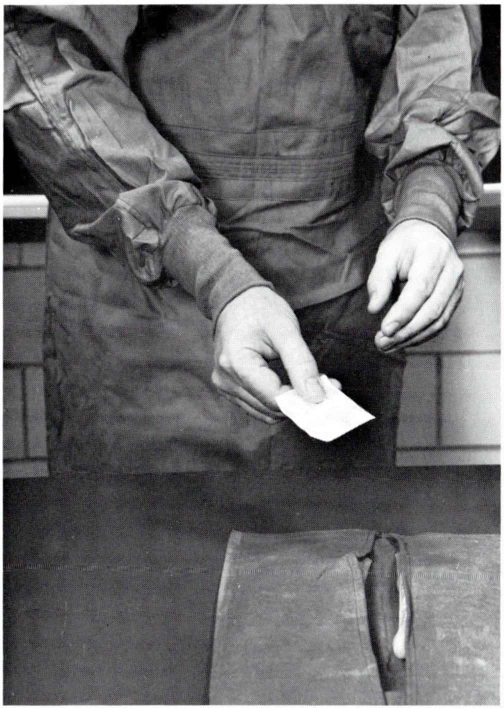

FIGURE 4–30.

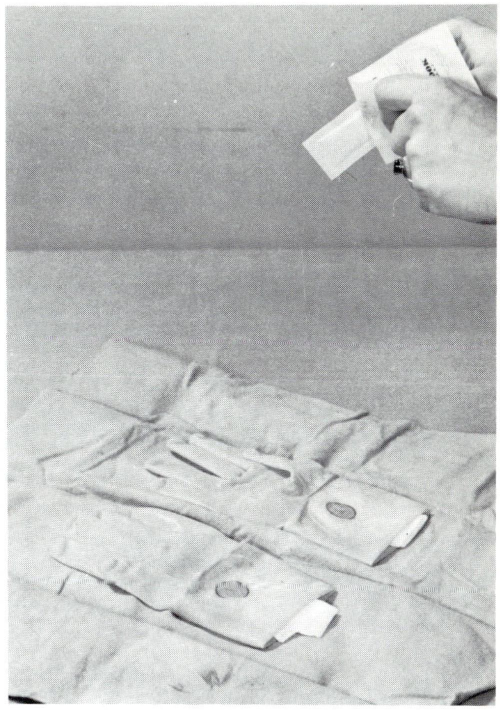

FIGURE 4–31.

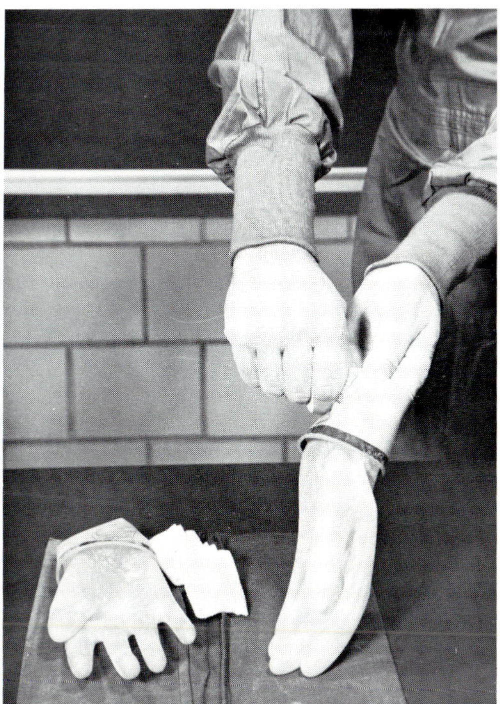

FIGURE 4–32.

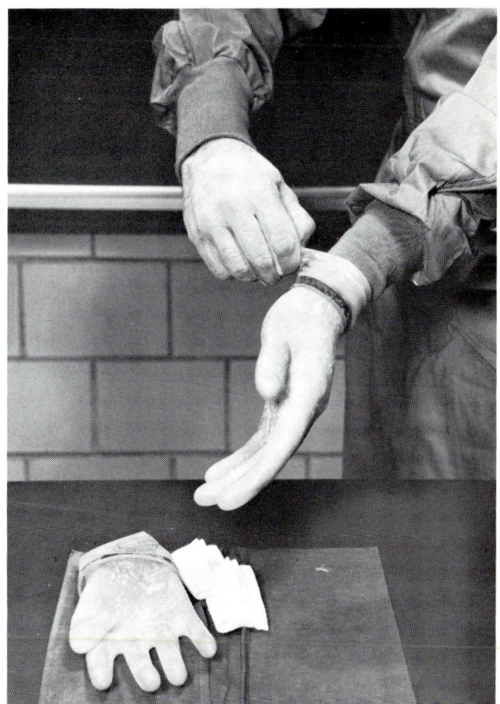

FIGURE 4–33.

The right glove is picked up by placing the fingers of the gloved left hand within the fold of the everted cuff, which is actually the outside of the glove (Fig. 4–34). The glove should be engaged on the palm surface, and the fingers of the left hand should be flexed (Fig. 4–35). Thumb pressure is not necessary. This glove is completely donned before leaving it. Make sure that the cuff covers the gown cuff completely.

The donning of the left glove is then completed by slipping the fingers of the gloved right hand beneath the fold of the everted cuff and stretching it over the gown cuff with a circular motion (Figs. 4–36 and 4–37).

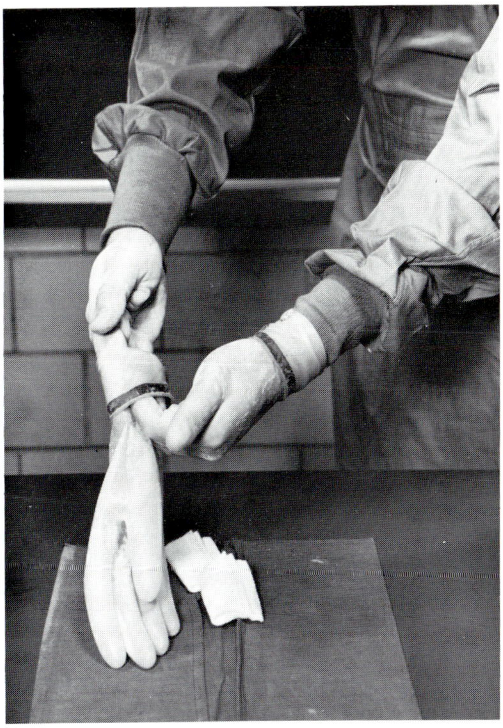

FIGURE 4–34.

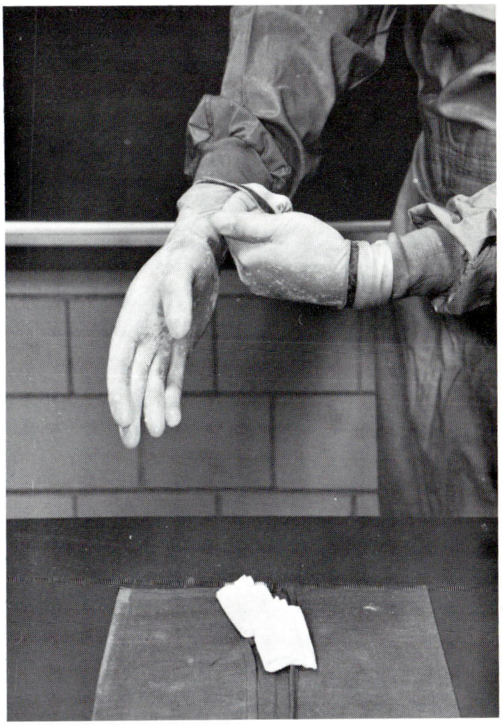

FIGURE 4–35.

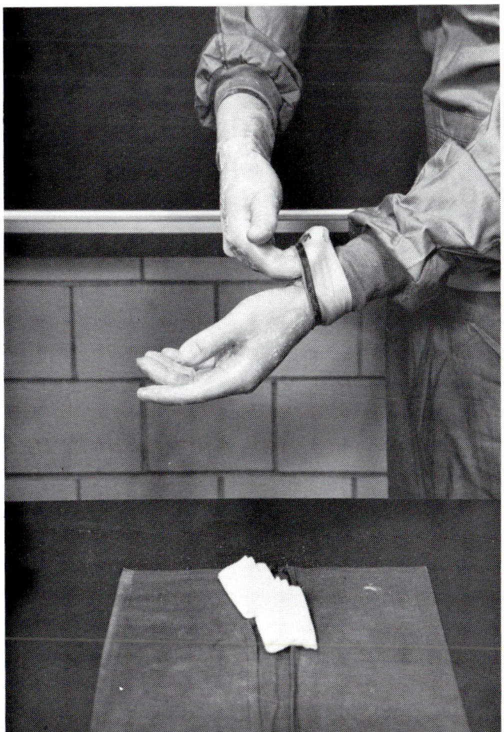

FIGURE 4–36.

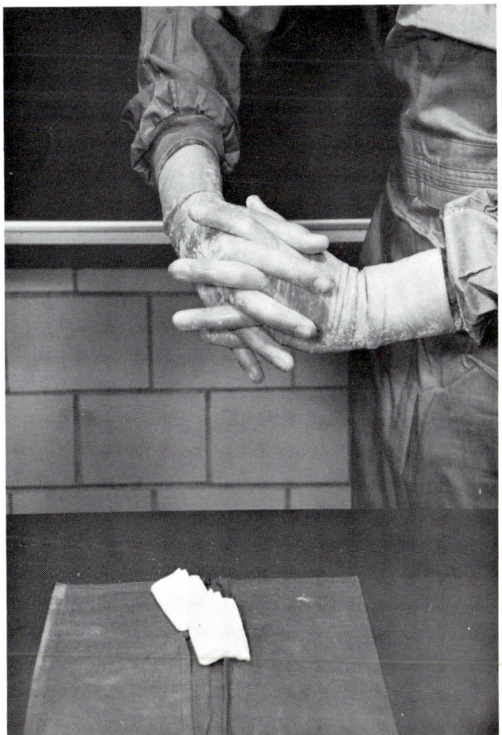

FIGURE 4–37.

THE PATIENT

The preparation of the patient should receive as much attention as that given to the surgeon. It should be thorough in every detail inasmuch as it is frequently the weakest link in surgical preparation. With few exceptions the work is best carried out under general anesthesia. Even under ideal conditions, the patient's skin is not sterile, but a good preparation without interference from the patient reduces the likelihood of contamination considerably.

ANESTHESIA

A complete description of anesthetics and their use is available in *Small Animal Anesthesia* by W. V. Lumb. Our description will be confined to the preliminary steps of induction preparatory to surgery. While the use of pentobarbital is quite general, one may wish to use an inhalant form of anesthetic. In either case an intravenous injection is usually made. This may be for total anesthetization or for preanesthetic purposes.

RESTRAINT

The patient should be put on a table of convenient height and controlled by one person while the other makes the injection. A venipuncture can be accomplished single handedly, but this should only be attempted as an emergency measure. Place the patient in sternal recumbency, and make sure that he is comfortable and relaxed.

Most dogs and cats do not require forceful restraint. Cats are especially refractive to excessive restraint measures. Once the confidence of the patient has been gained, very mild pressure is all that is required in order to negotiate a venipuncture.

There may be an occasional patient that requires muzzling or a cat that should be placed in stocks (Fig. 4–38) for the safety of the assistant as well as the patient (Fig. 4–39). These are the exception rather than the rule, however. If the anesthetist is planning on venipuncture of the right cephalic vein, the assistant takes up a position on the left side of the patient. His left hand is placed under the throat and his right hand is on the right forelimb of the patient. The limb should be between the thumb and forefinger. The thumb should be slightly flexed. Slight pressure is applied as the arm and hand are gently rotated clockwise toward the patient until the patient's elbow rests in the palm of the assistant's hand. The assistant can then bring his elbow and forearm to rest on the table. He is now in control of the patient, and the vein is properly distended for the anesthetist (Fig. 4–40).

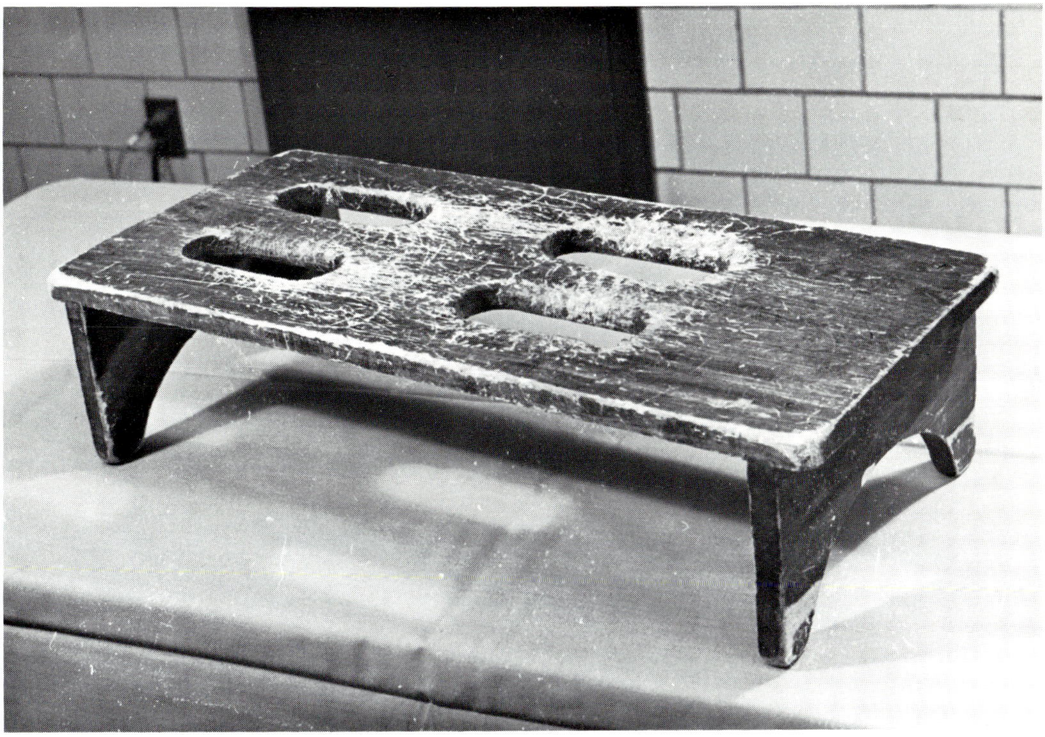

FIGURE 4–38.

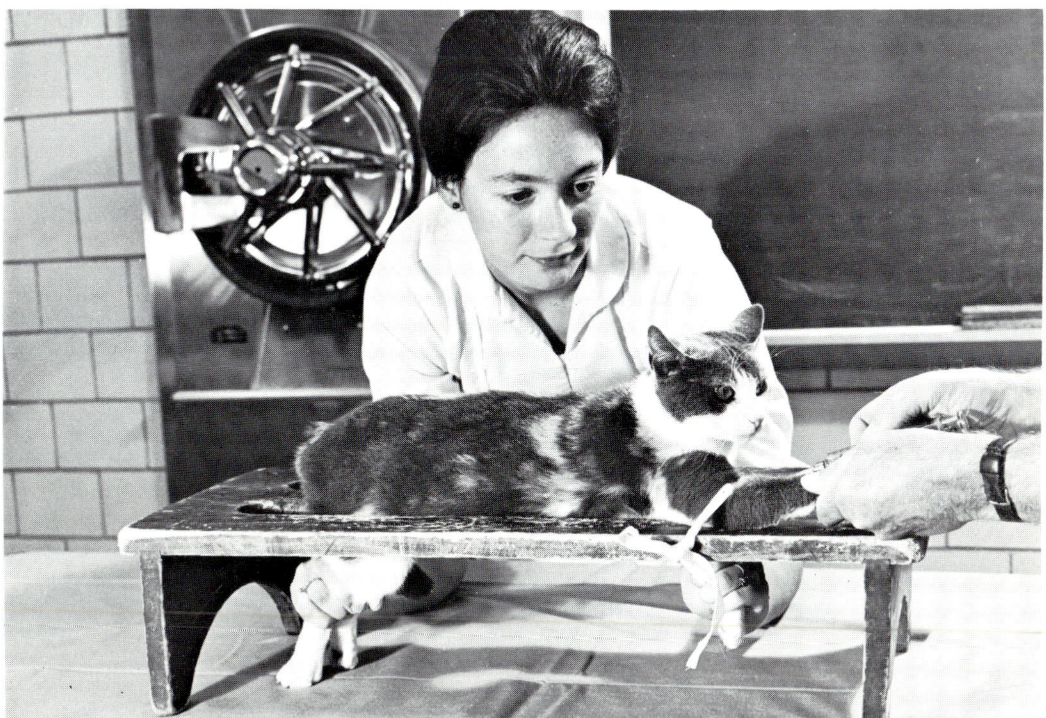

FIGURE 4–39.

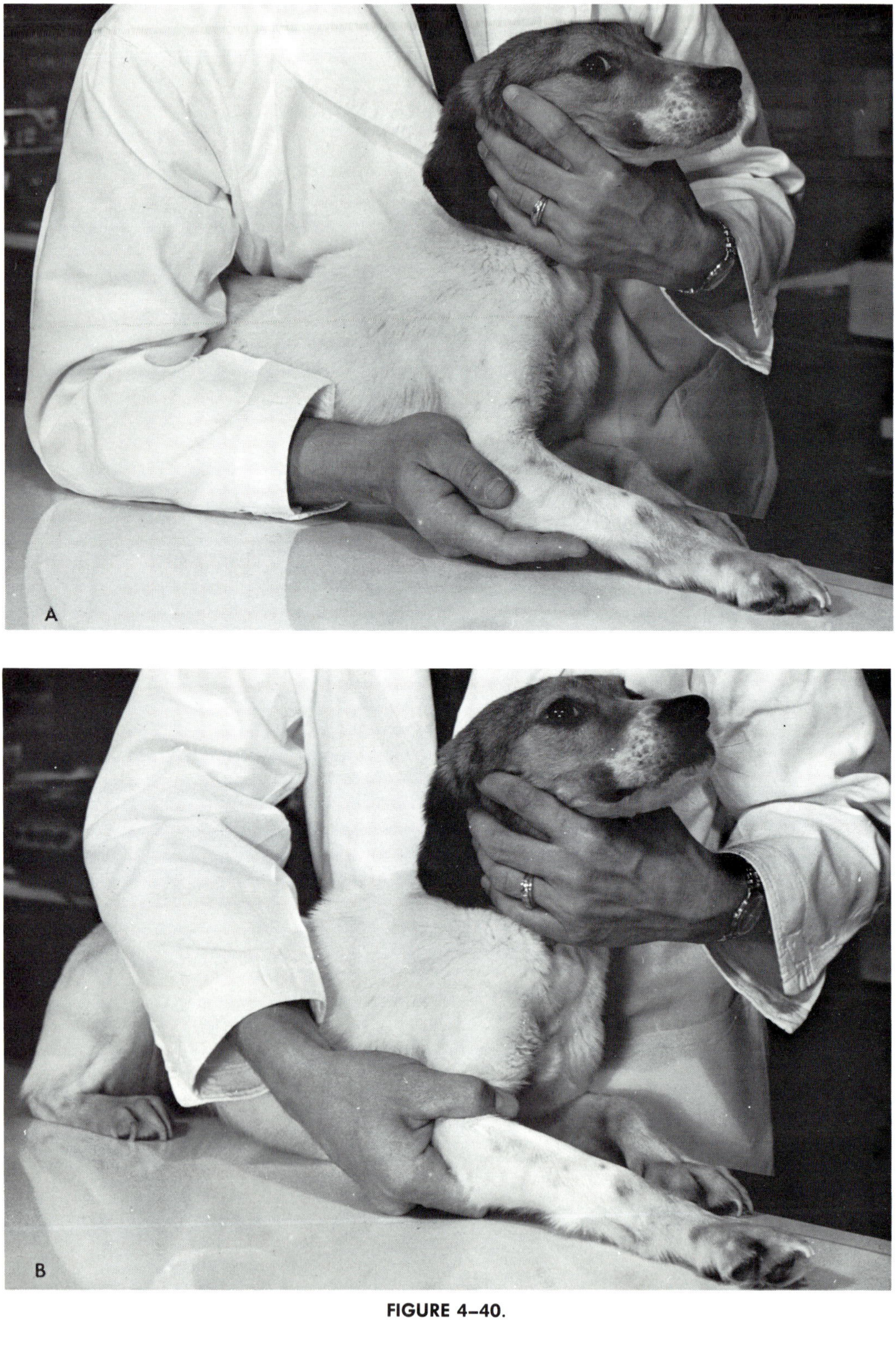

FIGURE 4–40.

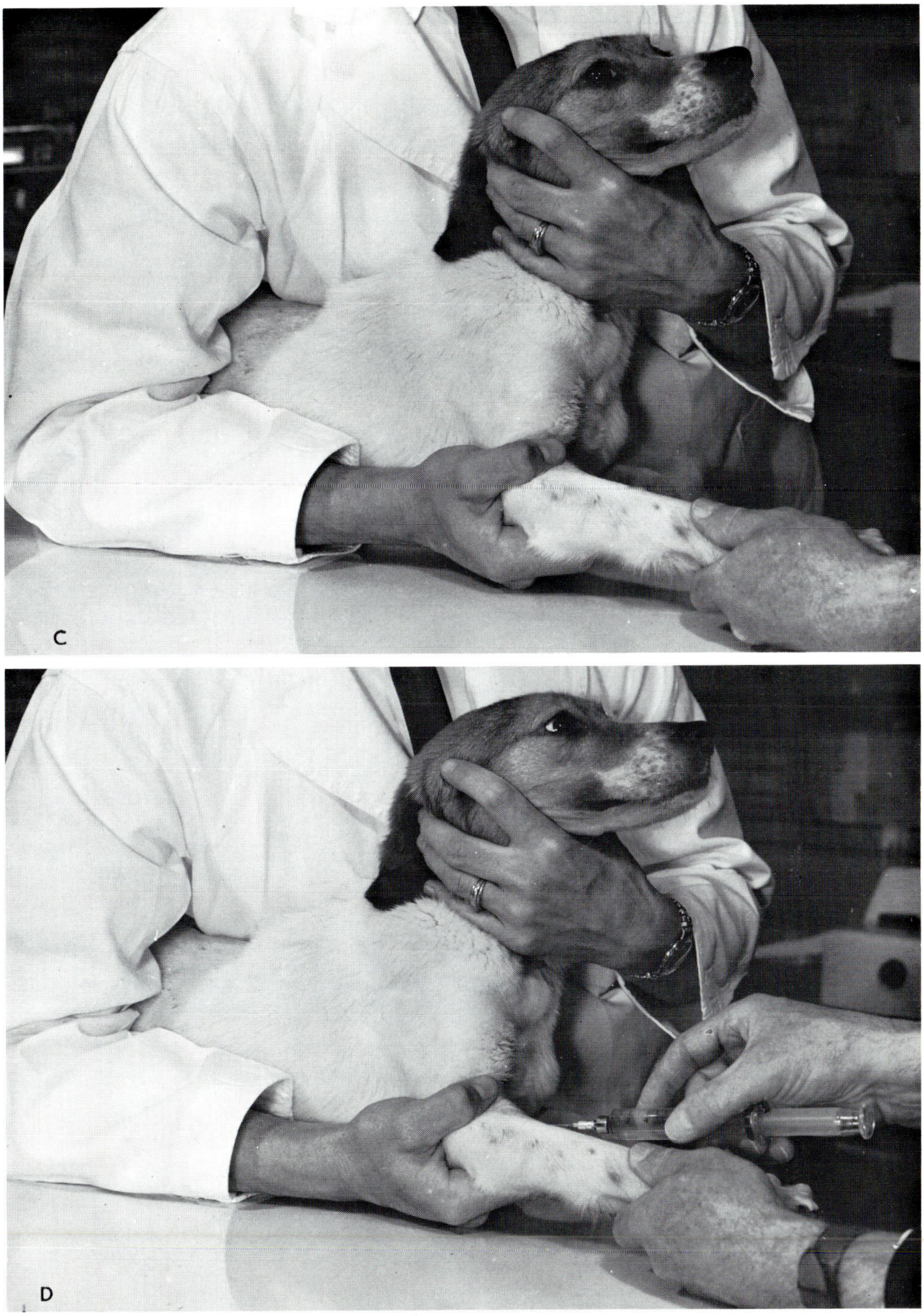

FIGURE 4–40. *Continued.*

VENIPUNCTURE

In the meantime, the anesthetist, having filled his syringe with the proper anesthetic, makes certain the bevel of the needle is aligned in the same plane as the graduations on the syringe. This serves the double purpose of rapidly locating the position of the bevel after the needle is under the skin and of keeping the graduations readily available when the bevel is in proper position.

As the assistant brings the extended forelimb into position, it is grasped by the anesthetist, who places the palmar surface of his hand against the palmar surface of the patient's foot. The hair and skin over the cephalic vein are thoroughly swabbed with alcohol or some suitable antiseptic. It is not necessary to clip the hair; in fact, it may be detrimental to do so.

The anesthetist applies pressure to the skin with his thumb and at the same time flexes it so that the skin is tensed over the vein. Holding the syringe lightly between the thumb and middle finger, with the index finger extended to balance it, he places the needle, with the bevel upward, on the skin at a point just medial to the midline of the vein (see Figure 4–41). The needle is then aimed along the axis of the vein and thrust into it.

As soon as blood appears in the barrel of the syringe, the assistant relaxes the tension of his right thumb and the injection is begun (Fig. 4–42). Pentobarbital is given to effect and not primarily by dosage. It is therefore important when using this anesthetic to watch the reflexes carefully. Usually the pupillary reaction is the first visible sign. The pupil dilates widely and then gradually contracts to pinpoint size. The palpebral reflex, which can be elicited by tapping gently medial to the inner canthus of the eye, gradually disappears. Finally, the pedal reflex, produced by pressure on the foot or toes, is lost, whereupon the injection of anesthetic is discontinued.

While the cephalic veins are commonly used in both the dog and the cat, other veins may be used. Both the medial and lateral saphenous are readily available and should be considered as the second choice. Lumb recommends the femoral vein in the cat. The jugular vein is ordinarily considered a third choice but is seldom used if other veins are available. The sublingual veins are not recommended because of the tendency to form large hematomas. This difficulty can be avoided if the needle is inserted into the muscle first and the vein approached from the dorsal side with the bevel of the needle away from the vein.

The intravenous route of injectable general anesthetics is the only one that can be recommended as safe and without tissue damage if properly performed. If some of the anesthetic is deposited outside the vein there may be an acute inflammatory reaction with sloughing (a very unsightly and embarrassing situation). At the time such an accident occurs, the area should be briskly massaged and injected with 2 per cent procaine hydrochloride. The massaging should be continued at intervals for at least two days.

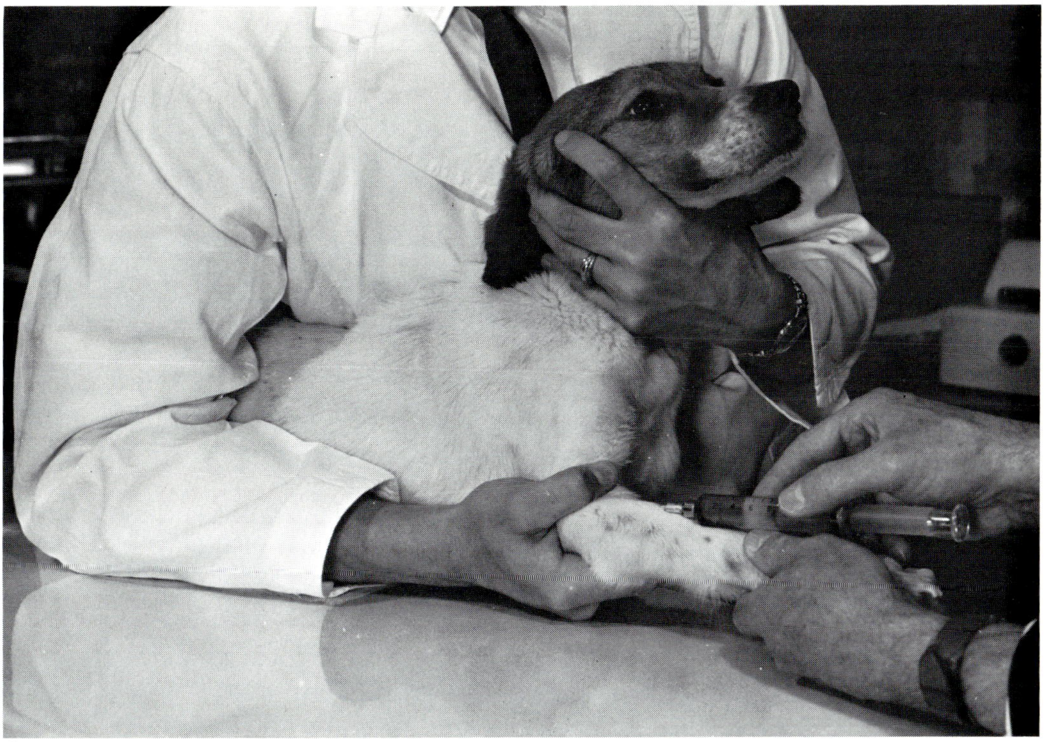

FIGURE 4–41.

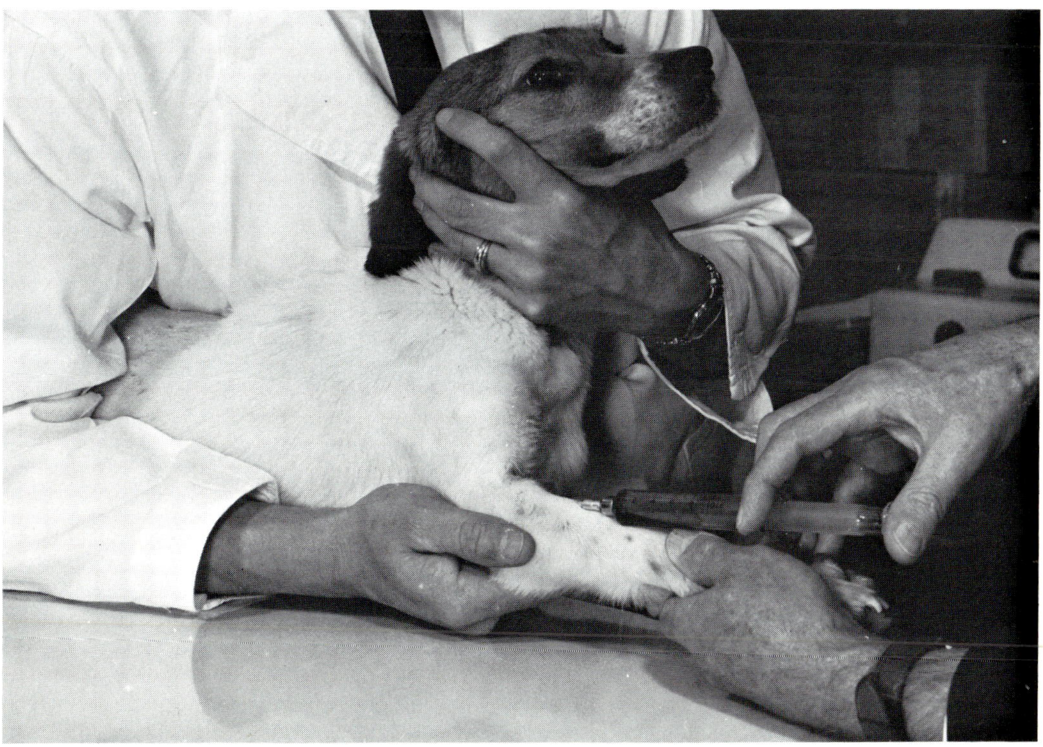

FIGURE 4–42.

INTUBATION

It is regarded as good practice to intubate all patients that are under general anesthesia. There are many advantages to such a procedure: an open airway is assured, the lungs are protected against regurgitated material, and a quick, easy means of resuscitation is provided. When an inhalant type of anesthetic is used, intubation is almost necessary for smooth administration. A short-acting barbiturate is commonly used for induction when the anesthetic is to be volatile.

Endotracheal tubes are made of plastic, rubber, or metal and are available in a variety of sizes. When selecting a tube for a patient, always choose one that approximates the inside diameter of the trachea. It should fit snugly but should not be forced. This gives an adequate airway and requires less inflation of the cuff.

The tube should be lubricated before passing. Water or certain water soluble jellies may be used, but oils and ordinary lubricating jellies are not recommended. After use the tube should be thoroughly cleaned with soap and water.

A laryngeal speculum is often used to restrain the epiglottis and open the glottis so that the endotracheal tube can be passed easily. One should also learn to pass the tube without the speculum, since the speculum may not always be available in a moment of emergency (Fig. 4–43). With the dog in sternal recumbency, the left hand is passed into the mouth so that the index finger can depress the epiglottis and touch the glottis (Fig. 4–44). The tube is then passed with the right hand, keeping the bevel up, between the left index finger and the epiglottis. When the tip of the tube touches the glottis, the tube is rotated one-quarter turn. The tube is now directed downward through the glottis by the tip of the left index finger (Fig. 4–45).

It is sufficient to insert the tube so that the cuff is just beyond the larynx. Inserting the tube to the tracheal bifurcation is dangerous (Fig. 4–46).

To ascertain correct positioning of the tube, the throat region is palpated. If two tubes can be palpated, it indicates that the endotracheal tube is in the esophagus. If only one tube is found, the positioning is correct, since the tube palpated is the trachea (Fig. 4–47). Placing the ear to the end of the tube and blowing into the tube are not reliable tests. Sometimes one can hear and feel air movement when the tube is in the esophagus, particularly if the respirations are deep and the stomach is slightly distended. It is also quite likely that the cough reflex will be abolished if the patient is properly anesthetized before intubation; therefore, blowing in the tube will give little indication of its location.

A simple way to anchor the tube so that it will not be dislodged is to tie a 1 inch bandage around it and then recross the ends under the tube and tie over the nose in a bow knot (Fig. 4–48). This holds the tube firmly against the roof of the mouth, yet it is easily released if necessary.

The cuff is next inflated with a small amount of air, usually 5 ml. or less. The tubing to the cuff is clamped with a rubber-shod forceps, and the forceps is tied to the anchor bandage over the nose so that it will not become entangled when the patient is moved.

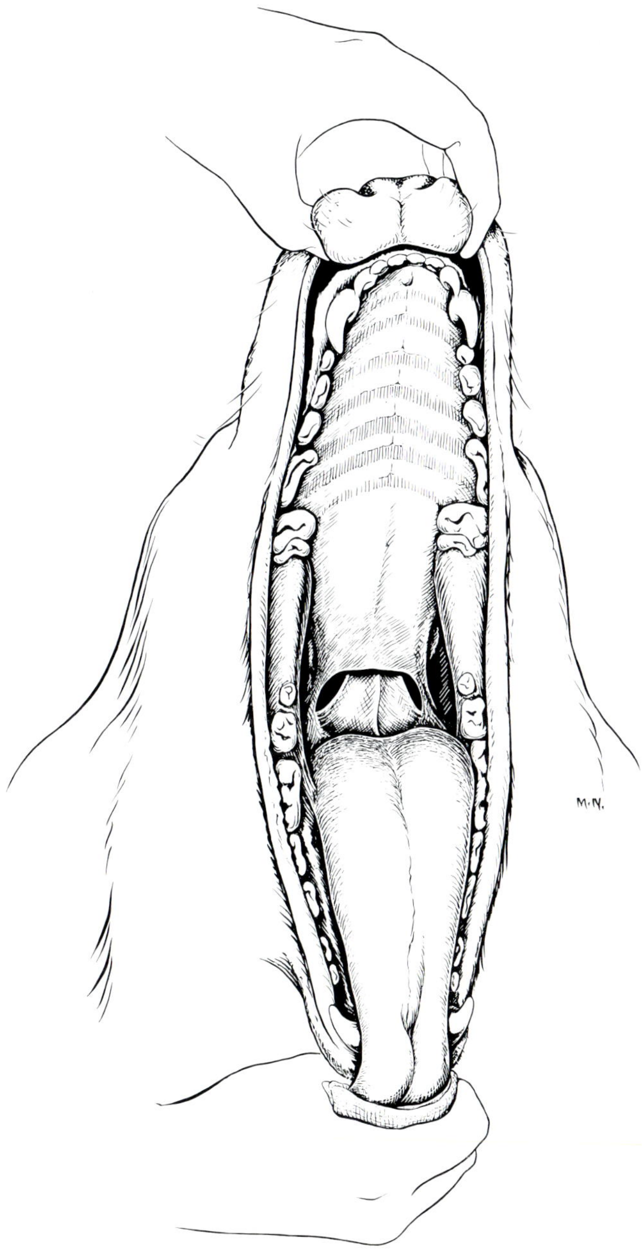

FIGURE 4–43.

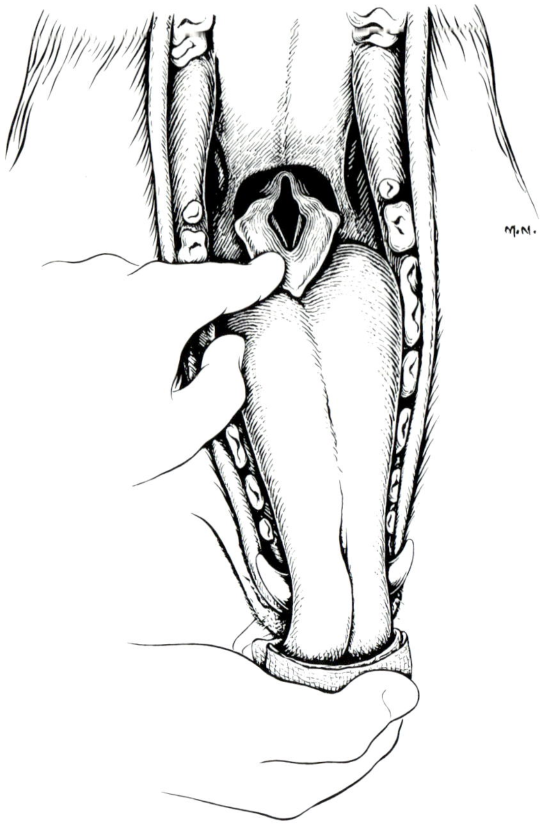

FIGURE 4–44.

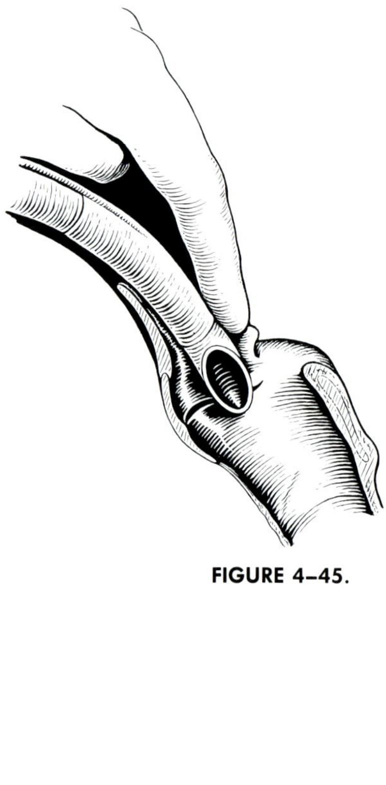

FIGURE 4–45.

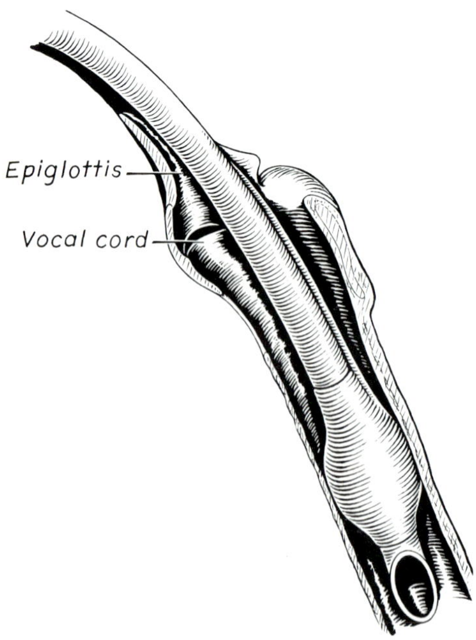

FIGURE 4–46.

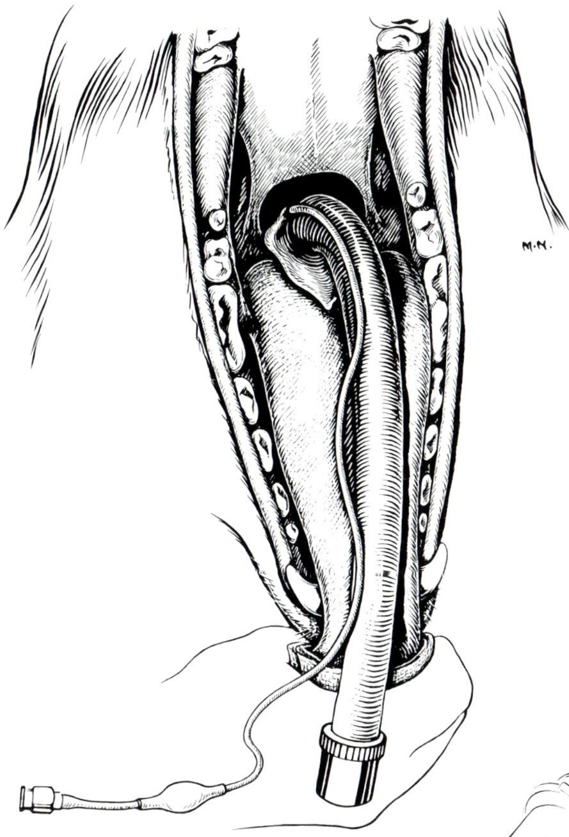

FIGURE 4–47.

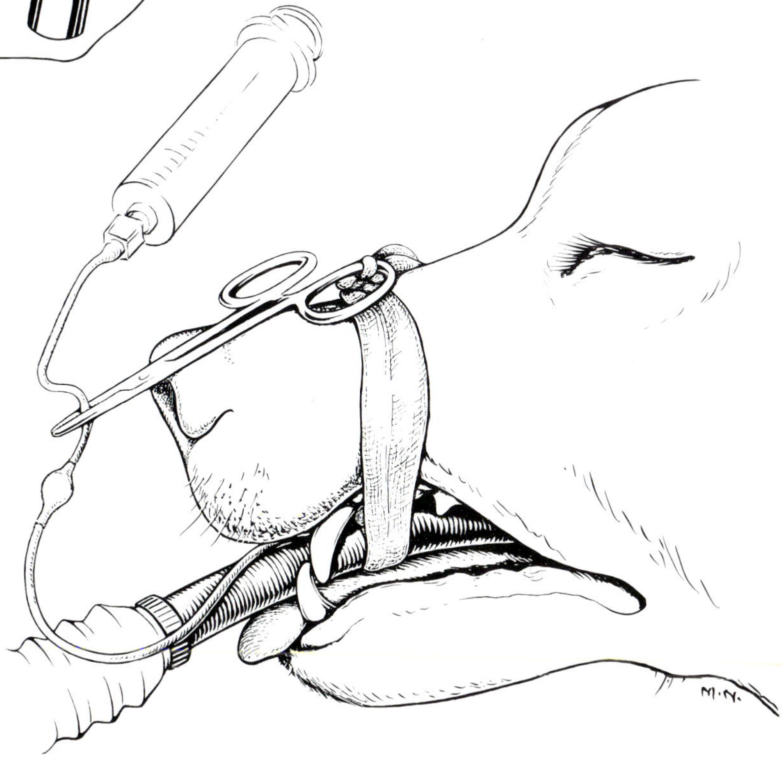

FIGURE 4–48.

SKIN PREPARATION

CLIPPING

Clipping should be done in an area away from the surgery, and care should be taken that all loose hair is kept out of the surgery. An Oster clipper with a No. 40 blade (Fig. 4–49) followed with a vacuum cleaner (Fig. 4–50) makes an excellent method of hair removal and disposal. The area clipped should be ample so that there will be no interference or contamination from hair during the preparation or the surgery.

SCRUBBING

The scrubbing procedure is best carried out on a rack placed over a tub so that the soapy water does not accumulate under the patient (Fig. 4–51). A thorough yet gentle scrub should be given to the surgical area and areas adjacent to it. The hand, not a brush, and a good surgical soap such as hexachlorophene are used to completely wash the skin (several times if necessary) until it is spotless. A brush is too irritating to a dog or cat's skin. When the wash is completed, the entire area should be dried with clean towels. This should include wet areas anywhere on the patient's body.

The removal of oily secretions from the skin is accomplished by using ether. Small pledgets of cotton soaked in ether are applied with a rubbing motion. The first stroke is over the proposed line of incision. Each stroke after that is applied progressively farther and farther from the first until the edge of the clean area is reached. The pledget is then discarded and a fresh one is used in the same manner. Always work from the cleanest area to the dirtiest, and never cover the same area twice with the same pledget. This step in the preparation is completed when the ether pledgets appear clean after use.

SKIN ANTISEPTICS

The skin is now ready for the final step in preparation, the antiseptic. This is applied in the same manner that has been described for defatting the skin. It may also be applied by using a circular motion. Starting at the incision site, move the pledget in ever increasing circles until the perimeter of the area is reached. This is repeated with a fresh pledget. The antiseptic used is a matter of choice. Some prefer antiseptics which leave visible evidence of their presence. U.S.P. tincture of iodine would satisfy this criteria. However, Lugol's solution is preferable.

Of all the antiseptics used in canine and feline surgery, alcohol is the most popular and the most efficient. The germicidal power of ethyl alcohol, however, varies according to its concentration. The optimum effect is obtained at 70 per cent by weight. This percentage is critical because the germicidal effect decreases rapidly in higher or lower concentrations.

Solutions above 80 per cent and below 50 per cent are of no practical value. A 70 per cent solution by weight can be made if 815 ml. of 95 per cent ethyl alcohol at 25° C. (77° F.) is diluted to 1000 ml. with cold distilled water.

Isopropyl alcohol, on the other hand, has the same germicidal effect in 30 to 50 per cent solutions. It is easily obtainable, tax free, and usually quite agreeable both to the surgeon and the patient. Since the optimum germicidal effectiveness covers a wider range of dilutions and is not as critical as ethyl alcohol, isopropyl alcohol is much more practical.

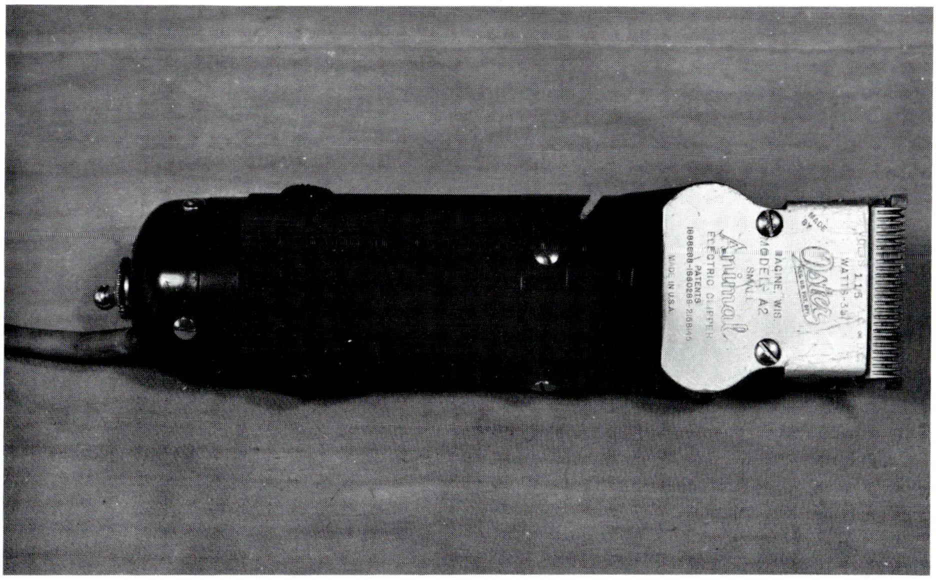

FIGURE 4–49.

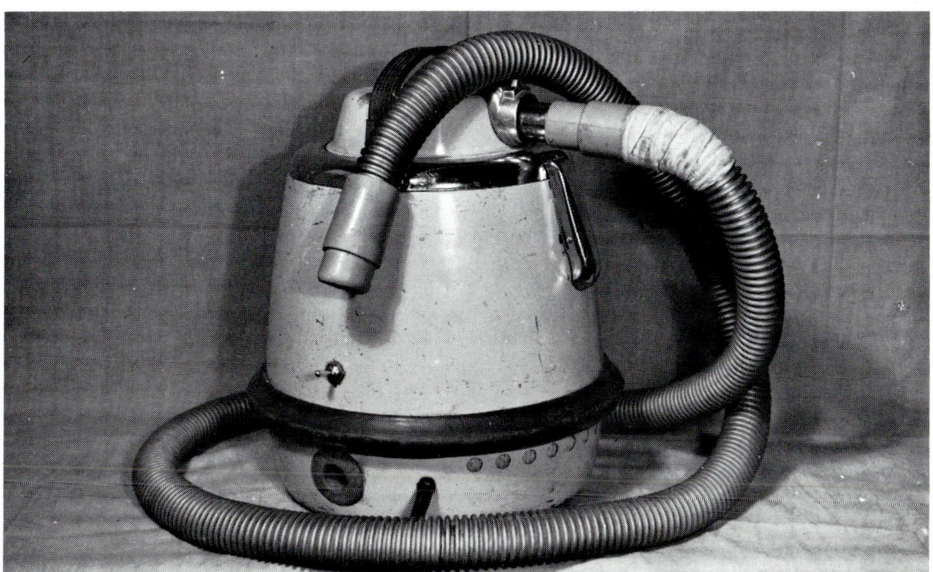

FIGURE 4–50.

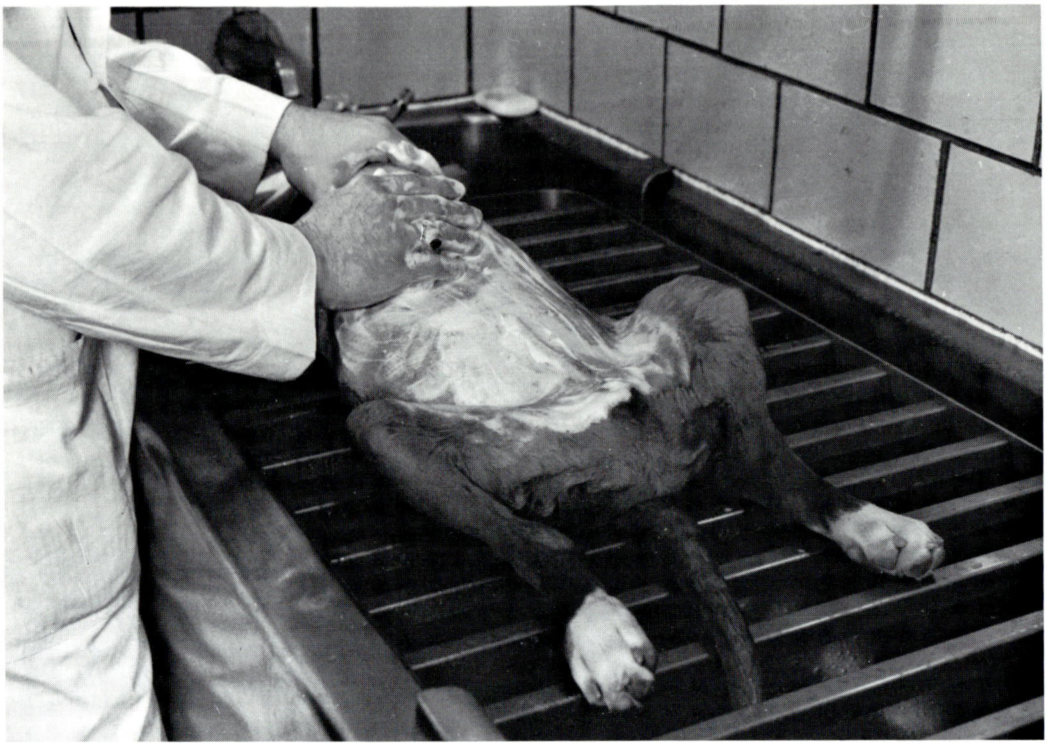

FIGURE 4–51.

REFERENCES

Blatt, R., and Maloney, J. V. *Surg., Gynec., and Obst.* 113:699–704, 1961.

Freeman, M. A. R., and Barwell, C. F. *Jour. Hygiene.* 58:337–345, 1960.

Lowbury, E. J. L., Lilly, H. A., and Bull, J. P. *Brit. Med. Jour.* May, 1963, pp. 1251–56.

Lumb, W. V. *Small Animal Anesthesia.* Philadelphia: Lea and Febiger, 1963.

Nealon, Thomas F., Jr. *Fundamental Skills in Surgery.* Philadelphia: W. B. Saunders Company, 1962.

Vitez, I. *Zbl. Bakt. I.* 184:531–537, 1962.

Walter, C. W., and Arlein, M. S. *J.A.V.M.A.* 111:41, 1943.

Walter, Carl W. *Aseptic Treatment of Wounds.* New York: The Macmillan Company, 1953.

Chapter 5

OPERATING ROOM PROCEDURE

The operating room is the scene of a constant battle against infection. Every safeguard must therefore be taken to reinforce the efforts of the surgical team. The room should be spotlessly clean from floor to ceiling. It should be as simple as possible with a minimum of equipment and cabinets to collect dust. The table should be easy to clean and should be used for surgery only. As a matter of fact, the whole room should be reserved for surgery only. There should be no traffic through the room, the windows should remain closed, and the movement of air should be minimized.

The scrub-up room should be adjacent to the surgery and should contain all the necessary equipment required prior to the gowning procedure. Gowns, gloves, drapes, and sterile operating bundles should be stored in the surgery.

PERSONNEL

The ideal staff for the operating room is made up of a surgeon, an assistant surgeon, a surgical nurse, and an attendant. Few hospitals are fortunate enough to have such a staff. An individual may be required to "wear several hats." In such cases the organization should be such that the work can be carried out in logical sequence. Let us consider the opposite extreme, in which the surgeon is working alone. The proper sequence for aseptic surgery would be:

1. Anesthetize the patient.
2. Prepare the patient.
3. Position the patient on the table.
4. If inhalation anesthesia is used, adjust the apparatus. A sterile towel may be used over the hand for adjustments during the surgery.
5. Lay out the instruments, sterile gown, and gloves.
6. Don cap and mask.

7. Scrub.
8. Don gown and gloves.
9. Drape the patient.
10. Perform the surgery.

For each additional staff member over one, the task becomes simpler, until, with the ideal group, many of the steps would be carried out simultaneously.

It is well for the surgeon or assistant surgeon to supervise the induction of anesthesia. Following this, the surgeon and his assistant begin their scrub. In the meantime the surgical nurse is laying out the instruments, and the attendant is preparing the patient. The attendant positions the patient on the table, assisted by the nurse if necessary. The surgeons may require help from the nurse in donning their gowns, or they may not. Usually nothing further is required of the attendant, since the nurse will be able to watch the anesthesia machine and get any extra instruments.

Naturally the number of personnel can vary, as has been shown, but for the purposes of discussion of operating room procedure, we will assume a group of three or four are available. They do not necessarily need to fall into the same categories that have been mentioned, but it is best to have more than one person available during surgery.

POSITIONING THE PATIENT

The position of the patient must be such that the surgeon has ample access to the region involved, but it should also be a position that is comfortable for the patient. Fastening limbs to the table is primarily for maintaining the body or limbs in a fixed position and ordinarily is not used for restraint. It is not necessary to fasten the limbs so tightly or in such grotesque positions as to cause edema of the distal appendage or temporary paralysis due to stretching a nerve. Often it is not necessary to tie the limbs, but if it is essential, they should be fastened in fairly normal positions. Restraint ropes should not be placed proximal to a venipuncture, because of the danger of producing a hematoma (Fig. 5–1).

The three principal positions are sternal, dorsal, and lateral. In any of these positions or variations of them the flat-top table provides the best support. A metal frame can be used to support deep-chested dogs in dorsal or sternal positions without undue traction on the legs. This frame consists essentially of a bar on which two metal loops slide and fasten at any required distance apart (Fig. 5–2). The patient's forelimbs are placed through the loops, and the loops are then pressed against the sides of the chest and fastened with thumbscrews. This leaves the body fully exposed for any type of surgery.

Whenever surgery of the head or neck is required, the Flexicast (Picker x-ray) is ideal for positioning and holding. This is an irregular rubber bag filled with plastic granules (Fig. 5–3). It can be pushed into any

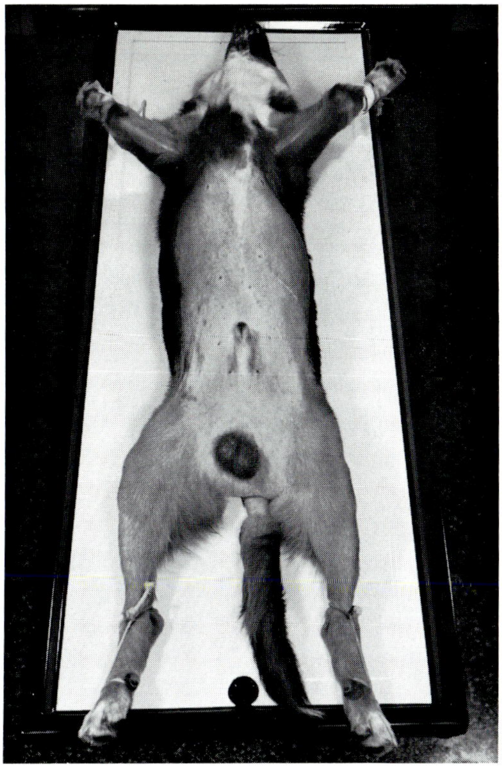

FIGURE 5–1.

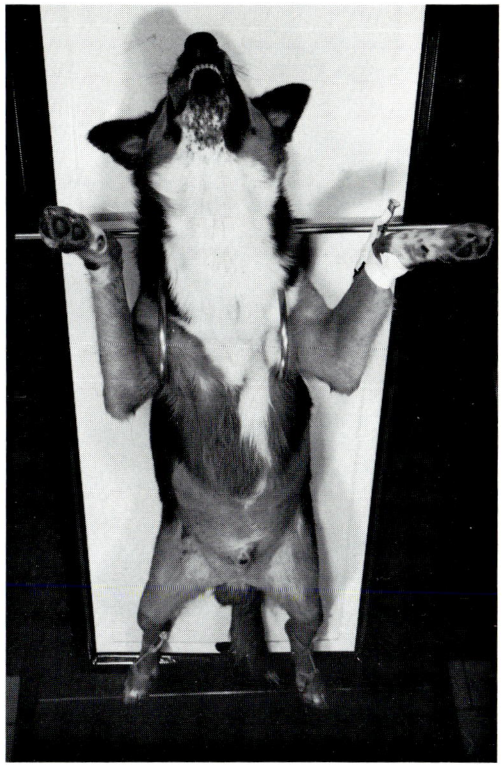

FIGURE 5–2.

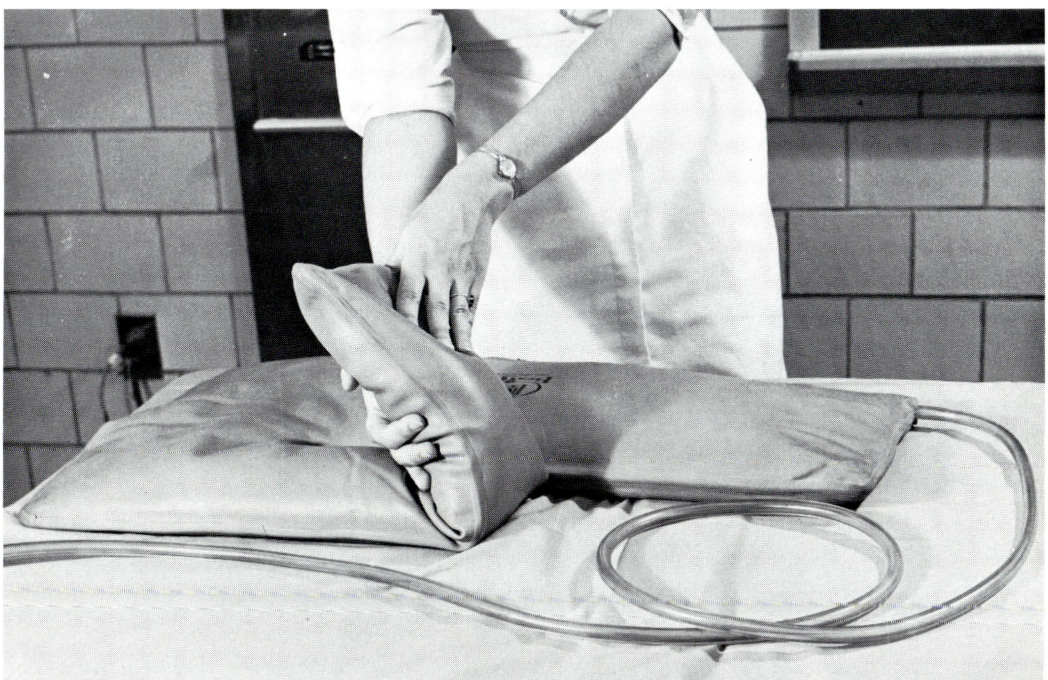

FIGURE 5–3.

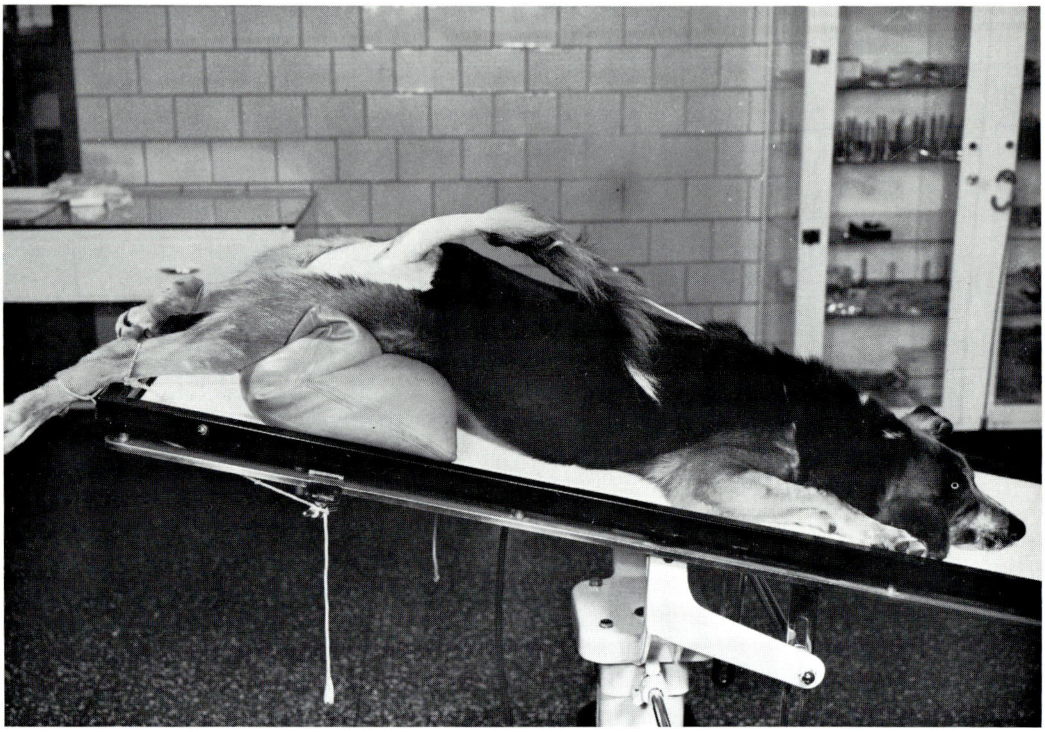

FIGURE 5–4.

shape, but when a pump is attached and the air exhausted from the bag, it becomes a solid hard block and will maintain the preset shape. The Flexicast can also be used to elevate the pelvis for surgery around the vulva and anus (Fig. 5–4).

DRAPING THE PATIENT

Single drapes with small openings are commonly used for simple surgery such as the spay, small tumors, small wounds, and ear cropping and frequently for more delicate surgery where only a small space such as the eye is involved. For more extensive surgery, a four-drape system is preferable. These drapes have been described in Chapter 2.

The sterile drape should only be handled during the draping process by those persons prepared to do sterile surgery. In removing the folded drape from the instrument tray, it should be picked up without unfolding (Fig. 5–5). When clear of the tray, a corner is grasped, the arm is extended and the drape is allowed to unfurl.

It is important that the sterile gloved hands be protected during the draping. Accordingly, the drape is first arranged to cover the hands. It is grasped at either end with the hands on the short sides about 4 inches from the corner. The arms are then extended laterally so that a fold forms

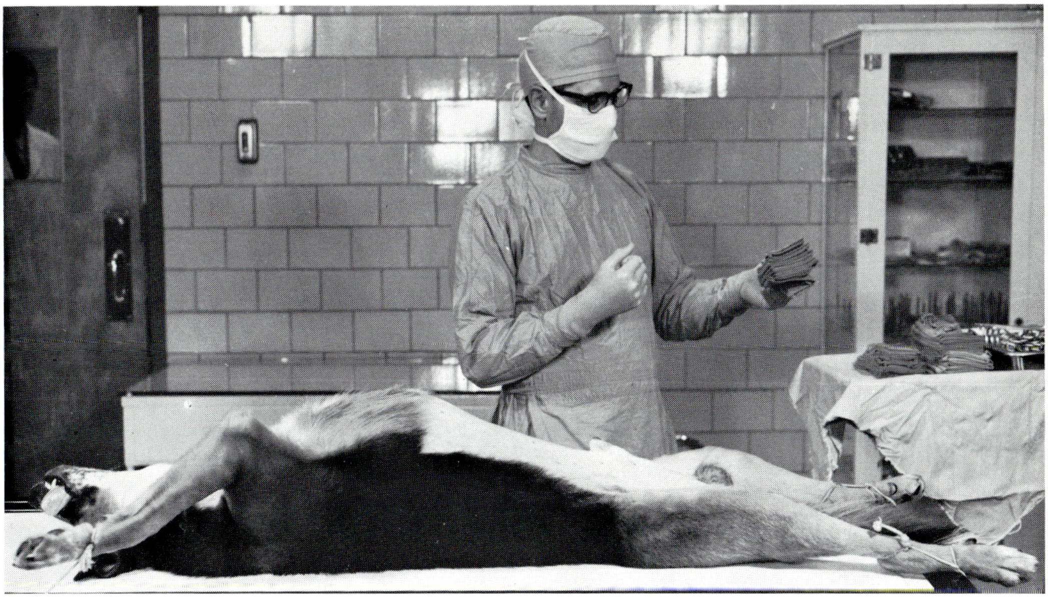

FIGURE 5–5.

along the long side, falling away from the operator and covering the fingers. The thumbs are on the side toward the operator. This position causes the wrists to be flexed. The wrists are extended and the palms are turned upward. The palms are then turned away from the body. As a result of this maneuver, the hands are covered with the drape and fully protected (Fig. 5–6).

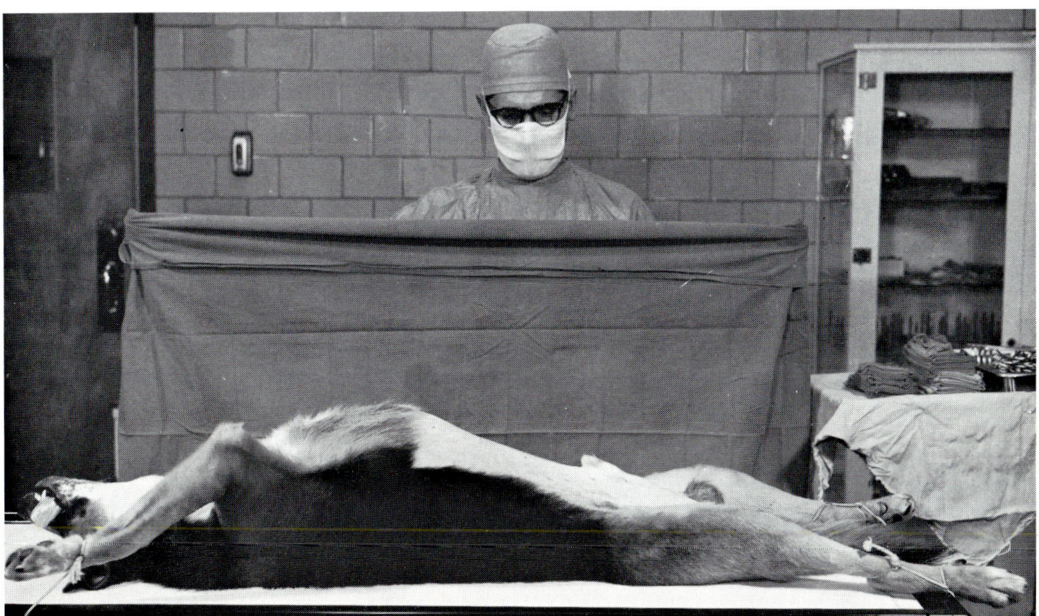

FIGURE 5–6.

Cross drapes are applied first, with the initial drape placed across the caudal parts (Fig. 5–7). The operator raises one hand and lowers the other so that as he lays the drape across the patient the folded edge will be toward the proposed incision site. The second cross drape is handled the same way and placed across the cephalic end of the patient, with the folded edge toward the operative area.

The longitudinal drapes are placed next by applying the third drape next to the operator and fastening it with towel clamps at the points of intersection with the cross drapes. The fourth drape can be placed by lifting it over the patient and dropping it into position on the far side of the incision site. This is fastened in a manner similar to the third drape. Protection for the hands is not so important with the fourth drape, since the entire area is practically covered at this point (Fig. 5–8).

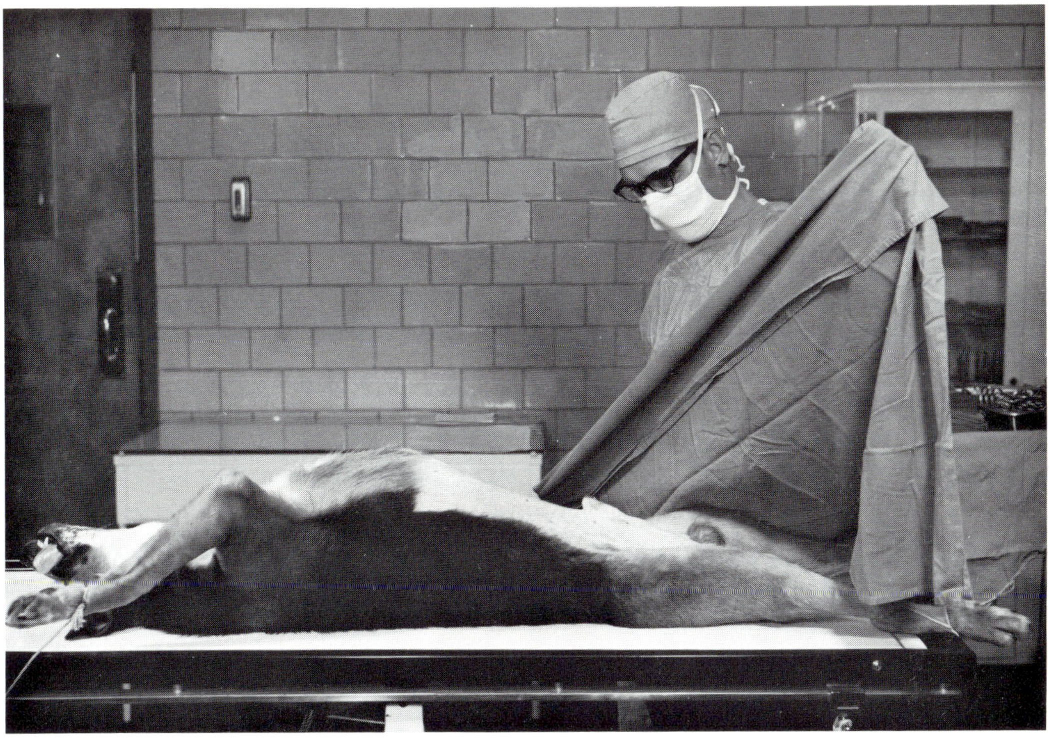

FIGURE 5–7.

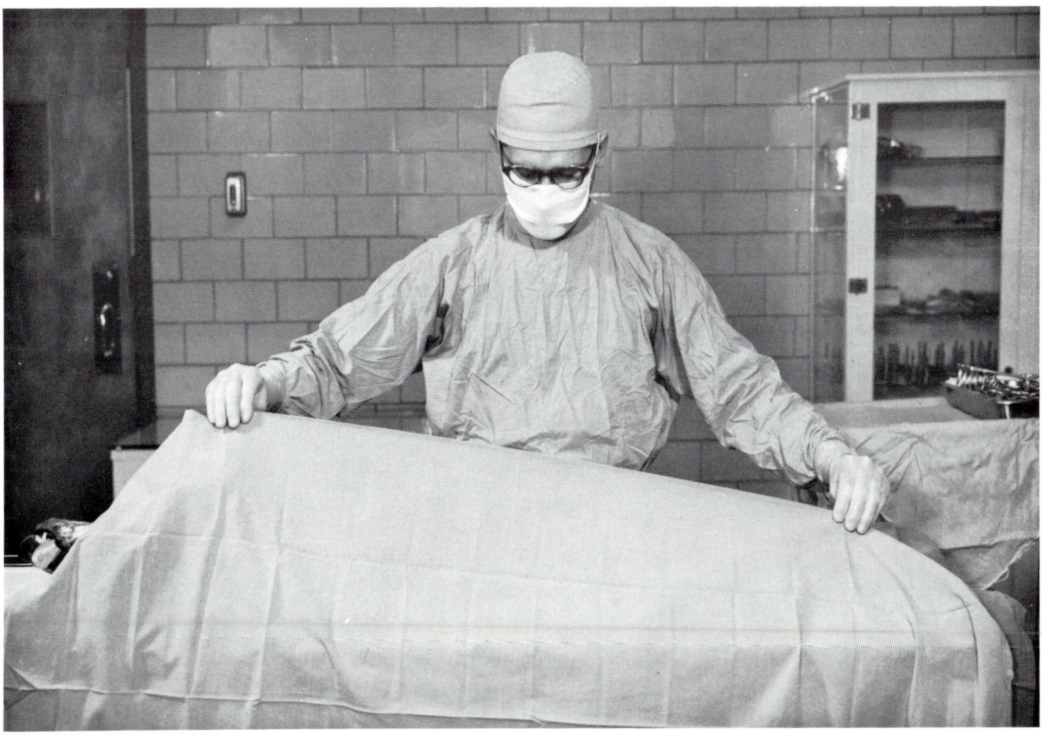

FIGURE 5–8.

It can readily be seen that such a system of draping is adaptable to many situations and can be modified to meet the requirements of most surgery. Draping to the incision requires two extra drapes, which are applied after the incision is made, or a plastic drape can be applied to the skin with adhesive prior to the standard draping. When drapes are applied following the skin incision, the first drape is laid on the side toward the operator, with the far edge approximating the far edge of the incision (Fig. 5–9). It is fastened to the edge of the skin by three or more towel clamps and then turned so that it falls to the side away from the operator. The second drape is placed on the side away from the operator, with the edge approximating the near edge of the incision. This is fastened in the same way and turned toward the operator. A towel clamp may be placed at each end of the incision to prevent the two drapes from separating where their edges adjoin.

If draping to the incision is done with plastic drapes, the incision can be made through both the drape and the skin in a single stroke. Skin sutures may also be placed through the draping material, which would then be left in place until the sutures are removed. The adhesive type of plastic drape is designed for flat, hairless surfaces and therefore does not work well in average dog or cat surgery.

There are many types of drapes. Some prefer heavy rubber or plastic because of its durability, while others favor light disposable ones in order to eliminate laundry and sterilizing problems. The type of drape used is immaterial as long as there is strict adherence to the principles of asepsis. Any "shortcut" in draping should be carefully studied for any "shortcuts" to sepsis.

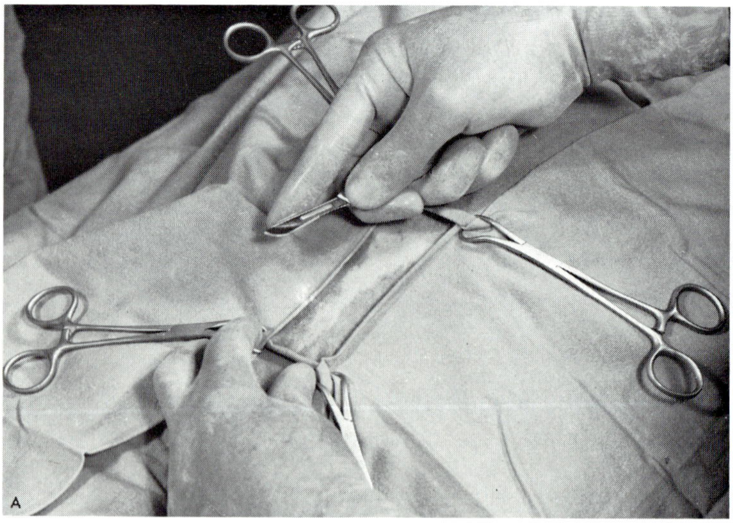

FIGURE 5–9.

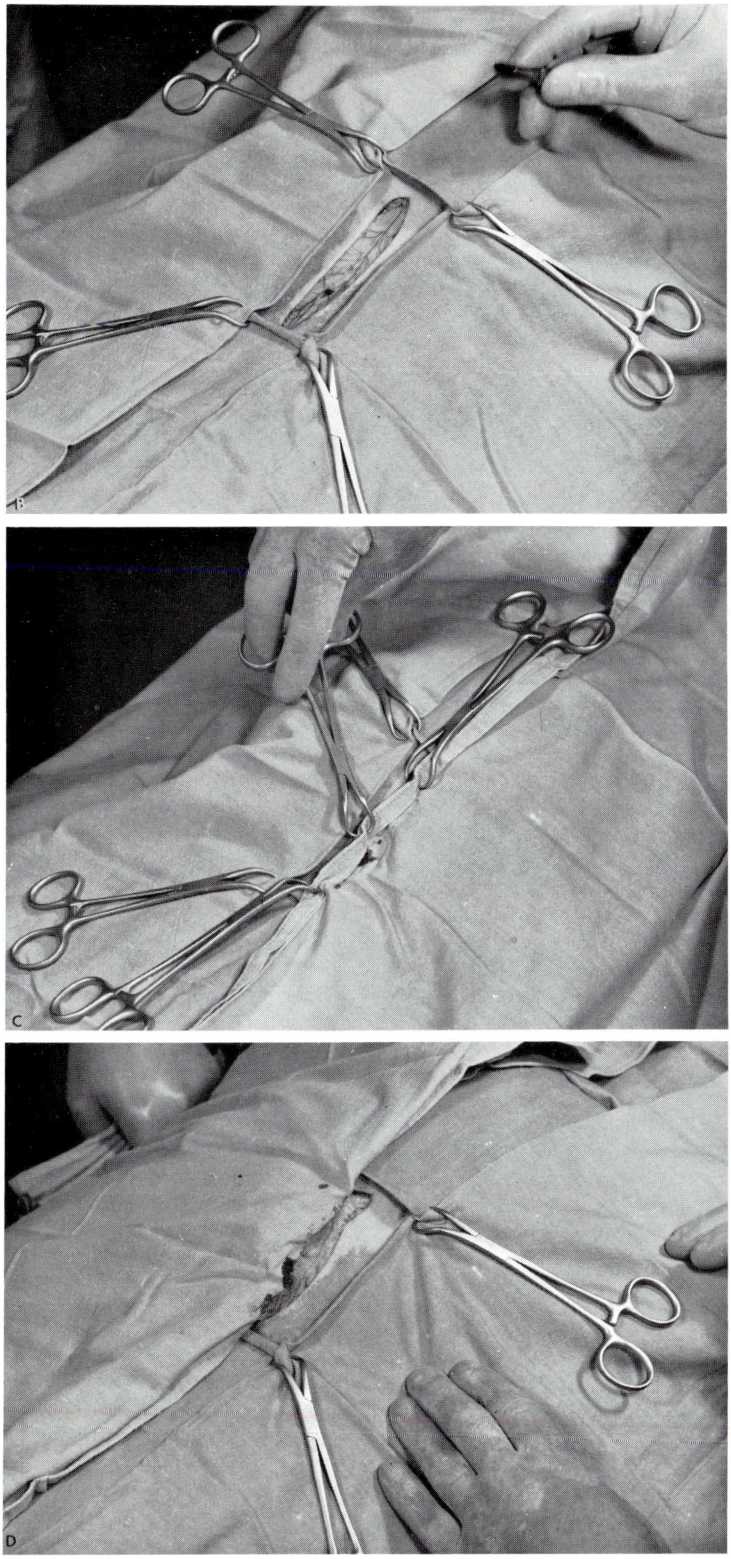

FIGURE 5–9. *Continued.*

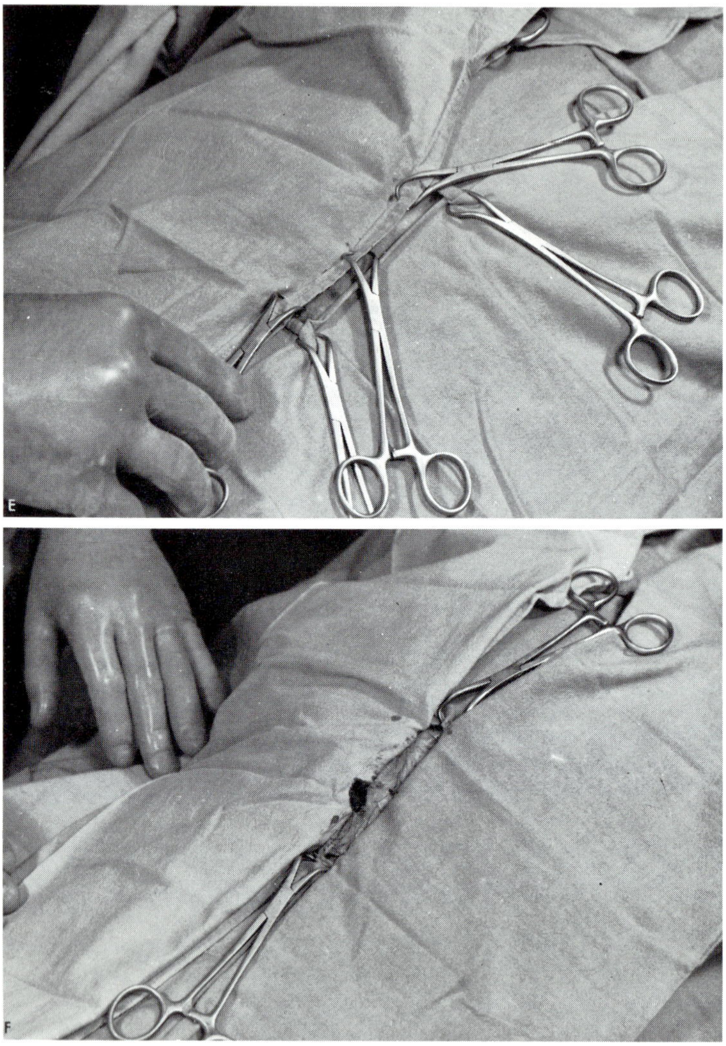

FIGURE 5–9. *Continued.*

ACCOUTERMENT LAY-OUT

Each instrument tray or bundle should be planned according to the needs of the operator. It is fairly common practice to have a standard tray of instruments which can be supplemented by individual instruments. This kind of system would also have trays of instruments for special purposes. For instance, there might be an orthopedic tray, an eye tray, or a cardiac tray. A simple standard tray might consist of a thumb or tissue forceps, a needle holder, four Allis forceps, 10 hemostats, six towel clamps, three angiotribes, a spay hook, suture material and needles, gauze sponges, and a small metal tray for fluids. Such a tray would serve for much of the general surgery, especially if supplemented by some of the individually wrapped special instruments. The special trays of instruments would be reserved for specific types of cases.

The instrument bundle is placed on the stand so that it is crosswise to the tray (Fig. 5–10). The wrapper is opened, thus exposing a sterile surface which entirely covers the tray (Fig. 5–11). The pan containing the instruments is moved to the back of the tray by holding the front corner of the underwrapper and pushing against the underside with the other hand (Fig. 5–12). A space is thus provided on the front of the tray for cutting instruments, catgut, (Fig. 5–13) and the drapes (Fig. 5–14).

An estimated amount of catgut is placed on the tray by opening the outside wrapper and allowing a dry sterile packet to drop without touching it. Leftover packets are bundled periodically and shipped to the manufacturer for repackaging. The cutting instruments are removed from the chemical sterilizing tray with transfer forceps and deposited on the tray. Any special instruments that are required are removed from their wrappers and placed on the tray or if necessary on an adjoining tray. Finally the bundle of drapes is opened and the drapes placed on the tray with transfer forceps.

This transfer can also be done by holding the bundle in one hand with fingers outstretched while it is opened with the other (Fig. 5–14). The wrapper is then grasped and held around the hand supporting the bundle while the sterile drapes are brought in contact with the tray. The stack of drapes is then turned upside down on the tray.

The bundle containing the gown and sterile towel is opened on a side table. If gloves are not provided in the bundle, a glove envelope is also opened. If glove powder is used, the envelope containing this should be in the pack. If Biosorb cream (Johnson & Johnson) is used, a packet should be opened and dropped on the open glove pack. (See Fig. 4–31.)

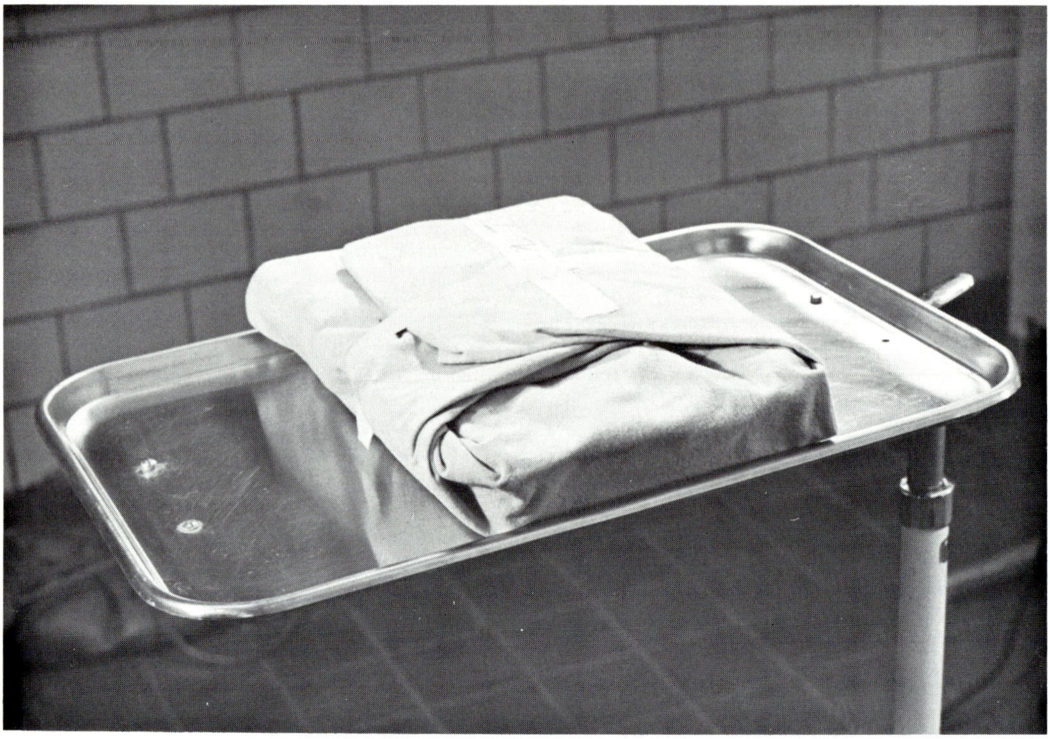

FIGURE 5–10.

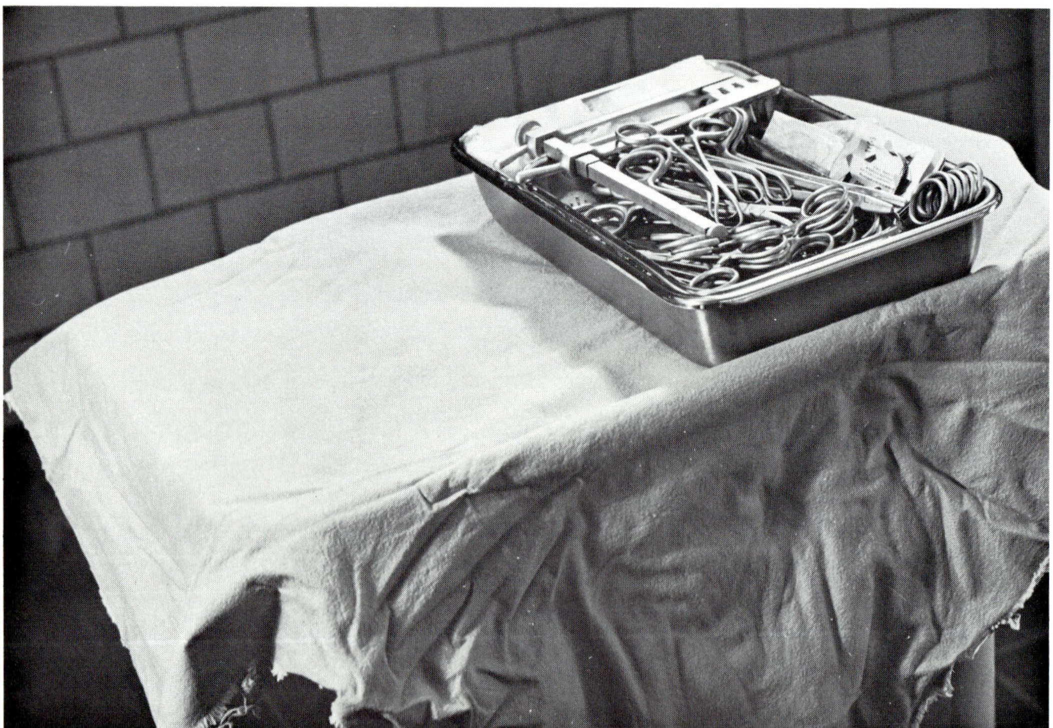

FIGURE 5–11.

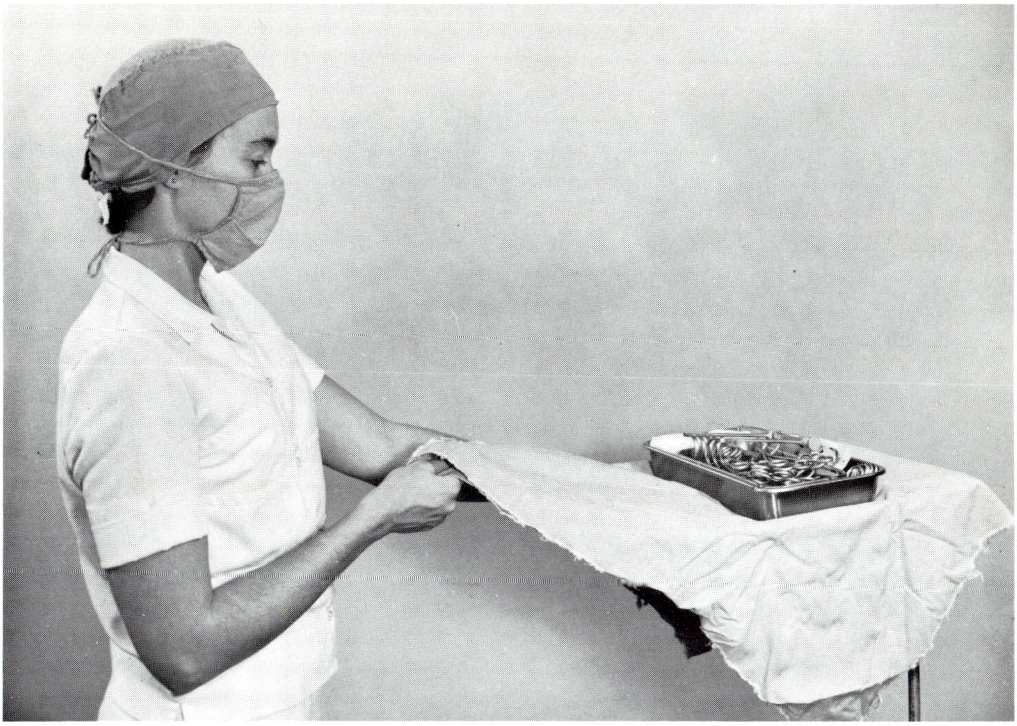

FIGURE 5–12.

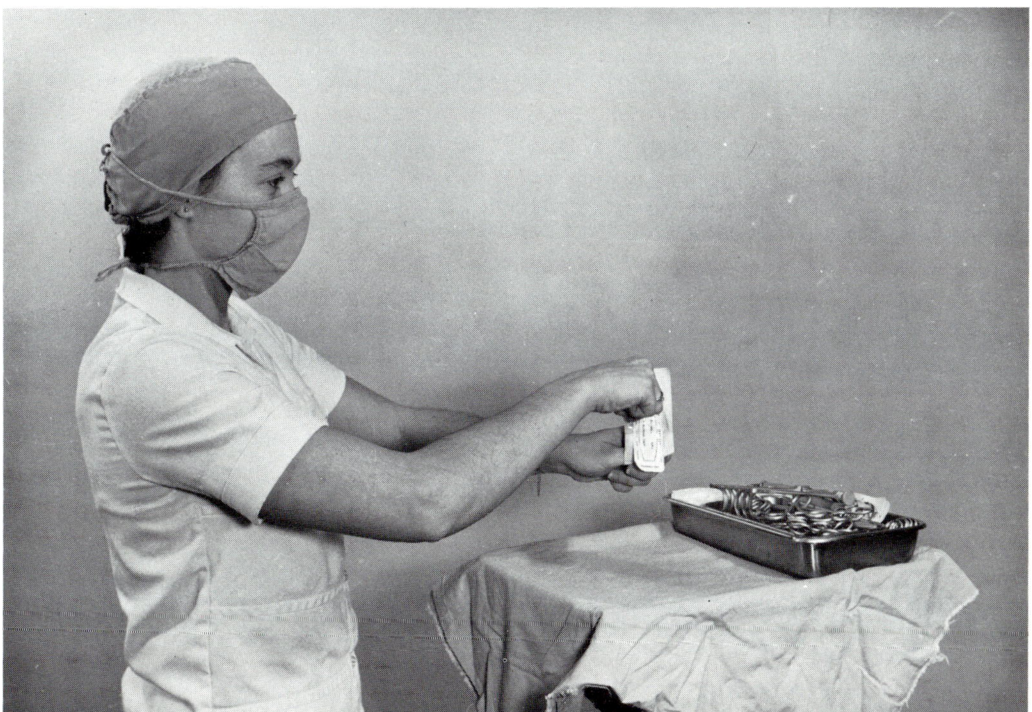

FIGURE 5–13.

ANCILLARY EQUIPMENT

First consideration should be given to a good operating room light. This does not have to be an expensive light or one that illuminates the entire room (Fig. 5–15). It should be capable, however, of providing good light in the operating area from any angle, and it should be as nearly shadow-proof as possible.

The anesthetic equipment has been well described in *Small Animal Anesthesia* by W. V. Lumb. This equipment should be as simple and foolproof as possible. Each individual must decide for himself the type of equipment that best suits his needs.

If the anesthesia equipment does not provide oxygen, it is essential that separate equipment for this purpose be available. The tank should be mounted on a dolly so that it cannot be tipped. A free tank is very dangerous because of the high pressure which could be released if the valve were broken. A reduction valve will be required in order to regulate

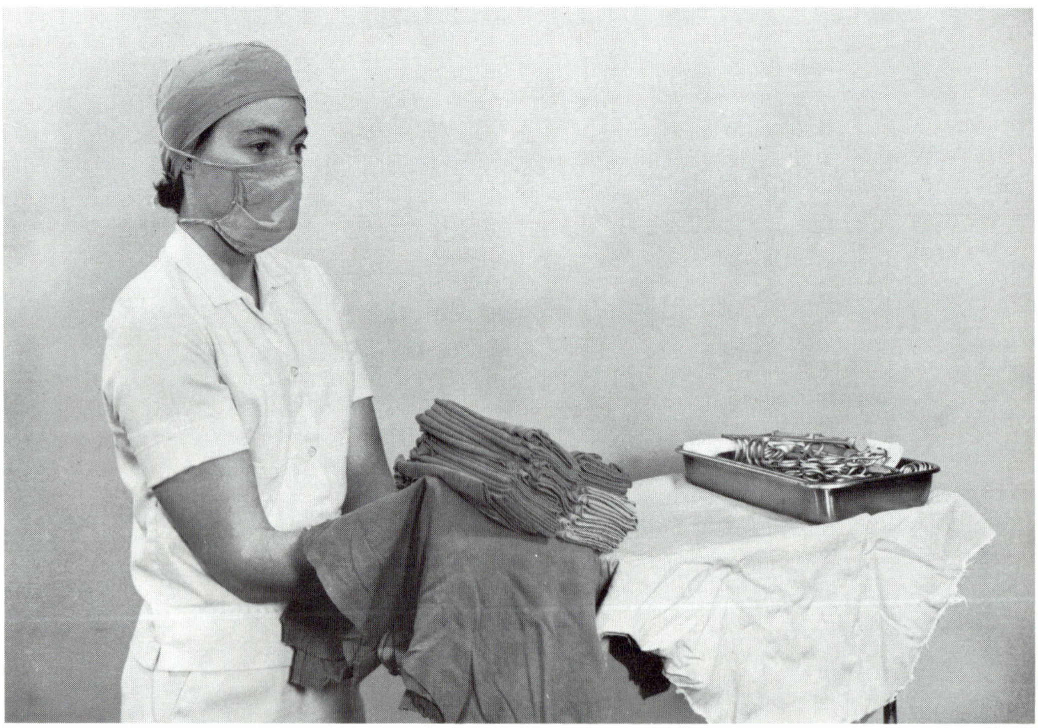

FIGURE 5–14.

the rate of flow. This should be connected to tubing with an adaptor so that the oxygen is immediately available if needed.

Many kinds of equipment for the use of oxygen alone or in combination with anesthetics are available. The reader is referred to Dr. Lumb's book.

A small electric motor with a suction pump is quite helpful at times when large amounts of fluid or transudate are encountered (Fig. 5–16). There are also certain hazards wherever electrical equipment is used in the operating room, particularly if an ether-oxygen mixture is being used as an anesthetic. Explosionproof switches will help, but there is still danger from sparks from the brushes unless the motor is set on a shelf at least 5 feet above the floor.

The suction tips and the connecting tubing for the suction pump should be sterile. Once the tubing and tip are connected to the pump, they should be anchored to either the operator or the patient to avoid slipping to the floor.

Electrosurgical equipment is superior for work around the mouth and throat because it makes the control of hemorrhage much easier. It is frequently used in general surgery but requires some experience to properly adjust for minimal tissue reaction. Most operators make the skin

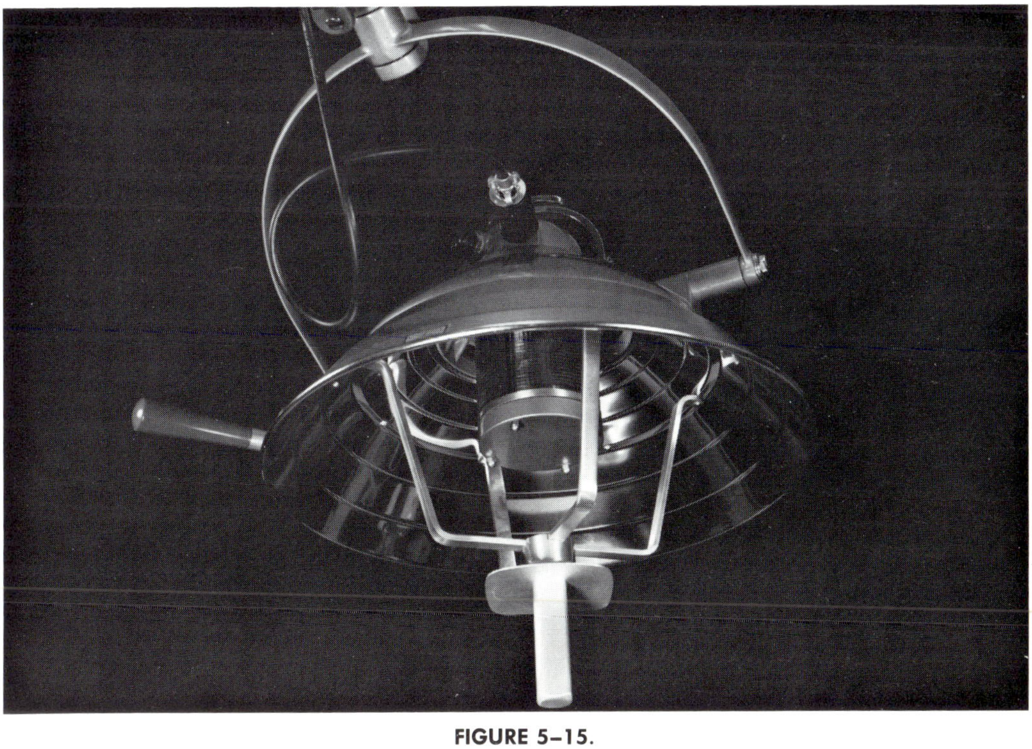

FIGURE 5–15.

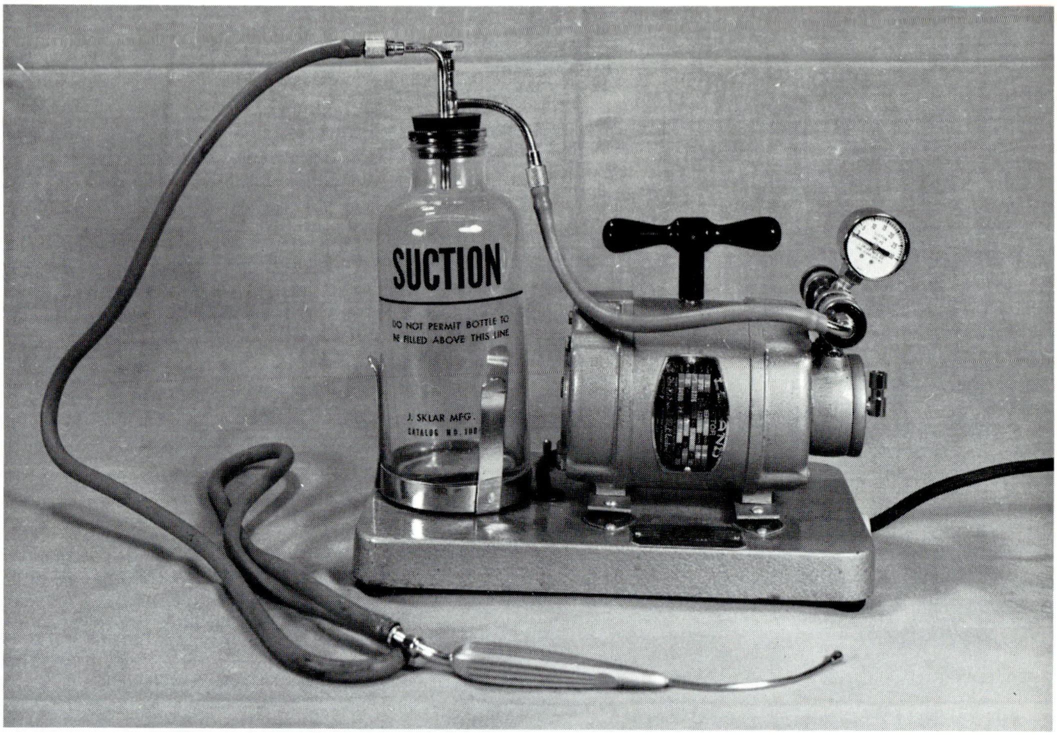

FIGURE 5–16.

incision with a scalpel and then continue the work with the electric knife.

Electrosurgery is not the same as electrocautery. Electrocautery is produced by preheating metal with an electric current. The hot metal is then applied to the tissue. Electrosurgery is the production of heat in the tissue through the passage of a high-frequency current by means of an electrode. The electrode remains cold.

There are two systems used in electrosurgery: one is bipolar and the other is monopolar. The bipolar system has an active electrode and an indifferent electrode which is considerably larger. The greatest heat is at the point of the active electrode, since there is dispersion over the skin and the indifferent electrode. Some warmth may be produced in the skin, but this is very mild.

The monopolar system depends on the body to absorb the heat. Large bodies are able to do this, but small bodies such as small dogs and cats are not always able to do so. In such cases it is helpful to place a hand on the animal's body so that some of the heat can be dissipated through the bulk of the human body.

In addition to cutting, the electrosurgical electrode can fulgurate, desiccate, or coagulate, depending on the electrode, the way it is used, and the type of current applied.

Fulguration is the destruction of superficial tissue by the use of high voltage and high milliamperage. The treatment consists of arcing over the surface to produce an eschar.

Coagulation is usually done with a ball electrode which is moved slowly over the surface.

Desiccation is deep tissue destruction with the use of the coagulating circuit but with a pointed electrode. The electrode is forced deeply into the tissue. The current is applied until the tissue around the electrode is coagulated. Usually several probings must be made. The result, which comes some days later, is a slough of the tissue desiccated.

The small machines commonly used in veterinary medicine usually have a single control for voltage and milliamperage, thereby producing a slight coagulating effect along with the cutting.

This type of equipment cannot be used when explosive mixtures of anesthetics are used.

REFERENCES

Annis, J. R., Lavignette, A. M., and Blakemore, J. C. Jr. *Allied Vet.* 36:13–16, 1964.

Archibald, J. *Canine Surgery.* 1st Archibald ed. Santa Barbara, California: American Veterinary Publications, Inc., 1965.

Berge, E., and Westhues, M. *Veterinary Operative Surgery.* 1st English ed. Copenhagen Medical Book Co , 1966.

Carter, H. E. *Vet. Record.* 76:147–148, 1964.

Graham-Jones, O. *Small Animal Anaesthesia.* New York: The Macmillan Company, 1964.

Hall, L. W. *Vet. Record.* 76:650–655, 1964.

Knowles, J. O., and Garcia, J. G. *Proc. World Vet. Congress, Hanover.* 1:43–46, 1963.

Linnell, M. R. *Calif. Vet.* 18:11–12, 1964.

Lumb, W. V. *Small Animal Anesthesia.* Philadelphia: Lea and Febiger, 1963.

Markowitz, J., Archibald, J., and Downie, H. G. *Experimental Surgery.* 5th ed. Baltimore: Williams and Wilkins, 1964.

Ormrod, A. N. *Vet. Record.* 75:1095–98, 1963.

Orr, T. G. *Operations of General Surgery.* 3rd ed. Philadelphia: W. B. Saunders Company, 1958.

Partipilo, A. V. *Surgical Technique and Principles of Surgery.* 6th ed. Philadelphia: Lea and Febiger, 1957.

Strande, A. *Jour. Sm. An. Pract.* 5:153–159, 1964.

Chapter 6

SURGICAL EXERCISES FOR THE BEGINNER

This section is devoted entirely to exercises designed to teach the basic maneuvers of surgery to the student who is undertaking aseptic surgery for the first time. These exercises are intended to give experience in the handling of various tissues, develop ability in surgical technique, and refresh the memory as to anatomical relationships. There are many mechanical details to be learned in order to carry out proper aseptic surgery. With the practice afforded in these exercises, the details will gradually become automatic, the appropriate degree of speed will develop, and the mind will be free to deal with the surgical problem at hand.

The student should begin by drilling himself in the mechanics of knot tying, scrubbing, donning the gown, and donning the gloves until he has reached a reasonable degree of proficiency. Correct operating room decorum should be maintained at all times, and since the surgeon in each team is the leader, it is his responsibility to see that each member observes the rules and carries out his assignment.

Good surgery is the result of a combined effort to treat the patient with gentleness and attentiveness. The surgeon is not a healer. He simply assists nature by providing the proper environment for healing. The following "ten commandments" enumerate the steps which lead to a good surgical result:

1. Produce good surgical anesthesia.
2. Practice strict asepsis.
3. Make incisions large enough for adequate exposure.
4. Avoid rough handling of tissues.
5. Practice good hemostasis.
6. Develop good dexterity and posture.
7. Be thoroughly acquainted with anatomical relationships.
8. Cooperate in organized teamwork.
9. Maintain intellectual integrity in all procedures.
10. Be diligent in the aftercare of the patient.

Surgery is a rigid and demanding discipline. Failure to observe the "ten commandments" leads to difficulties for the surgeon and sometimes loss of life for the patient.

If the proper plane of surgical anesthesia is not maintained, the patient suffers pain or expires from anoxia. When anesthesia is light, the surgeon is impeded by lack of proper muscle relaxation.

If asepsis is broken, the resulting infection may ruin the surgical repair or bring death to the patient.

Inadequate exposure leads to traumatized tissues and organs, not to mention the limitations placed on the surgeon's performance.

Rough handling of tissues is inexcusable and only adds to the burden of repair by producing edema and even necrosis.

Poor hemostasis interferes with the visualization of the operative site, causes excessive blood loss to the patient, and often leaves an excellent breeding ground for infection.

Dexterity and posture are often overlooked as contributing factors toward a good surgical result, but the bungler who whittles away at tissues with hands in all manner of awkward positions and face in close proximity to the surgical site seldom produces a good result. The most consistent result of poor posture is an aching back.

A thorough orientation in anatomical relationships creates a mental map of the structures and organs in the surgical area, thereby reducing trauma produced by excessive handling and searching.

Cooperative teamwork contributes much toward the surgical result. The efficiency of an assistant is just as important as that of the surgeon. The chain is no stronger than the weakest link. Therefore, the surgeon should have patience with the assistants and the assistants should feel the responsibility of the surgeon.

Intellectual honesty is of paramount importance. Bacteria do not recognize excuses for breaks in asepsis. The surgeon is under the surveillance of the most rigid police force in the world, i.e., pathogenic organisms. Any time the laws of asepsis are broken, either intentionally or unconsciously, the patient will suffer. The difference between life and death for the patient, therefore, may depend on the honest thinking of the surgeon and his assistants.

Finally, neglect of the needs of the patient following surgery can, at times, be as disastrous as a poor surgical performance. Good nursing completes the picture of a good surgical achievement. Kind humane treatment pays large dividends and is the mark of a compassionate and dedicated professional man.

LAPAROTOMY

The purpose of this exercise is to acquaint the student with the abdomen of the live dog and to help him learn the first steps of surgery. These are the making of a proper incision, the correct way of handling soft tissue, the control of bleeding, and a correct method of closure after examining the abdominal organs.

After the dog has been anesthetized and prepared for surgery, it is placed on the table in dorsal recumbency and draped. The draping is done by the assistant surgeon, who has previously prepared himself for asepsis.

Abdominal incisions in general are either cranial midline, caudal midline, right or left paramedian, or right or left paracostal (Figs. 6–1 and 6–2).

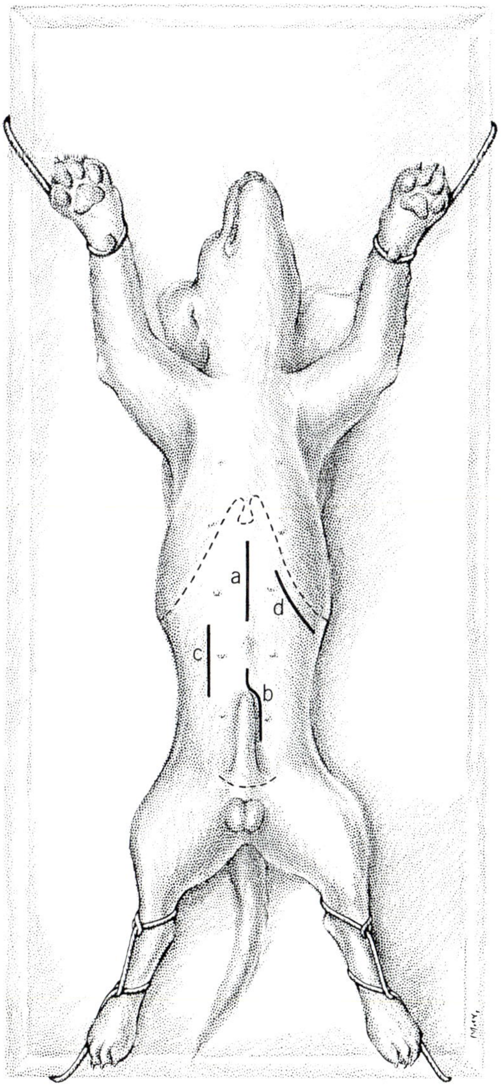

FIGURE 6–1. *a,* Cranial midline incision. *b,* Caudal midline incision. *c,* Paramedian incision. *d,* Paracostal incision.

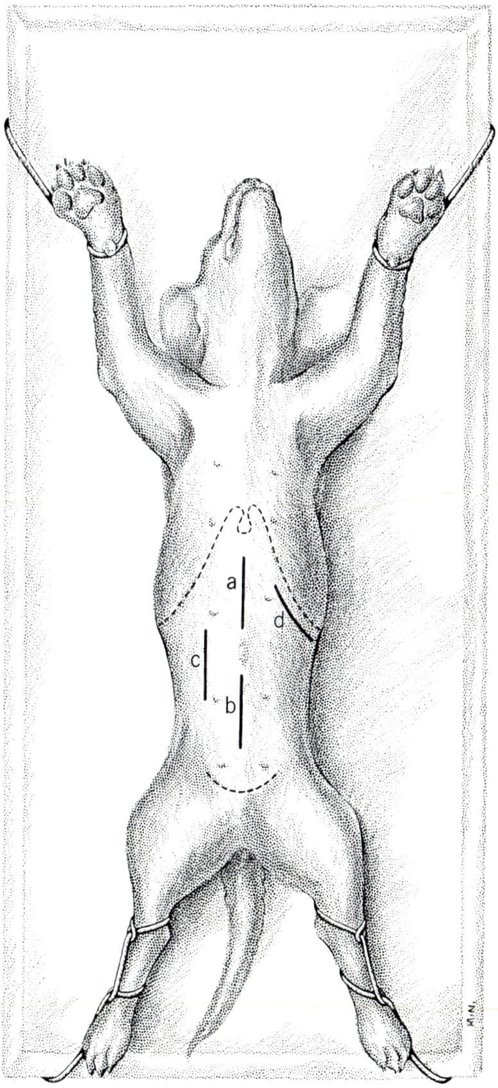

FIGURE 6–2. *a,* Cranial midline incision. *b,* Caudal midline incision. *c,* Paramedian incision. *d,* Paracostal incision.

The site of the incision is chosen according to the purpose of the abdominal exposure. For simple laparotomies, a midline or paramedian incision is usually made.

A hand's breadth incision should be made. The dimension of the incision is so stated because it must be large enough to admit the surgeon's hand. Since all hands are not the same size, it is impossible to state the size in specific linear measurement.

The surgeon should hold the knife handle firmly in the palm of his hand, with the forefinger extended along the rib of the blade (Fig. 6–3). This is not a pencil to be dangled from the fingertips, but a tool that should be held securely and under complete control. The opposite hand is used to tense the skin by pressing with the thumb and forefinger. With the knife blade pressed firmly against the skin and the elbow aligned with the incision line, the skin is parted in one clean sweep. The elbow is kept elevated until the skin incision is completed so that a straight line is made. If the elbow is allowed to drop, there is a tendency for the operator

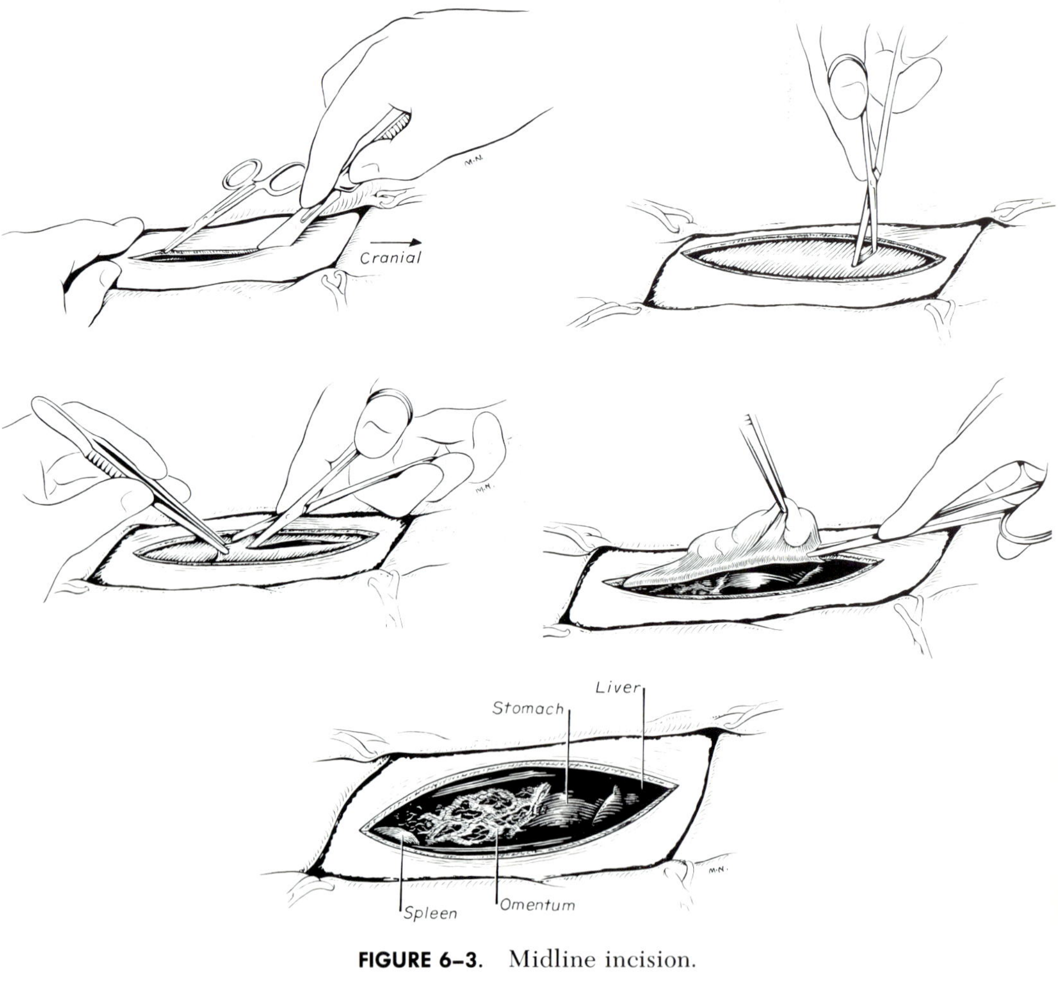

FIGURE 6–3. Midline incision.

to draw the knife toward himself, thereby making the incision in a slight arc. As the knife proceeds, the skin should open behind it like the wake made by a boat. If this does not happen, there is too little pressure on the blade.

As soon as the skin incision is completed, the knife is discarded and the tissues are further divided with scissors. Wherever possible the dissection should be along natural lines of cleavage. A small opening is made in the

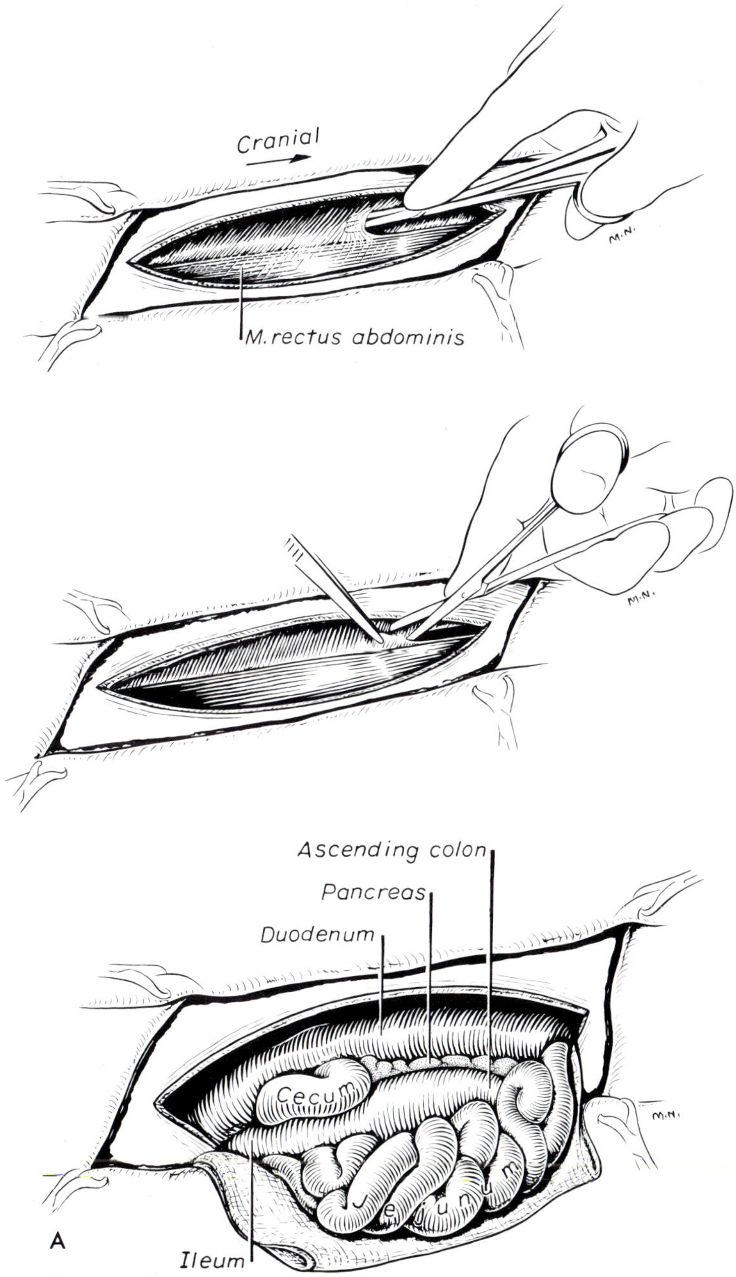

FIGURE 6–4A. Right paramedian incision.

fascia. The closed blades of the scissors are inserted and then opened to bluntly separate the tissues. The surgeon is thereby able to examine the tissue and take whatever precautionary steps, such as ligating, he deems necessary before cutting. The midline incisions will present a heavy layer of fascia, or aponeurosis. This is the linea alba, or white line, and cannot be separated as described. One can carry out blunt dissection by moving 1 or 2 mm. to either side.

One other structure is encountered in the cranial midline incision. This is the falciform ligament. This structure is a fold of peritoneum enclosing a varying amount of fat. It presents a serious hazard insofar as healing is concerned and frequently is the cause of eventrations. The student often mistakes this structure for the omentum. The omentum, however, can be drawn freely from the incision, while the falciform is firmly attached on either side and can only be elevated a very short distance.

The falciform should be divided with scissors and each half reflected outward and laterally. With slight traction, the demarcation between parietal peritoneum and that covering the fatty mass will become evident. By cutting along this line, one can remove the falciform, leaving a clean firm edge of peritoneum for closure (Fig. 6–3).

Once the abdomen is open, a careful inspection of the contents should be systematically undertaken. This does not mean the pawing and mauling of organs so commonly seen and often referred to as "gut-puddling." The examination should be gentle and without undue rubbing and handling of organs. One should quickly learn the physical relationship of one organ to another so that by identifying one organ the others can be found readily.

Let us assume, for example, that we are looking for the cecum. One way to find it is to drag intestinal loops through the incision until the cecum appears. A much easier way, however, is to remember its relationship to other organs. We know that it should be on the right side and just beneath the duodenum (Fig. 6–4A). The duodenum can be identified by the presence of the pancreas within its loop. It is therefore very simple to reflect the omentum, lift the duodenal loop, and expose the cecum. Other organs and structures can be found in the same way. It eliminates trauma and saves time.

The peritoneum is closed with a continuous or running stitch (Figs. 6–4B and C). The needle holder is used for placing all sutures, but the tying should be done by hand. The fascial layers are approximated by interrupted stitches (Fig. 6–4D). The midline incisions will have a single layer of aponeurosis. A subcutaneous layer of interrupted stitches may be required in order to bring the skin edges within 5 mm. of each other (Fig. 6–4E). The skin should not be sutured until the edges are almost approximated. Close the skin with simple interrupted stitches (Fig. 6–4F).

Return the patient to the postoperative quarters. A daily check should be made as to the physical condition of the patient and the surgical wound. The care and feeding will be done by the attendant.

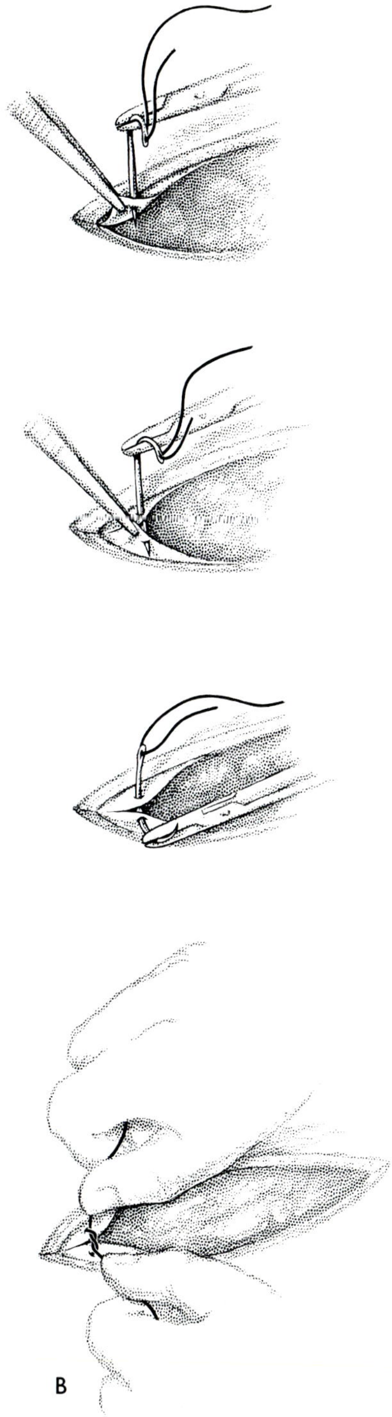

B

FIGURE 6–4B. Beginning of the peritoneal suture and setting of the knot.

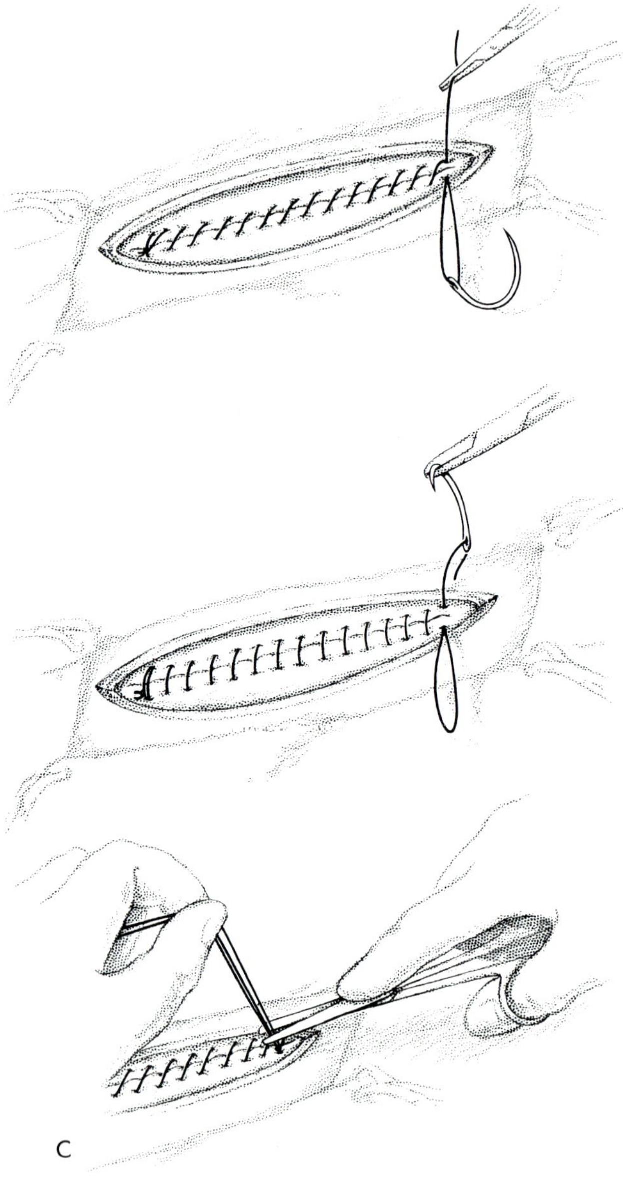

C

FIGURE 6–4C. Two methods of stitching and tying the peritoneal suture.

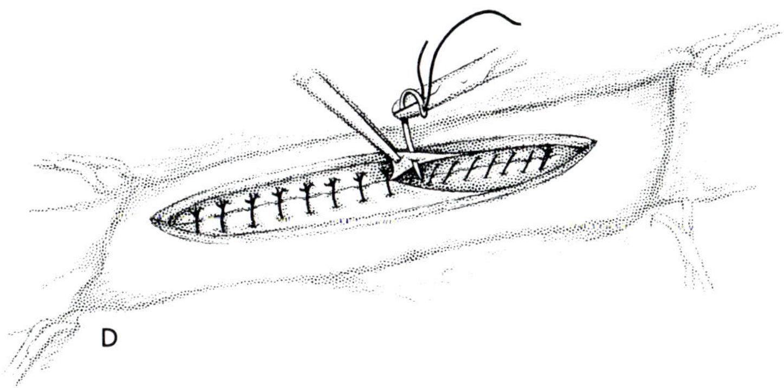

D

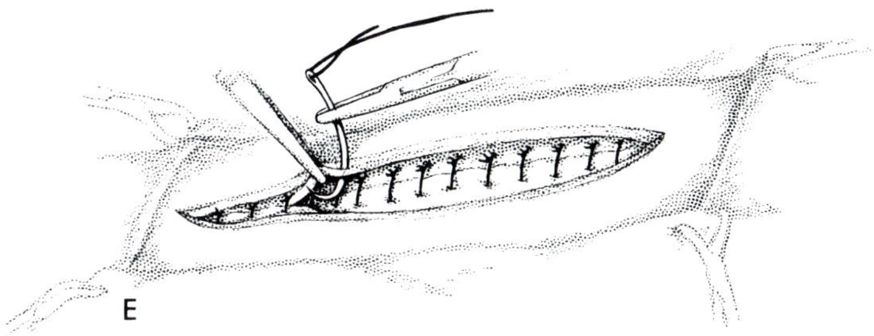

E

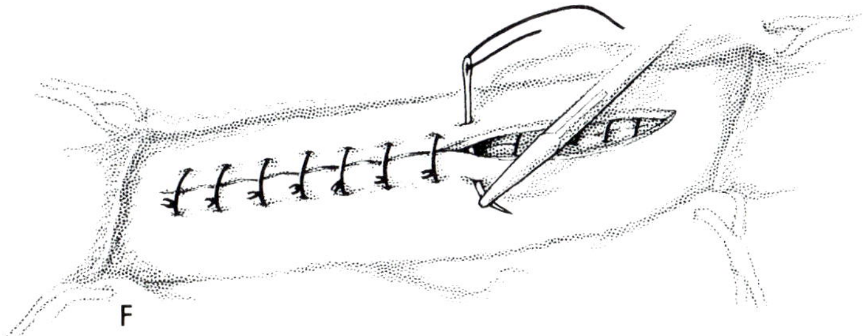

F

FIGURE 6–4D. Use half-circle needle and interrupted stitches to suture fascia.
FIGURE 6–4E. Use half-circle needle and interrupted stitches to suture subcutaneous tissue.
FIGURE 6–4F. Use half-curved needle and interrupted stitches to suture skin.

NOTES

SPLENECTOMY—AN EXERCISE IN LIGATION

The preparation of the patient for splenectomy is the same as for laparotomy. Draping, however, is slightly modified. The cross drapes are applied diagonally so that they will parallel a paracostal incision. The longitudinal drapes are placed as usual.

A left paracostal incision is made parallel to and about 2.5 cm. caudal to the costal arch. It should be a hand's breadth in length and extend to within approximately 12 mm. of the midline. The scalpel is discarded and the incision completed with scissors. Note which muscles are incised.

The spleen is attached to the omentum, which presents when the incision is opened. Using the index finger as a hook, lift the omentum, bringing the spleen with it. Turn the spleen so that the hiatus faces the assistant surgeon.

A classic splenectomy would call for ligation of the splenic artery, followed by milking as much blood as possible from the spleen, and ligation of the splenic veins. Since this is an exercise in ligation, we are more interested in making many ligations. Double ligate all vessels,

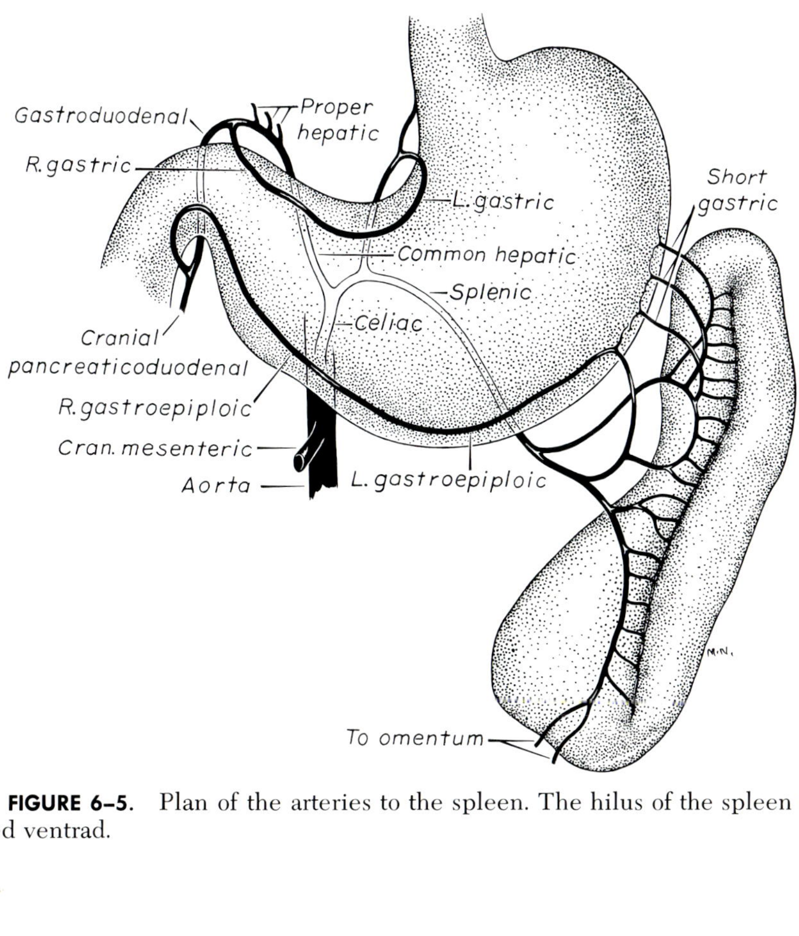

FIGURE 6–5. Plan of the arteries to the spleen. The hilus of the spleen is rotated ventrad.

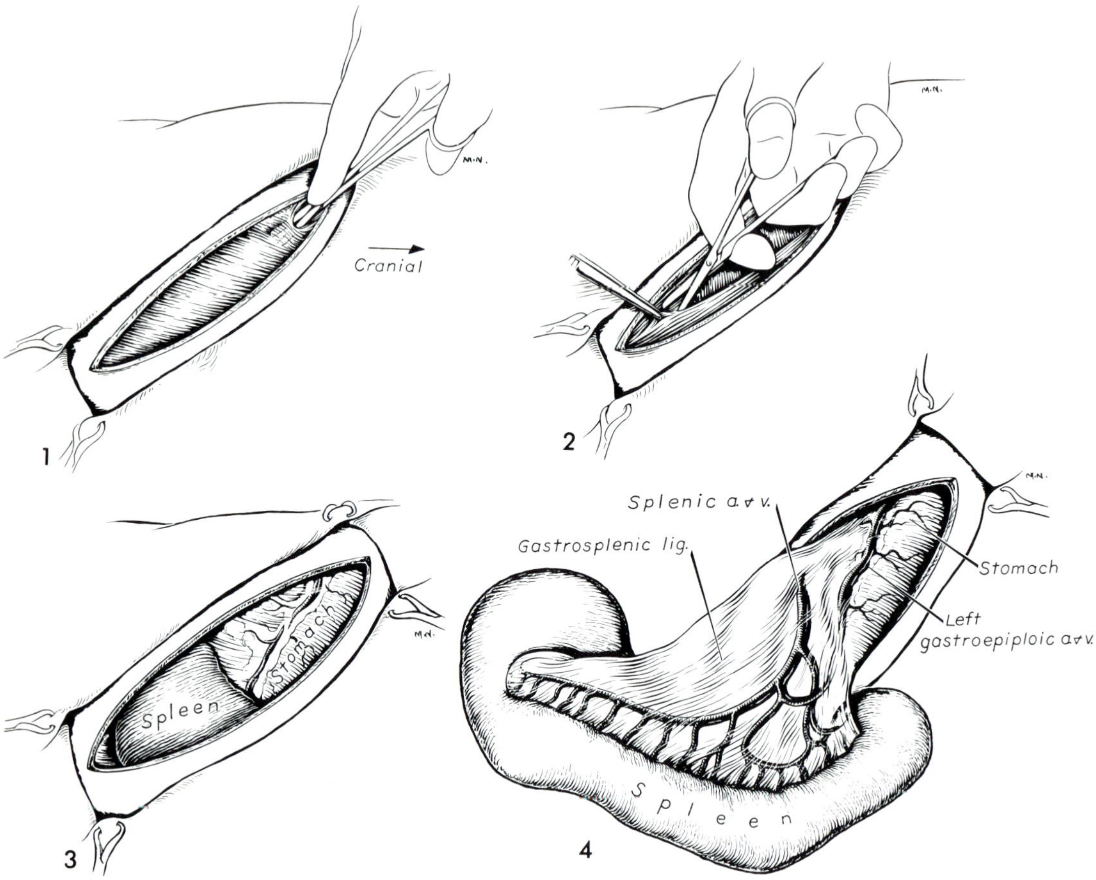

FIGURE 6–6.
Step 1. Left paracostal incision exposing m. obliquus externus abdominis.
Step 2. Separate m. obliquus internus abdominis from m. transversus abdominis.
Step 3. Enter peritoneal cavity through the m. transversus abdominis for splenic exposure.
Step 4. Deliver spleen from abdomen.

---

placing one ligature close to the spleen and the other about 12 mm. distal. The omentum and vessels are then divided between ligatures. This operation will require approximately 30 ligatures.

The peritoneum is closed by a continuous stitch. Interrupted stitches are used to approximate the fascial layers as well as the skin incision. The aftercare of the patient is the same as the previous exercise.

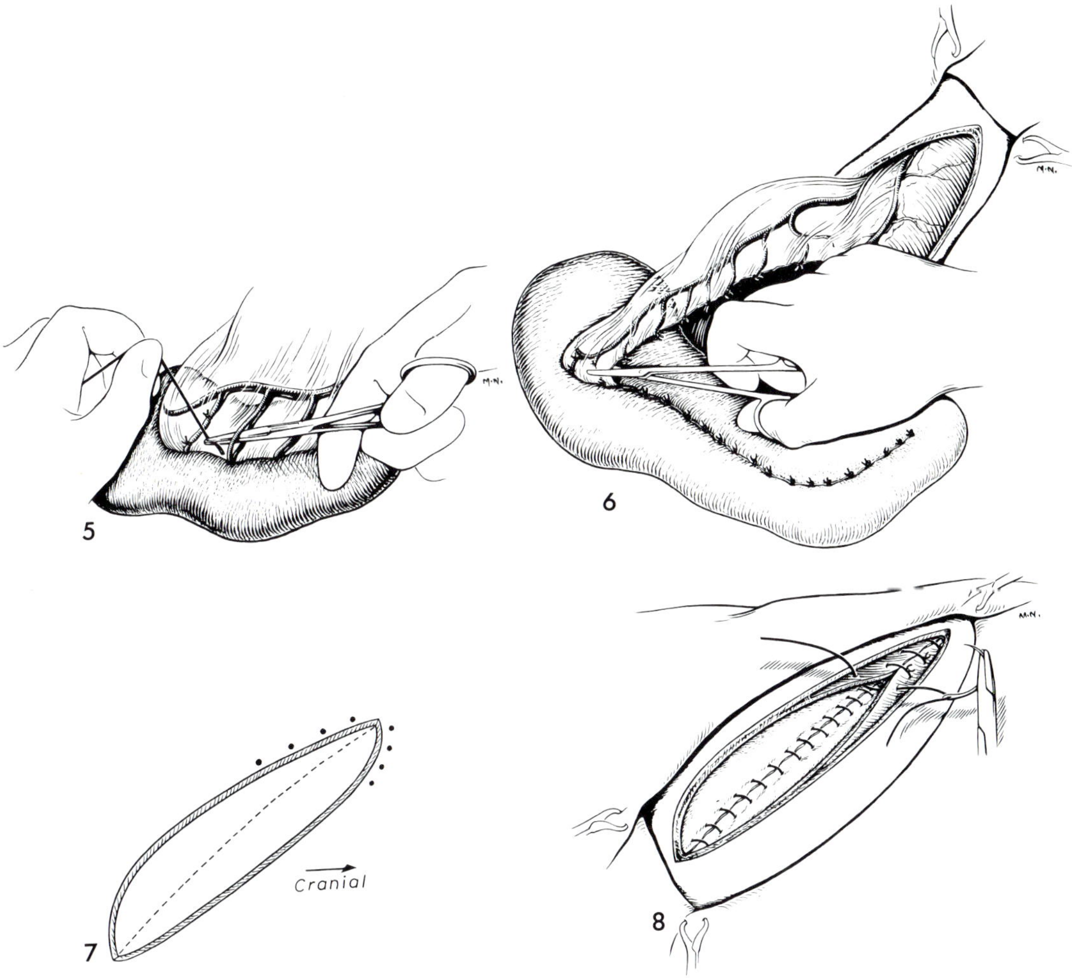

FIGURE 6–6. *Continued.*
Step 5. Double ligation of blood vessels.
Step 6. Transection of gastrosplenic ligament and blood vessels.
Step 7. Diagram showing suture placement for proper approximation. Broken line represents original incision.
Step 8. Closure of peritoneum and muscles.

NOTES

GASTROTOMY

This exercise is designed to acquaint the student with the surgery of hollow organs of the abdomen. The muscular coats of the digestive tract of the dog are much stronger than in most species and therefore the mucosa everts. This problem makes surgery of the alimentary tract slightly more difficult. The stomach has been selected because it presents the largest and broadest surface of any of the hollow organs and offers the least danger from contamination of any segment of the digestive tract. Because of the gastric acidity in carnivores, bacterial flora is rather sparse.

The usual preparations are made, and the patient is draped for a left paracostal incision. A cranial midline incision could be used, but the exposure is not as adequate.

Grasp the stomach wall with a dry sponge between the thumb and index finger. Apply traction toward the midline. This will expose more of the wall, which is grasped in like manner with the opposite hand. The traction continues toward the midline so that a rotating motion of the stomach is achieved. Direct traction on the stomach does not deliver the stomach as easily as the rolling motion. When enough gastric wall has been exposed, the assistant surgeon grasps it with dry sponges and holds it toward the surgeon.

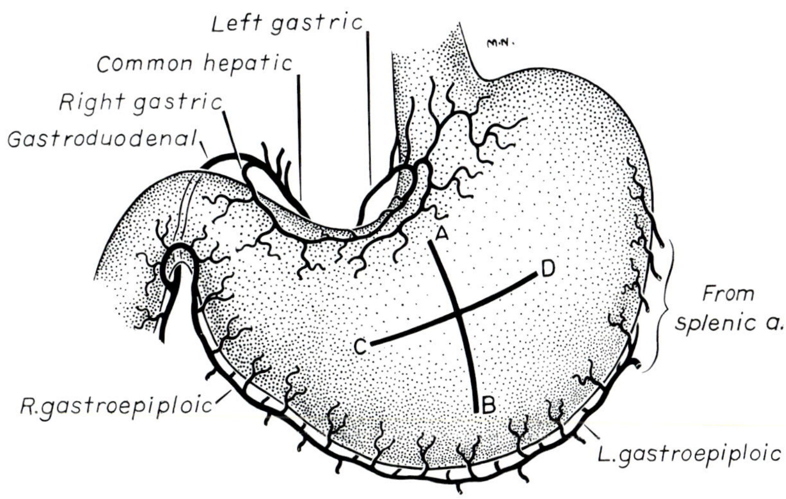

FIGURE 6–7. Scheme of gastric arteries and gastrotomy incisions (either *A B* or *C D*) that avoid the larger gastric arteries.

An incision about 7 to 8 cm. in length is made with a fresh scalpel. This incision may be either parallel or at right angles to the greater curvature, but it should be about 2 cm. distant. An area should be selected that is comparatively free of large blood vessels. Incise with the scalpel through the serosa, muscular coats, and submucosa. At this point the mucosa will bulge from the incision. Scissors should be used to incise the mucosa, and they should be discarded as soon as the incision is completed because they are contaminated. The mucosal opening is made by snipping a small hole and then quickly enlarging it. Any pressure or gas in the stomach may cause the contents to spurt through a small opening. It is therefore important to release any pressure rapidly. *Avoid spilling any of the stomach contents.* Discard any instruments or drapes that become contaminated. Make certain that the gastric incision is kept outside the abdominal incision and in a position where the abdominal contents will not be contaminated should spillage occur.

Two rows of sutures are used to close the stomach. The first row should be a continuous Lembert stitch, and the second row an interrupted Lembert. The first row should be started 1 to 2 cm. distal to the end of the gastric incision. Each bite of each stitch should be deep enough to include the submucosa. Increased resistance to the needle indicates contact with the submucosa. A narrow strip of tissue should be inverted with each row of sutures. Avoid large tissue inversions lest the final row of sutures become entangled in the vessels of the greater curvature (Fig. 6–8).

The paracostal incision is closed the same as for the exercise in splenectomy. If the midline incision is used, the closure is the same as for laparotomy.

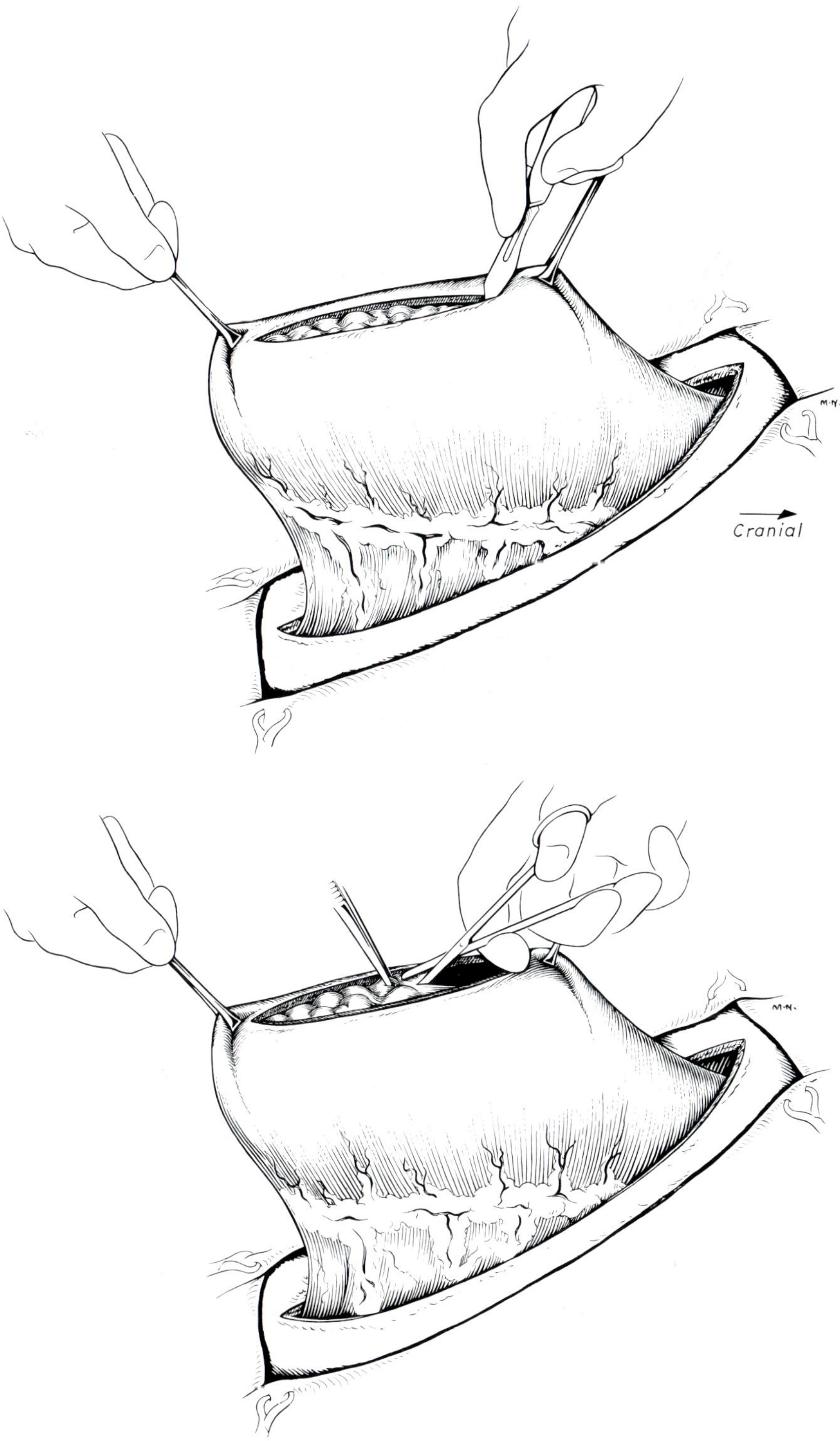

FIGURE 6–8.
Step 1. Gastric incision deep enough to allow mucosa to bulge.
Step 2. Mucosal incision by means of scissors.

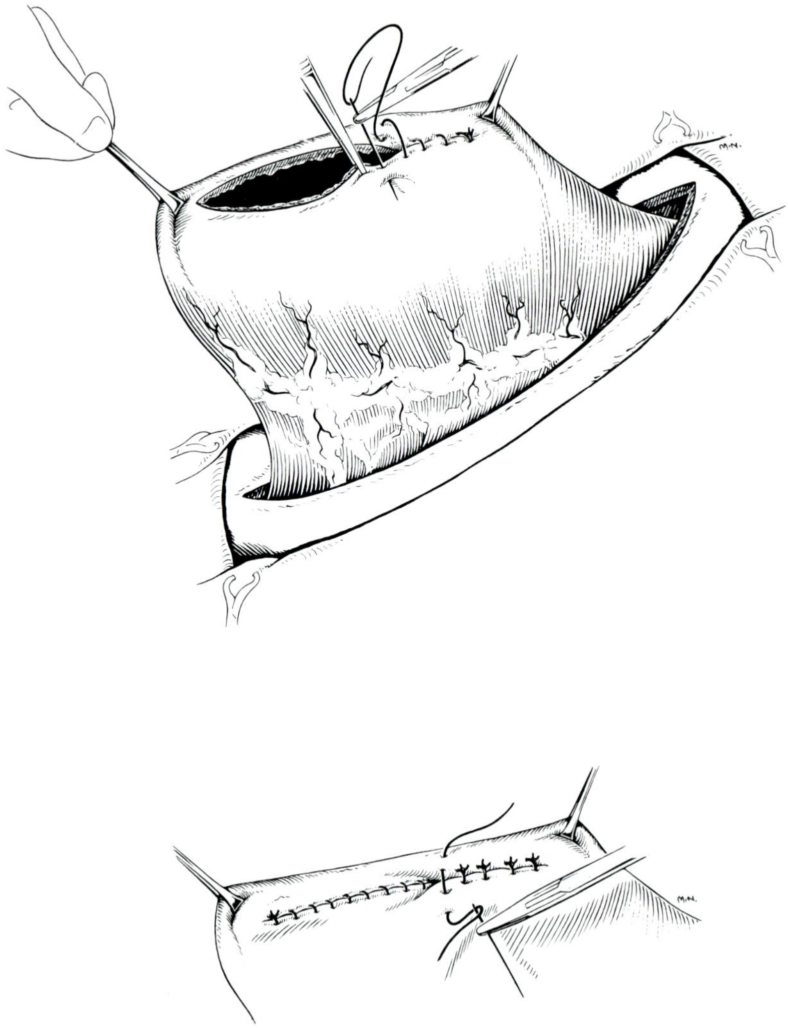

FIGURE 6–8. *Continued.*
Step 3. Closure by the use of Lembert continuous stitch.
Step 4. Closure of second row by the use of Lembert interrupted stitches.

NOTES

FEMUR EXPOSURE

The object of this exercise is to help the student understand the surgery involved in orthopedics through exposure of joints, bone, and structures related to locomotion. The exposure will be greater than is required for most classical operations in this area. It affords the student opportunity to study structures in the two most important joints in the body. This exercise also demonstrates the method of exposing the femoral shaft and illustrates how muscles can be separated in making a deep incision.

The leg is prepared by completely clipping from the hock to the dorsal midline. It is held in the vertical position during the final step in preparation and while the dog is being placed on the operating table. While the leg is thus held by the anesthetist, the assistant surgeon begins the draping by placing the first drape longitudinally so that it falls between the thighs and covers the opposite leg. Then, holding the second folded drape in one hand with about 1 foot unfolded in the other, the assistant surgeon allows the anesthetist to deposit the leg on the unfolded drape so that the foot and hock can be wrapped with the drape. After two or three wraps it is fastened.

The wrapped foot can then be lowered to the first drape without contamination. The two remaining drapes are placed diagonally so that they cross at the dorsal midline above the trochanter major. A towel clamp is placed at the intersection, and the leg is lifted so that the drapes can be brought together and fastened on the medial side.

Using the trochanter major and the patella as landmarks, the surgeon begins the skin incision near the dorsal midline and extends it over the trochanter major along the lateral side of the thigh. It should curve slightly caudal to pass through a point 2 to 3 cm. caudal to the patella and end at the head of the tibia (Fig. 6–9).

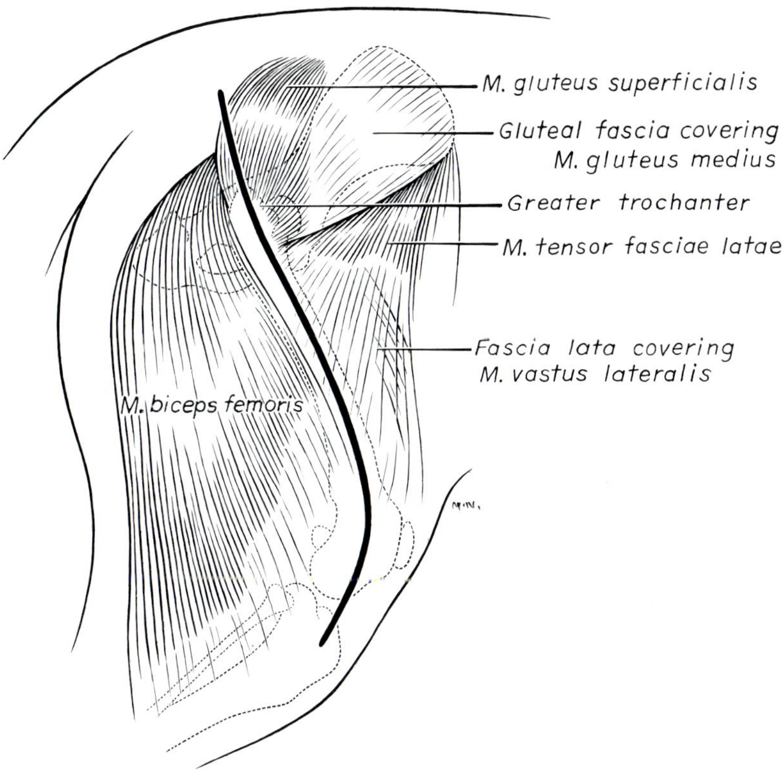

FIGURE 6–9. Line of incision and superficial muscles of the area. Bones are indicated by broken lines.

The fascia lata and the tensor fascia are separated with scissors close to the cranial border of the skin incision. The vastus lateralis and the biceps femoris are separated bluntly by using the scissors technique of spreading the tissues. By careful blunt dissection, the structures around the hip and stifle can be exposed and identified. The path of the sciatic nerve should be gently explored, especially in the region of the hip joint. One should be able to demonstrate the trochanter major, the gluteal muscles (superficialis, medius, and profundus), the sciatic nerve, the patella, the lateral condyle of the femur, and the shaft of the femur.

The fascial layers are closed with interrupted stitches by using an instrument tie. Each layer should be securely apposed so that no dead space will remain. When all layers have been closed, it may be necessary to place interrupted subcutaneous stitches before the skin edges will be close enough for proper closure. Interrupted stitches are also placed in the skin.

If the surgery has been properly done, the dog should walk without difficulty the day following surgery.

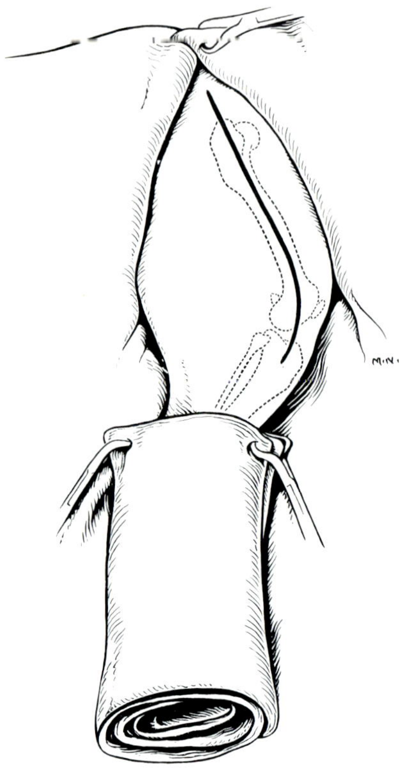

FIGURE 6–10. Line of incision in relation to right femur and tibia.

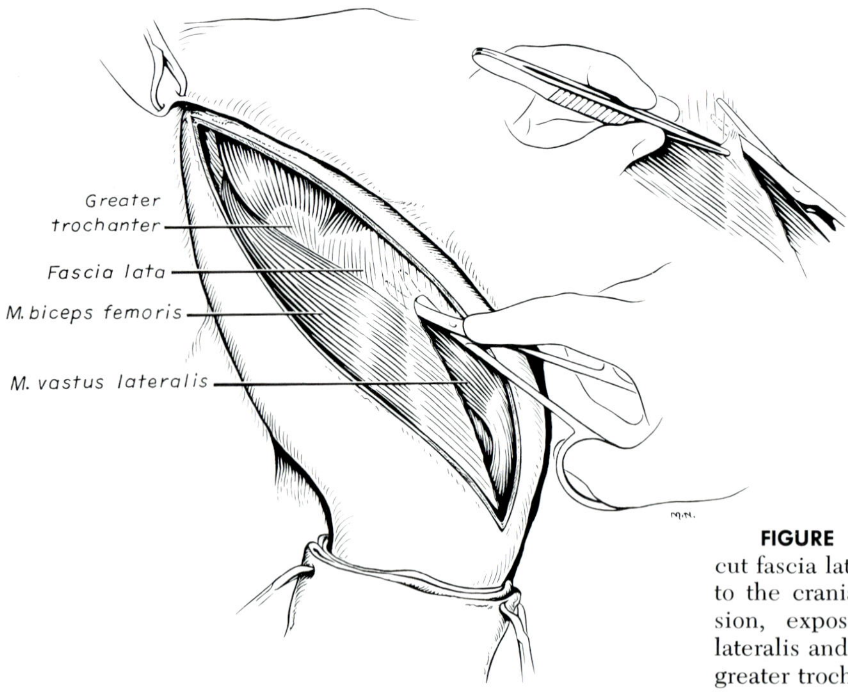

FIGURE 6–11. Spread and cut fascia lata with scissors close to the cranial edge of the incision, exposing the m. vastus lateralis and continuing over the greater trochanter.

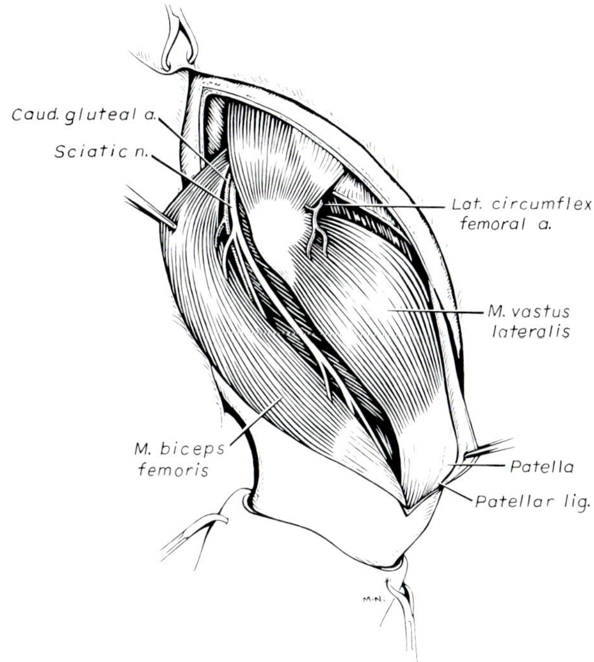

FIGURE 6–12. Reflect the m. biceps femoris to demonstrate the sciatic n. and caud. gluteal a. Reflect skin to demonstrate the patella and patellar ligaments.

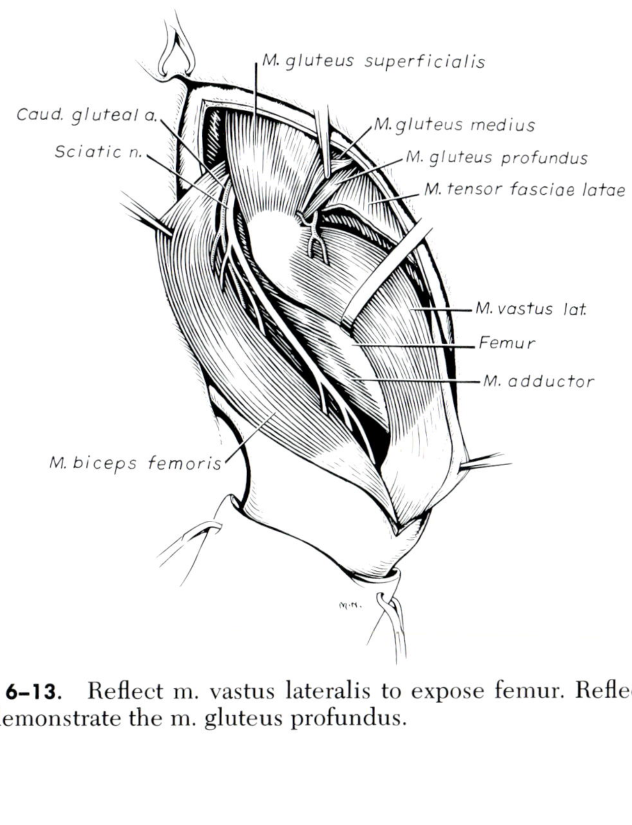

FIGURE 6–13. Reflect m. vastus lateralis to expose femur. Reflect m. gluteus medius to demonstrate the m. gluteus profundus.

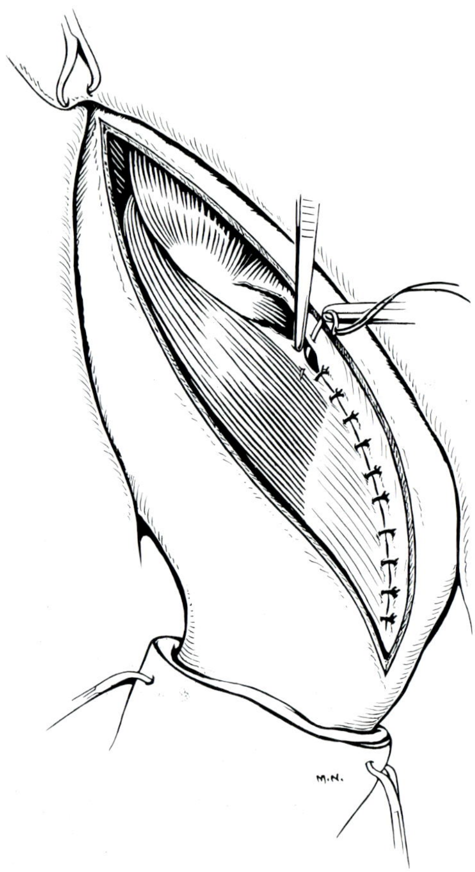

FIGURE 6–14. In suturing fascia lata and subcutaneous tissue, apply interrupted stitches with a half-circle needle; in suturing skin, apply interrupted stitches with a half-curved needle.

NOTES

THORACOTOMY

The purpose of this exercise is to give the student experience in opening and closing the chest. It also serves as an exercise in thoracic orientation.

Chest surgery requires some means of maintaining respiration. This equipment does not necessarily have to be elaborate. All that is required is a method whereby there can be an exchange of oxygen and carbon dioxide. Before any surgery of the chest is undertaken, the student should become completely familiar with the ventilation apparatus in use.

Following anesthetization, the patient is intubated. Directions for this procedure may be found in Chapter 4. The left side of the chest is clipped and prepared for surgery.

The patient is placed in right lateral recumbency and draped in the usual manner, with the surgical opening at the seventh intercostal space.

An incision is made from the middle of the latissimus dorsi to the costochondral junction midway between the seventh and eighth ribs (Fig. 6–15). Carry the incision by blunt dissection down to the pleura, making certain to avoid the intercostal blood vessels on the caudal side of the seventh rib. If the incision is properly made, the pleura will be exposed along the entire length of the incision.

The pleura is punctured and the opening extended for complete exposure (Figs. 6–16 and 6–17). The retractors are inserted and expanded so that the chest organs are properly exposed (Fig. 6–18). This may require some traction, but it is necessary in order to make an adequate field.

As soon as the retractors are in place, the respiratory apparatus is coupled to the trachea tube and adjusted for proper lung ventilation. From time to time it may be necessary to temporarily disconnect so that the lungs can be deflated for better visualization. Such a procedure is only done for very short periods of time and only when absolutely necessary.

It will be noticed that, if the lungs are hyperventilated with oxygen and all the carbon dioxide is depleted, respiratory movements will cease, even though the tissues remain a bright pink and the heart continues to beat normally. Such a phenomenon will continue until the carbon dioxide has returned to normal levels.

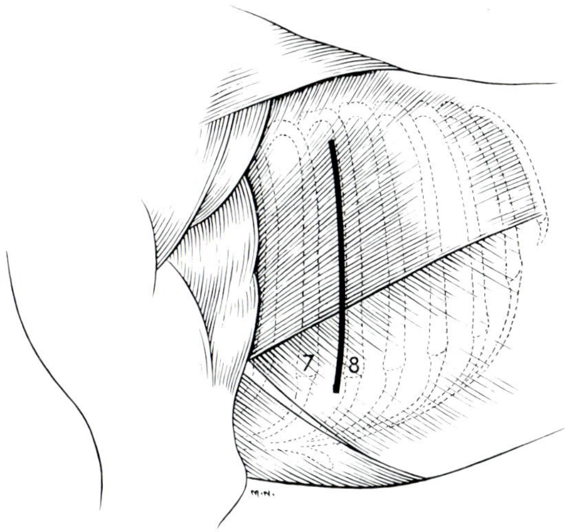

FIGURE 6–15. Line of incision.

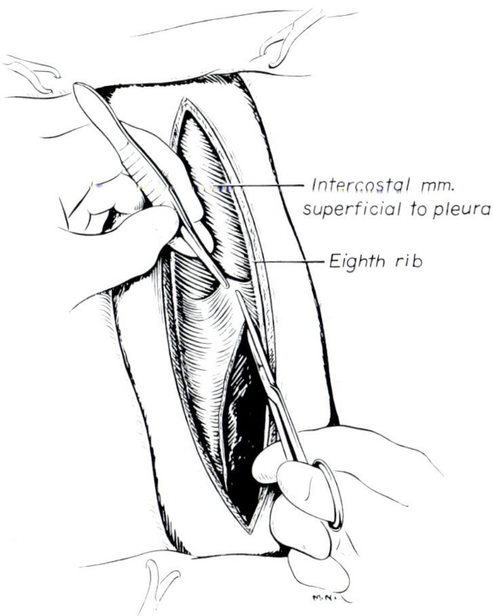

FIGURE 6–16. Enter pleural cavity close to cranial edge of eighth rib to avoid intercostal vessels and nerves. Transect intercostal mm. and pleura with scissors.

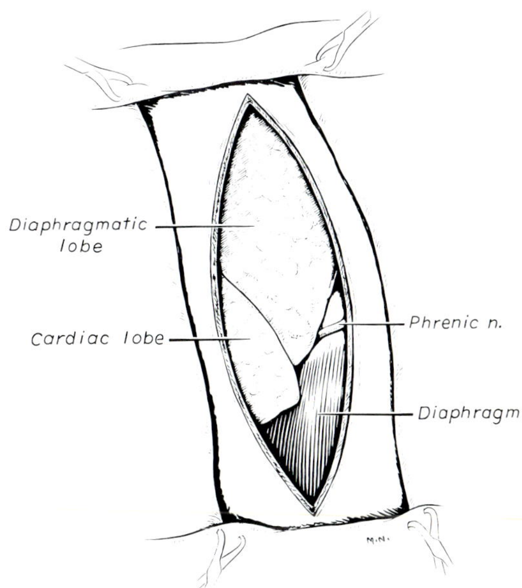

FIGURE 6–17. Left lung and diaphragm exposed.

Examination of the chest should include the lungs, the heart, the diaphragm, the phrenic nerves, the sympathetic trunk, the aorta, the intercostal vessels, and the ventral longitudinal ligaments over the intervertebral discs and their relationship to the heads of the ribs (Fig. 6–19).

A simple but secure method of closing the chest incision is to place monofilament stainless steel wire around the two adjacent ribs. The retractors are removed. Three 20 cm. strands of wire are placed equidistant along the incision. The needle should be inserted from within outward to avoid injury to the lung (Fig. 6–20). Since the intercostal vessels are on the caudal side of the rib, the wire may be passed close to the cranial side of the seventh rib but must make a wide excursion around the caudal side of the eighth. Only the two ribs and the inner and outer intercostal muscles are included in the loop. When all wire loops are in readiness, the anesthetist adjusts the respiratory equipment so that the lungs are expanded to the full capacity of the chest. The wire ends are crossed. The surgeon and assistant surgeon tighten the wires by grasping them with crossed hands (Fig. 6–21). Traction is first applied to draw the ribs together and then the wires are twisted. When all loops are secure and there is no evidence of leakage, the twisted ends are cut about 0.5 cm. long and turned inward against the rib. As soon as the chest is securely closed, the ventilation apparatus may be disconnected at the coupling to the trachea tube. The tube should not be removed until the patient is returned to its quarters.

To complete the closure, the fascia is closed by layers with interrupted stitches and finally the skin is closed with interrupted stitches (Figs. 6–22 and 6–23).

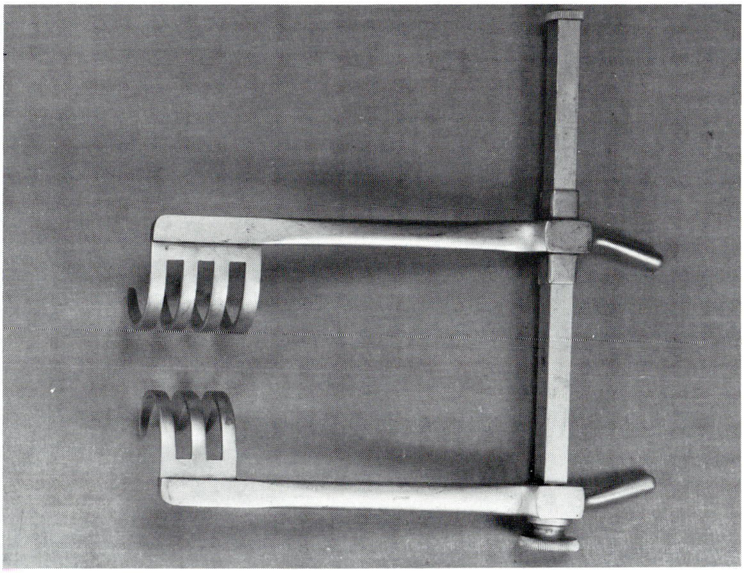

FIGURE 6–18. Frazer laminectomy retractors.

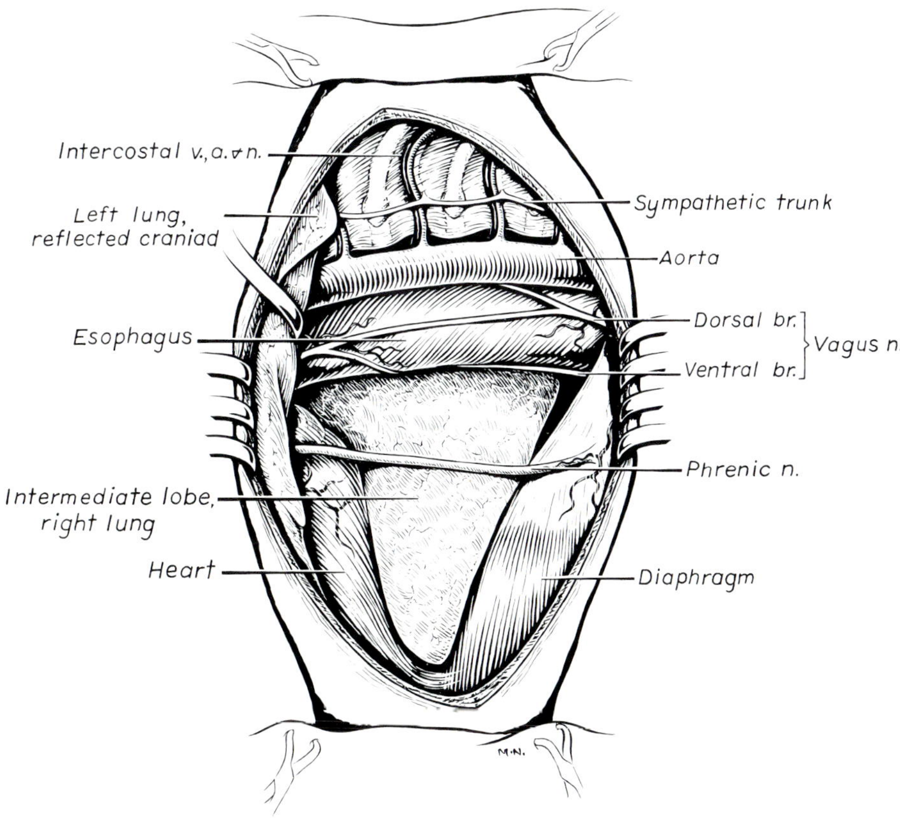

FIGURE 6–19. Incision opened and left lung retracted.

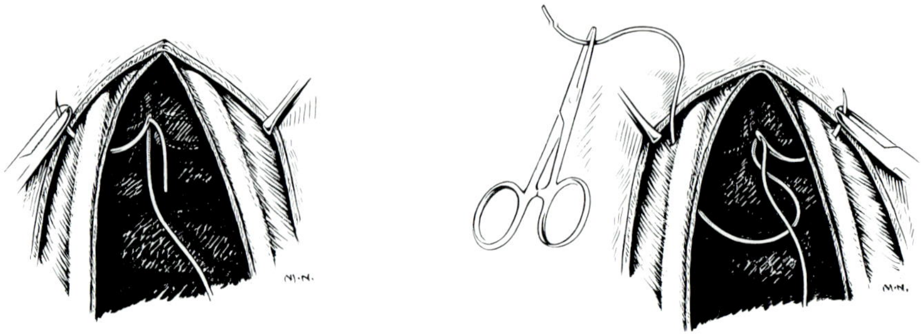

FIGURE 6–20. To close, reflect skin and external muscles. Place three wire stay stitches internal to external on the far side of the ribs. Avoid the intercostal vessels on the caudal side of each rib.

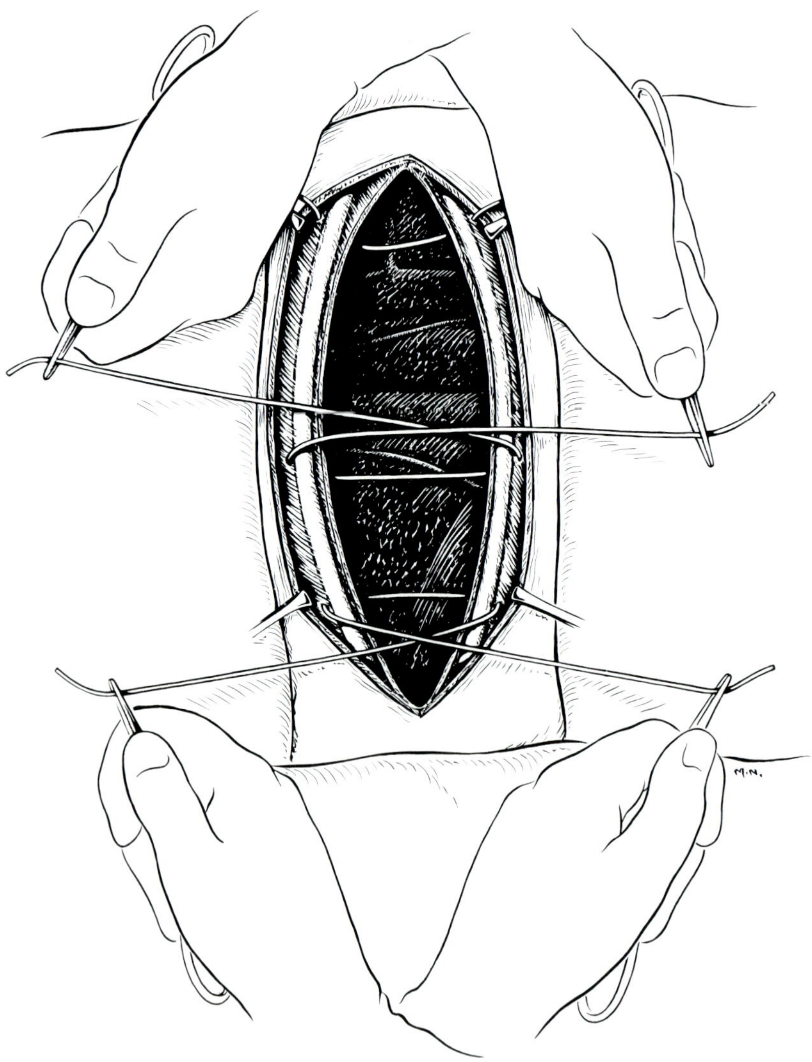

FIGURE 6–21. Closure.

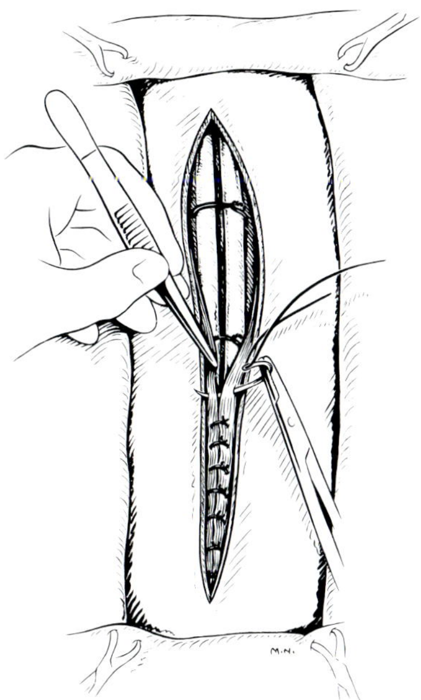

FIGURE 6–22. Ribs are approximated with wire. Use interrupted stitches for muscles and fascia.

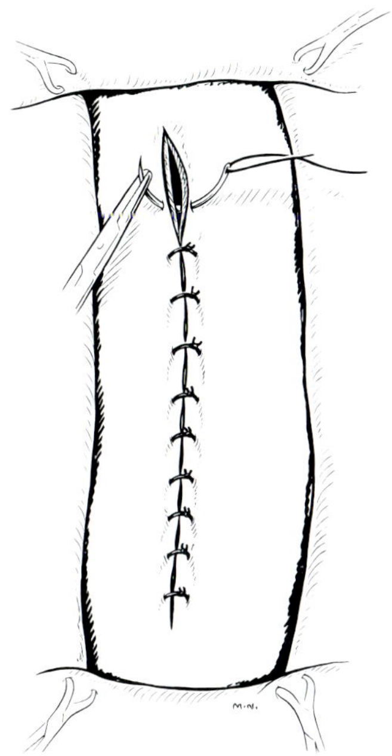

FIGURE 6–23. Interrupted stitches for skin.

NOTES

Chapter 7

COMMON SURGICAL PROCEDURES IN SURGERY OF THE DIGESTIVE TRACT

The common major and minor operations used along the alimentary canal will be presented so that the student may study each procedure in some depth. The steps will be as detailed as possible, with a minimum of repetition. Procedures for the correction of less common conditions will not be dealt with in the following descriptions.

CHEILOPLASTY

While this operation is mostly involved with the integumentary system, it is included because it also involves the lips to a degree. The principal objective is to obliterate the "flue," or skin sulcus, which is responsible for the cheilitis.

A large area of skin is prepared in the mandibular region. A single drape with an opening of sufficient size is placed over the area to be excised and fastened securely.

The first incision is made the depth of the skin along the mucocutaneous border. It should extend slightly beyond the edges of the excoriated skin. At the rostral end of this incision, another incision is begun and carried obliquely ventrocaudally beyond the ventral border of the lesion. Two more incisions are made parallel to the first two. This produces a parallelogram that runs obliquely across the mandible. The island of excoriated skin should be undermined with scissors and removed. It is not necessary to include any tissue beyond the depth of the skin (Fig. 7–1).

Closure is made by using interrupted stitches of 32 gauge stainless steel. The dorsal and caudal edges are joined to the rostral and ventral edges so that the furrow is entirely obliterated.

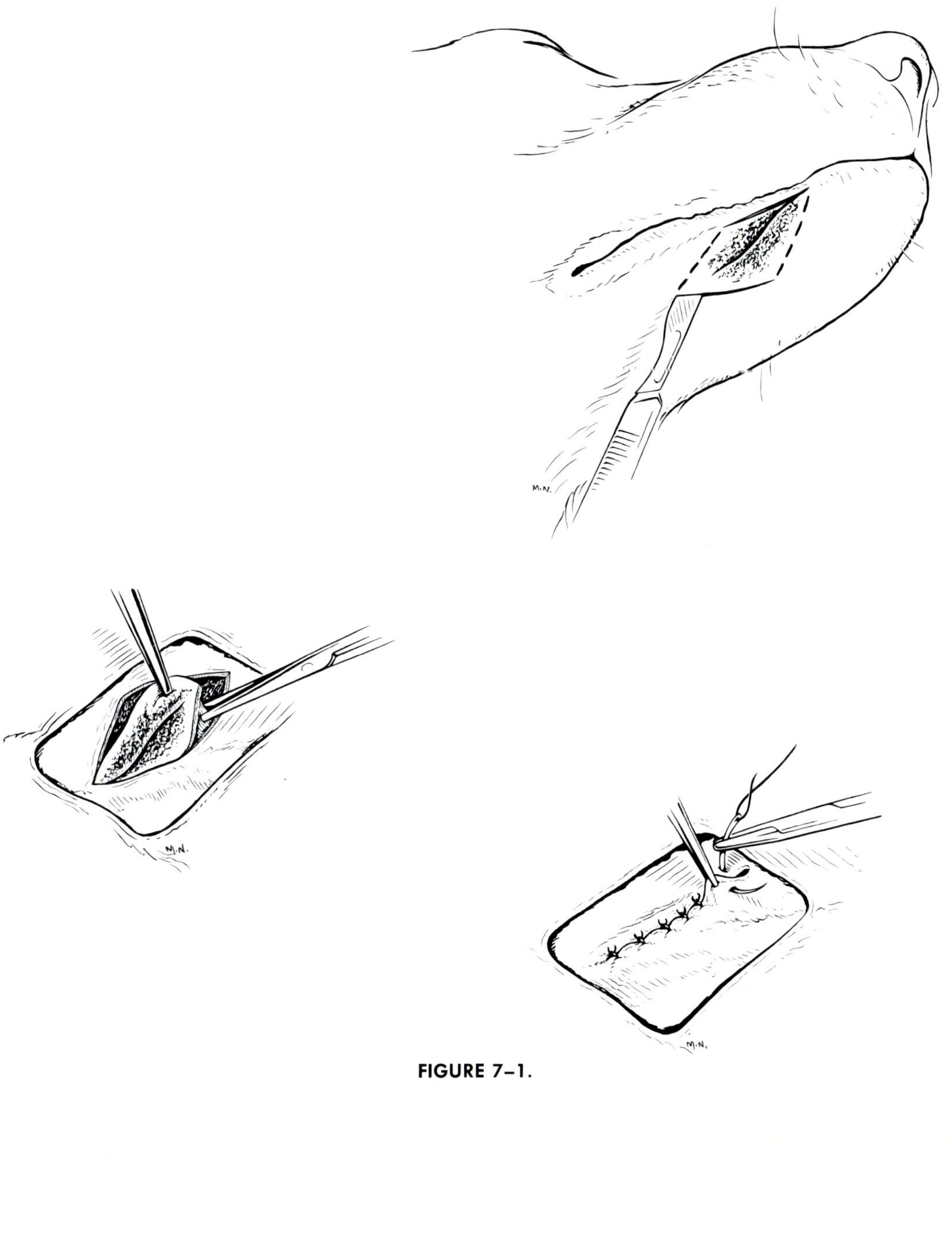

FIGURE 7–1.

UVULECTOMY

The patient, almost invariably a brachycephalic type, is anesthetized with either a short or long-acting barbiturate intravenously. The usual position is sternal recumbency with the head elevated. A mouth speculum is inserted and the jaws are spread as widely as possible (Fig. 7–2).

At this point it is often possible to see the uvula drawn into the glottis with the epiglottis rostral to it. If this is the case, the spot on the uvula opposite the tip of the epiglottis should be marked. A small cotton swab dipped in an antiseptic dye or tincture of iodine is adequate. The tip of the electrosurgical electrode may also be used to burn a small mark. In cases where the uvula is rostral to the epiglottis, the two organs should be repositioned so that the guide mark can be made.

An endotracheal tube is then passed and, in this case, anchored to the mandible with a 1 inch gauze bandage. If a short acting barbiturate has been used, the anesthesia can be continued by using a volatile anesthetic administered through the tube. As a precautionary measure, the cuff is inflated so that fluids collecting in the mouth will not be inhaled.

The tip of the uvula is grasped with an Allis forceps and slight traction is applied in the rostral direction. The electrosurgical knife is used to describe an arc from the lateral edges, with the marked point as the top of the arc. The cutting should be done slowly, with coagulation as the cut progresses. There should be very little hemorrahge with this method. It ordinarily does not require ligating or suturing.

A liquid diet for two postoperative days is all the aftercare required.

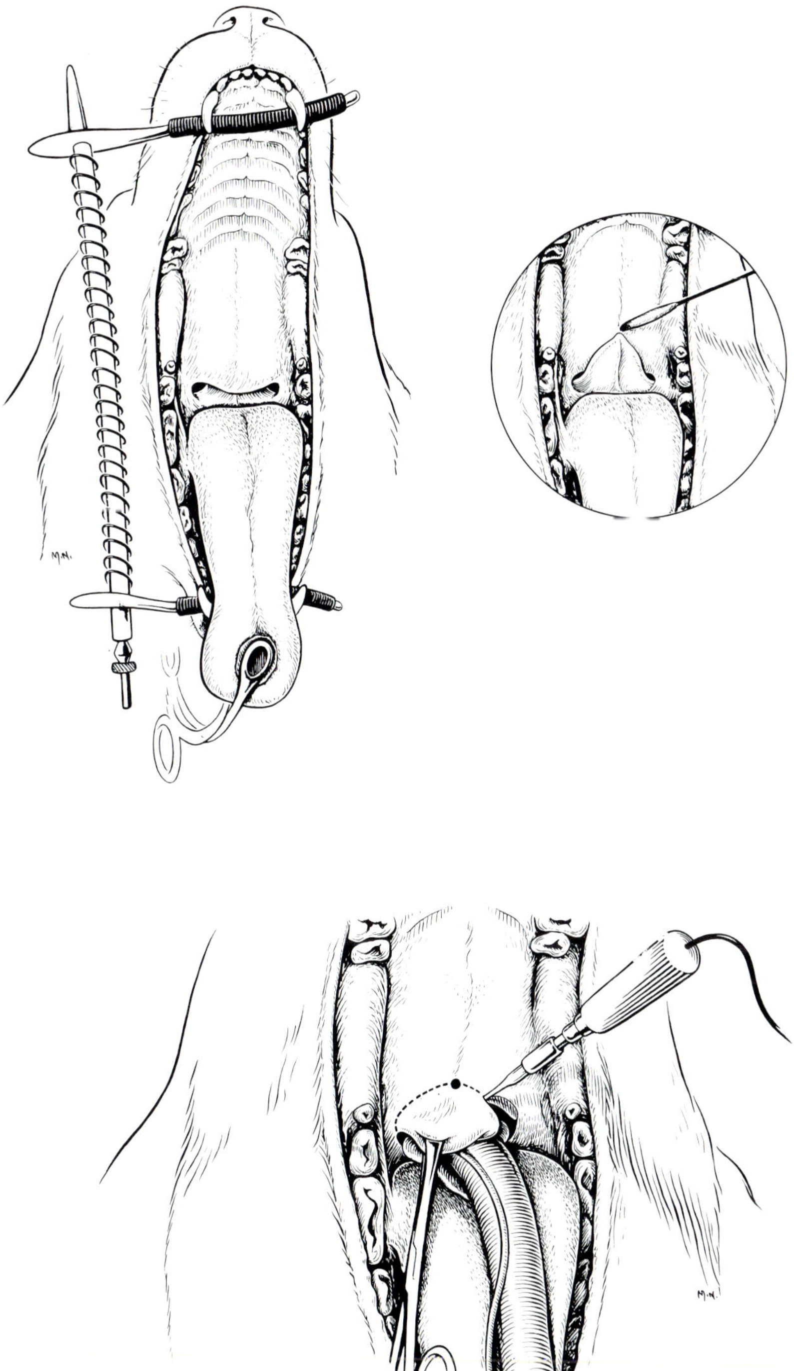

FIGURE 7–2.

TONSILLECTOMY

This operation is performed under general anesthesia, and the use of a trachea tube is optional. However, if a volatile anesthetic is used, it is safer to employ a tube so that the administration is constant and smooth.

Positioning is also optional. In large dogs, dorsal recumbency with the head elevated or sternal recumbency with the head elevated seems most satisfactory. In small dogs, dorsal recumbency with the table tipped to a vertical position and the forelegs fastened over the end of the table affords an excellent exposure, but this should only be used by an experienced operator who can complete the surgery quickly.

A speculum is used, and traction is applied to the tongue. An assistant may retract the tongue or a weighted tongue forceps may be used when the patient is in the upright position.

The tonsils lie in a tonsillar sinus on either side of the pharynx, and unless they are grossly enlarged or swollen, it may be necessary to depress the tonsillar fold of tissue in order to expose them. This lymphatic tissue is quite friable. Using an Allis forceps, gently lift the tonsil from its sinus. The forceps should be placed so that it grasps around the tonsil and not into it. Traction should be approximately in the middle of the major tonsil. A deeper minor portion will follow as the major portion is retracted.

Beginning at one pole of the tonsil and progressing across the fold of mucosa forming its attachment, extirpate the tonsil by scissors, guillotine, snare, or cautery. The cautery has many advantages. Because of its fulgurating action, the bleeding is minimized while the desiccating action ensures complete removal of the lymphatic tissue. Whatever method of extirpation is used, it is well for the operator to keep in mind the three branches of the tonsillar artery which enter the tonsil near the middle. The surgery should also be as shallow as possible so that the main tonsillar artery is not severed (Fig. 7–3).

Usually pressure in a lateral direction with a sponge placed on the tip of the index finger will control any oozing from the sinus. If bleeding is severe, the artery should be located and ligated. In moderate bleeding, the sinus may be sutured with catgut by using a continuous stitch.

All cases should be checked frequently until they have regained consciousness. A fluid diet for 48 hours is desirable.

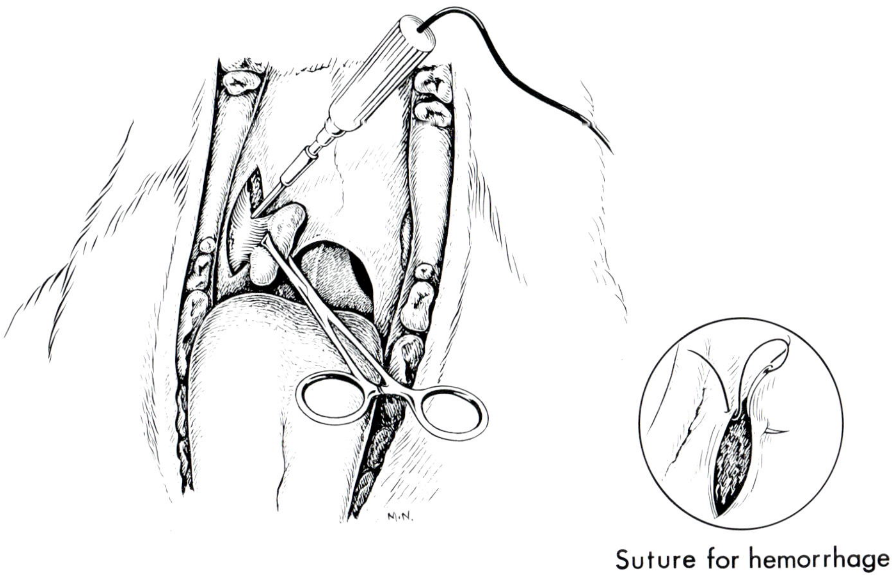

FIGURE 7–3.

SIALOADENECTOMY

MUCOCELE

A general anesthetic that the operator considers suitable is administered. The side to be operated is determined previously by observation, palpation, or sialography. A large area of skin beneath the ear and over the region of the cyst is prepared. The incision site is located by pressing on the jugular. This will distend the internal and external maxillary veins which lie just caudal to the angle of the mandible. The mandibular salivary gland can often be palpated in this region (Fig. 7–4).

The patient is positioned in lateral recumbency and draped so that an incision about 8 cm. long can be made over the mandibular gland.

The skin incision is made with a scalpel in a craniocaudal direction, and the fibers of the platysma muscle are separated with scissors. Since the muscular fibers run in the same direction as the incision, it is seldom necessary to divide this muscle. The depressor auricularis muscle may require cutting in order to get adequate exposure of the gland. This muscle is not large. After separation of the connective tissue, the capsule is exposed and incised.

Within the capsule will be found the buff-colored, waxy mandibular gland as well as the monostomatic portion of the sublingual gland. The latter can be distinguished by its darker color. By blunt dissection the glandular tissue is freed from the capsule. The blood supply will be found on the medial side of the gland and should be carefully ligated before separation. If the gland is lifted gently from the capsule, there should be no problem. The ducts are followed in a rostral direction to the medial border of the mandible. At this point a small grape-like lobule of the sublingual will be found. This, too, is separated bluntly and a ligature placed around both ducts just anterior to the free glandular tissue. The ducts are severed caudal to the ligature and the glands removed (Fig. 7–5).

The cervical cyst may be treated in one of three ways:

1. Remove the redundant skin by making an elliptical incision near the base of the cyst. This, together with as much of the cyst wall as possible, is removed. The area is thoroughly cleansed with sponges and sterile saline and the wound closed with interrupted stitches.
2. The cyst is lanced at its most pendent part, and after draining the contents, it is swabbed with Lugol's solution and allowed to remain open.
3. A large needle or trocar is used to drain the cyst, and no further treatment is given.

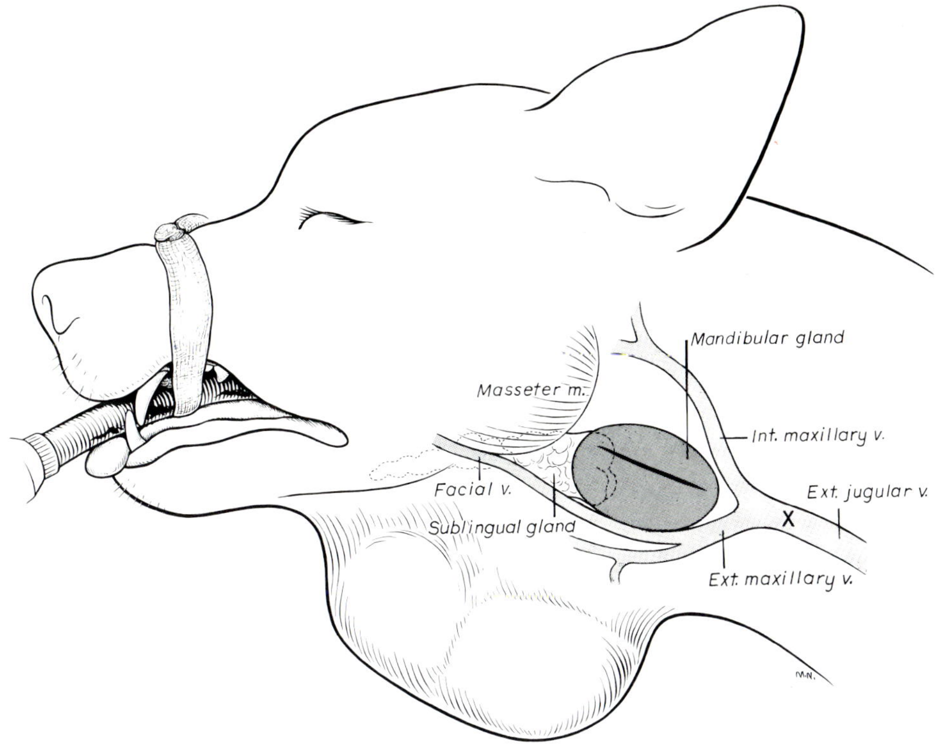

FIGURE 7–4. Incision is between the external and internal maxillary veins and over the mandibular gland.

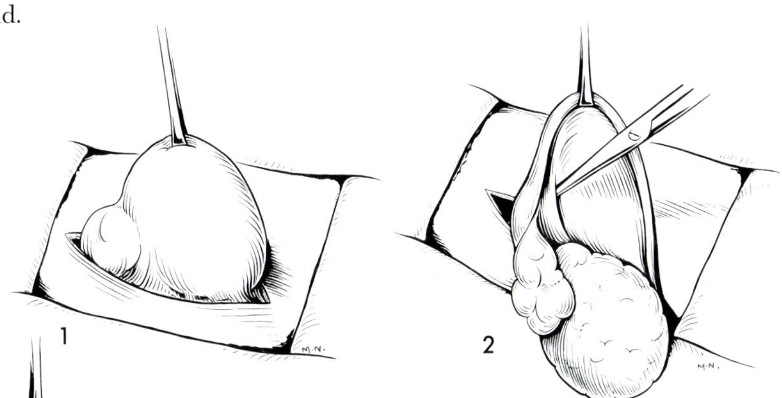

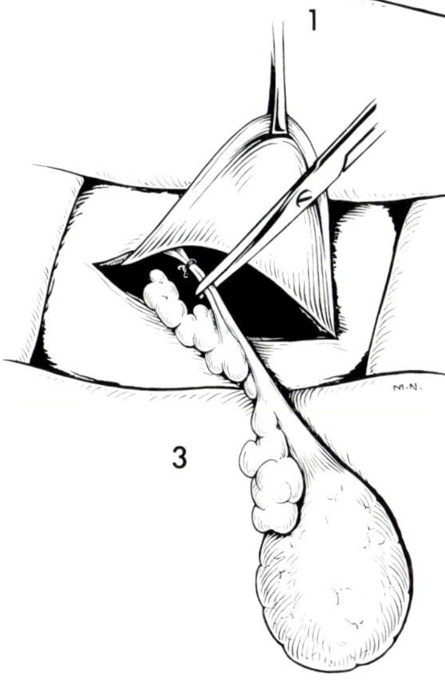

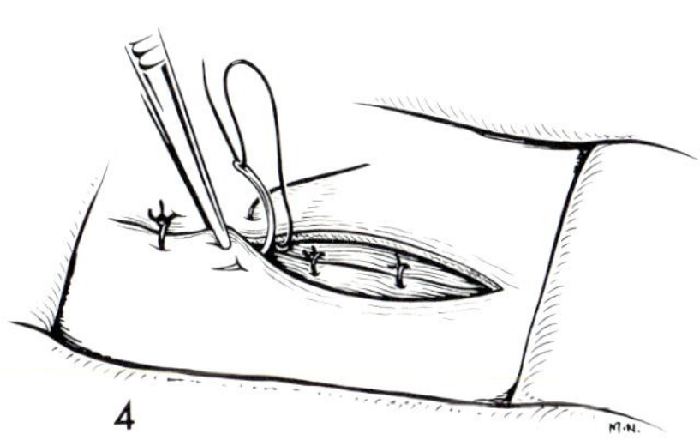

FIGURE 7–5.
Step 1. Capsule encloses mandibular gland and monostomatic part of sublingual gland.
Step 2. Separate capsule from glands by blunt dissection.
Step 3. Ligate and transect ducts. Remove glands.
Step 4. Closure.

RANULA

The same type of surgical procedure recommended for the mucocele has been recommended for the ranula, since it is believed that the ranula is a pathological condition of the sublingual duct and the mucocele is a pathological condition of the mandibular duct. It is also not uncommon for both conditions to occur simultaneously. Removal of the monostomatic portion of the sublingual gland therefore seems logical.

In cases of simple ranula, however, it is possible to grossly extirpate the cyst so that it will not recur. This requires the removal of all mucous membrane involved so that there is no possibility for closure until salivary drainage is well established. A simple incision or lancing of the cyst will not suffice. All free mucous membrane along the frenulum and base of the tongue must be debrided (Fig. 7–6).

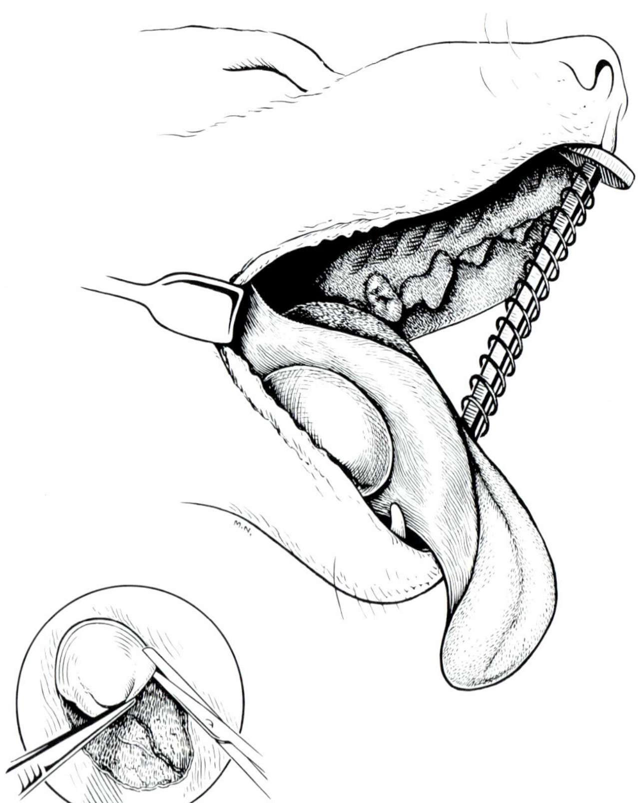

FIGURE 7–6.

ESOPHAGOTOMY

The esophagus presents more surgical problems than any other segment of the digestive tract. Poor healing due to excessive movement often leads to disruption, which can frequently terminate fatally. The limited circulation requires that great care be given to the vascularity at the incision site. The muscular coats do not retain sutures well, but fortunately the mucosa is extremely tough and is much more amenable to suturing than the mucosa of the stomach or intestine. Leakage at the incision site is far more frequent in the esophagus because of the absence of proper serosa or other fibrin-producing tissues, such as omentum, with which to seal off the suture line.

Strictures are common in esophageal surgery. Because of the stenosis caused by postoperative swelling or the presence of a permanent stricture, vomiting is extremely common. If the stenosis is temporary (postoperative swelling), the vomiting will abate after about seven to 14 days. Strictures, on the other hand, are quite likely to produce persistent vomiting.

CERVICAL ESOPHAGUS

After anesthetizing the patient, an endotracheal tube should be inserted as a precautionary measure. The trachea must be manipulated during the surgery and may require reinforcing in order to maintain a patent airway. The surgery could possibly invade the chest through the thoracic inlet and thereby require chest ventilation.

Preparation of the patient should include passing a stomach tube to the operative site and attaching it to a suction apparatus. The skin over the ventral aspect of the neck from the larynx to the manubrium of the sternum and laterally to the angle of the mandibles cranially and the points of the shoulders caudally should be prepared.

A dorsal recumbency with the head tied forward and the forelegs tied in a caudal direction places the patient in a good position. A small pad or sandbag under the middle of the neck may improve the positioning. Draping should leave a long narrow opening on the midline of the neck.

The skin incision should be on the midline and extend from the region of the larynx to the thoracic inlet. Once the blood vessels in the skin have been ligated, there should be very little trouble from bleeding. Blunt dissection on the midline between the paired sternothyroideus and sternohyoideus muscles will expose the trachea. During this exposure it may be necessary to ligate one or two small branches of the tracheal artery which cross the incision line. The trachea is moved to the right so that the esophagus, which lies either left dorsal or left ventral to it, can be fully exposed. The Frazer laminectomy retractors are inserted between the trachea and the left sternohyoideus muscle and gently expanded. Care should be taken not to injure the recurrent laryngeal nerves, which are clearly visible beneath the proper fascia of the trachea (Fig. 7–7).

At this point in the surgery, the involved area of the esophagus should be plainly visible. If the problem is a laceration, the surgical site has already been chosen, but more often obstruction is the reason for surgery. In such a case, the surgical site should be cranial or caudal to the obstruction so that the tissue involved in the closure will be reasonably healthy.

The esophagus is gently separated from the fascia investing the carotid, the vagosympathetic nerve trunk, and the internal jugular and packed off with gauze sponges. Surrounding tissues must be protected from spillage, and the surgical area of the esophagus should be positioned to the best advantage for the operator.

A longitudinal incision is made, preferably over the stomach tube, since it imparts some firmness to the esophagus. The stomach tube is then withdrawn enough to remove it from the incision, and blunt forceps are inserted in the direction of the obstruction. Spreading the jaws of this instrument will help to dilate the esophagus and perhaps free the lodged foreign body. Care must be taken in retrieving the foreign body that the surrounding tissues are not contaminated. The suction will be of considerable help in removing contaminating fluids. Sterile sponges held with forceps are also useful. Any contaminated material should be discarded.

Before beginning the closure, it may be helpful to stabilize the esophagus by gently clamping with rubber-shod forceps. Intestinal clamps or Allis forceps with rubber tubing covering the blades can be placed about 3 to 6 cm. from either end of the incision and closed very lightly. The tissue which must carry the heaviest burden is the mucosa, since the submucosa, the two spiral muscular coats, and the adventitia are quite friable and do not hold sutures well. Various methods of inverting or everting the coats of the esophagus have been proposed, but the simple two-layer closure seems safest, since it causes the least circulatory interference. The mucosa is closed with 5-0 surgical silk, using simple interrupted stitches about 2 mm. apart with the knots tied in the lumen of the esophagus. Great care should be taken with this suture line because it is the key to a successful operation. The stitches should not be too tight but should hold the mucosa in firm apposition. A second row of interrupted stitches is placed so that the submucosa and muscular layers are apposed. The use of 3-0 chromic catgut is recommended for this closure.

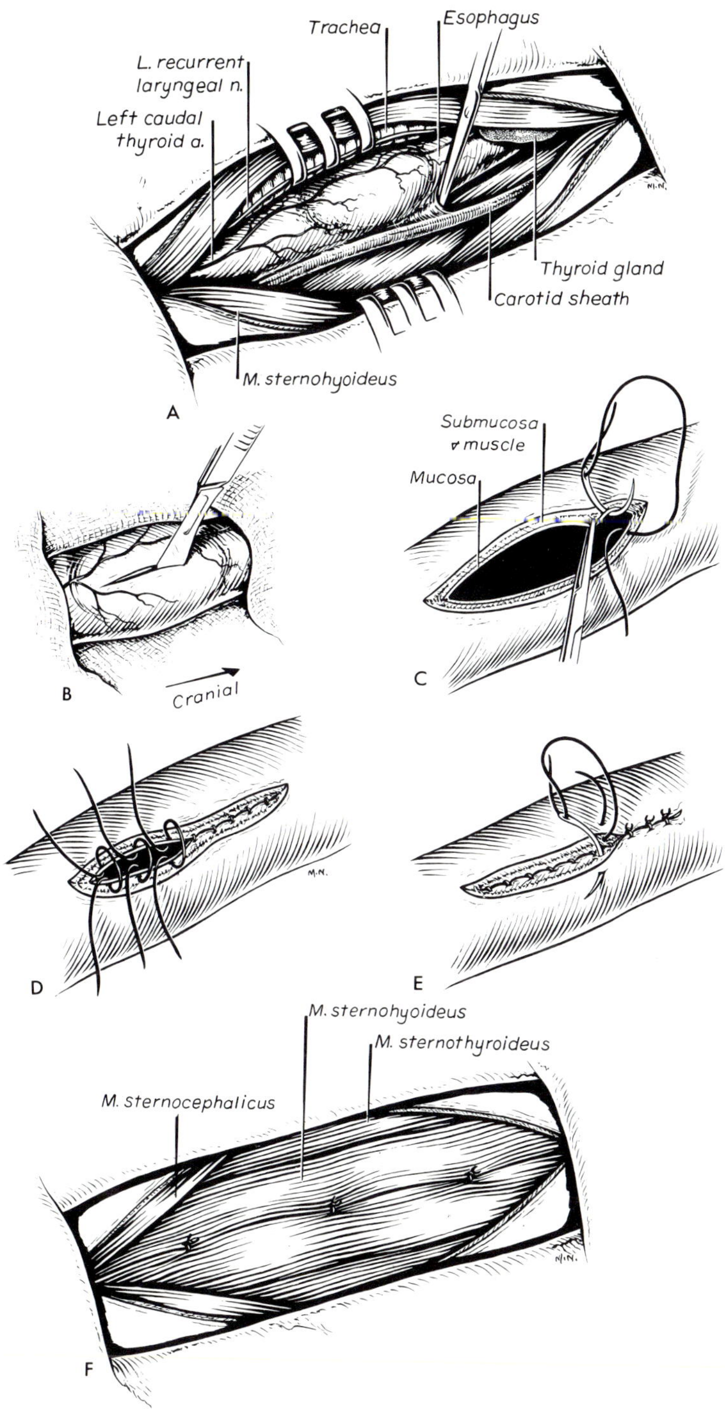
Trachea
Esophagus
L. recurrent laryngeal n.
Left caudal thyroid a.
Thyroid gland
Carotid sheath
M. sternohyoideus
A
Submucosa & muscle
Mucosa
B
Cranial
C
D
E
M. sternohyoideus
M. sternothyroideus
M. sternocephalicus
F

FIGURE 7–7.

THORACIC ESOPHAGUS

If an esophagotomy is to be done on the thoracic portion of the esophagus, some form of lung ventilation is required. Anesthetization and intubation is carried out as previously described under the cervical esophagus. Depending on the location of the lesion, either the left or right side of the chest is prepared for surgery. If the surgical site is to be the cranial portion of the esophagus, the preparation should be for an incision at the fifth intercostal space on the left side. The more likely area would be the caudal portion, which requires an incision at the seventh intercostal space on the right side.

The patient is positioned in lateral recumbency and draped for the appropriate intercostal incision. The incision is made according to the description under Thoracotomy, but it may require some modification if it is in the cranial portion of the chest because of the presence of the latissimus dorsi muscle. It may be necessary to transect part of this muscle in order to obtain adequate exposure. This should be done with scissors and with care, ligating any bleeding vessels and transecting only as far as necessary. Each tissue layer should be completely separated before proceeding to the next, so that the final exposure will not be delayed unduly after the lungs have been collapsed.

The endotracheal tube should be coupled to the respirator as soon as the retractors are in place. A lobe of the lung overlying the esophagus is reflected and packed off with saline moistened towels. The esophagotomy area can be seen through the mediastinal pleura (Fig. 7–8). In the left cranial area, the left vagus will traverse the left side of the esophagus, while in the right caudal area the left and right branches converge to form one trunk on the dorsal side of the esophagus. This nerve must be handled carefully and retracted from the surgical field.

The surgery for esophagotomy of the thoracic portion is the same as for the cervical portion, except that, once the esophagus is repaired, the chest must be closed. This is best accomplished by using the technique described under Thoracotomy in Chapter 6.

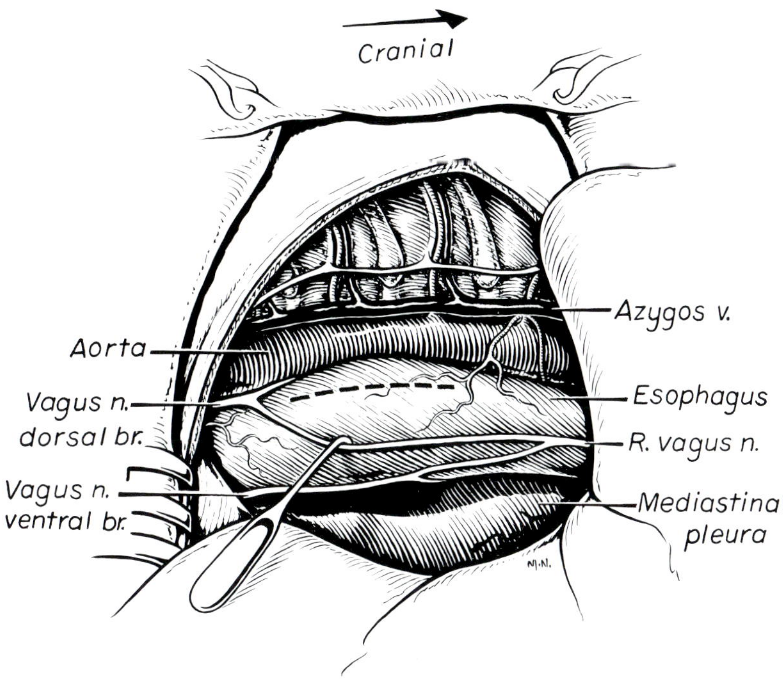

FIGURE 7–8. Exposure of the caudal esophagus from the right side.

ESOPHAGEAL RESECTION

Although an anastomosis of the esophagus is usually performed on the caudal portion of the thoracic esophagus, the technique would be the same throughout its length provided the resected portion is not too great. Removal of a section of esophagus over 6 cm. in length is hazardous because of the tension put on the suture line and the arterial supply to the organ.

The preparation and approach is the same as described for esophagotomy of the caudal thoracic portion. After the esophagus has been freed from endothoracic fascia and the vagus nerve carefully retracted from the field, the esophagus is gently clamped with rubber-shod clamps placed an adequate distance apart. The area is then packed off with sponges or towels to reduce the possibility of contamination. Forceps are placed at the limits of the portion to be resected. A section is removed by cutting close to the outer edge of the forceps with a scalpel. The section, along with the forceps and scalpel, is discarded (Fig. 7–9).

Suturing is begun on the side away from the operator. Simple interrupted stitches of 4-0 chromic catgut are placed with great care, precision, and gentleness through all layers except the mucosa. An assistant holds all sutures as they are placed in the far third of the esophageal wall. When all are in place, gentle traction is applied to appose the tissues, and the stitches are tied with the knots outside the adventitia. These stitches should be small and close together. When the far side has been closed, it is well to have the assistant place some tension on the rubber-shod clamps so that the suture line is free of strain. A line of simple interrupted stitches of 5-0 silk is next placed in the mucosal layer by beginning at the far side and working to the near side. The sutures should be placed about 2 mm. apart and 2 mm. deep with the knots inside the lumen. When the mucosa is completely closed, the outside row of sutures is then completed.

The mediastinum is tacked into place with two or three sutures and the chest closed in the usual way.

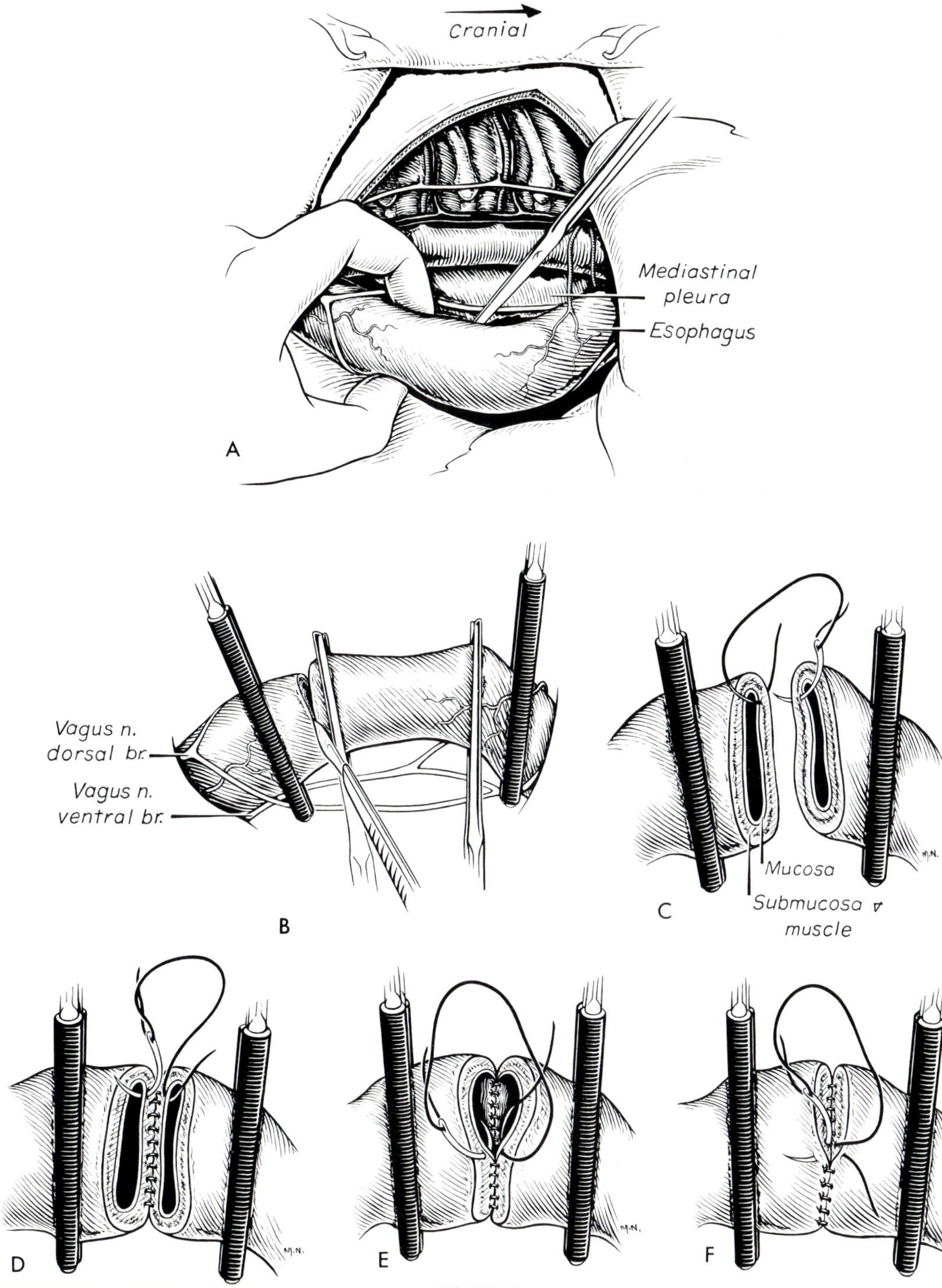
Cranial
Mediastinal pleura
Esophagus
A
Vagus n. dorsal br.
Vagus n. ventral br.
B
Mucosa
Submucosa & muscle
C
D
E
F

FIGURE 7–9.

Aftercare following esophageal surgery is extremely important. No food should be given by mouth for the first five days and only liquids and very thin gruels for the next seven days. The patient should be kept in a very quiet spot so that there is no excitement, and the temperature should be moderated to avoid panting. Food or the sounds of feeding stimulate salivation, and this should be avoided as much as possible. Most patients will vomit if solid food is given during the first week and sometimes two weeks. An everting method of closure has been suggested as a way of avoiding this difficulty.

Since stricture is the common cause of postoperative vomiting, it is well to bear in mind the factors which contribute to stricture formation: (1) Tension on the suture line creates excessive inflammation and granulation. (2) If an inverting type of anastomosis is used, there should be a very small amount inverted. Eversion is said to be superior in this respect and is seldom the cause of stricture and vomiting. (3) A fistula caused by leakage of the suture line can usually be avoided by very careful suturing and proper aftercare of the patient. (4) Infection causes inflammation, swelling, and necrosis. It usually is very damaging and often fatal. (5) Tissue reaction to suture material can cause a temporary stricture but is the least important factor involved in the vomiting syndrome.

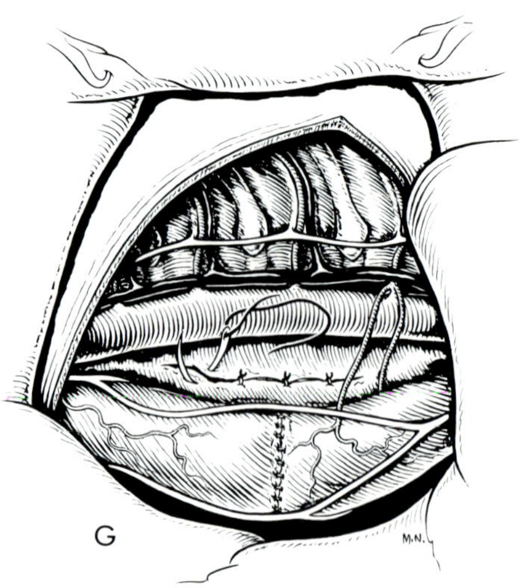

FIGURE 7–9. *Continued.*

GASTROPEXY

Whenever gastric torsion occurs with dilatation, it must be corrected surgically. The surgery is very simple, but it must be done with dispatch and with certain safeguards, since the condition is peracute. The patient is in shock and therefore deep anesthetization is not only unnecessary but dangerous. A small dose of chlorpromazine and atropine combined with halothane or methoxyflurane or with a local anesthetic is usually all that is required. Oxygen should be used during the procedure to control the hypoxia. Regardless of the method of anesthetization or the use of oxygen, an endotracheal tube should be inserted and the cuff inflated to prevent inhalation of regurgitated stomach contents following torsion correction.

Preparation is made for a left paracostal incision. The position of the patient should be right lateral recumbency. The draping should allow for at least a hand's breadth incision but preferably more to allow ample room for manipulation.

Once the skin incision is made, the muscles are separated and divided with scissors. Muscles involved in this incision are the obliquus externus, obliquus internus, and rectus and transversus abdominis. As soon as the peritoneum is divided, the stomach will bulge into the incision.

With a clockwise rotation, the greater omentum will cover the stomach. This must be divided so that the stomach can be tapped. With a counterclockwise rotation, the omentum may be torn free so that the stomach wall is exposed. In this case the stomach will appear congested but not as dark as it appears with clockwise rotation (Fig. 7–10).

A 12 or 14 gauge needle with free tubing or tubing coupled to a suction apparatus is used to tap the stomach so that gas and fluid can be removed. As soon as the stomach is deflated, a close examination of the cardiac end and the esophagus is made to determine the direction of the torsion. By rotating the pylorus around the cardia in the opposite direction to the twist in the esophagus, the torsion can be relieved; however, if this is attempted before reducing the pressure within the stomach, there is great danger of fluid regurgitation.

It is important that the gastrosplenic ligament of the greater omentum be inspected to see that the splenic vessels are not occluded. Once both stomach and spleen have been returned to normal position, the stomach should be palpated to determine the amount and consistency of the ingesta. Frequently it is necessary to perform a gastrotomy to remove excessive solids. A description of this operation is found under Gastrotomy in Chapter 6. Great care must be taken to avoid contaminating the abdomen when the stomach is opened.

After the gastrotomy has been closed, the stomach is sutured to the cranial edge of the abdominal incision with interrupted stitches of 2-0 catgut. The suture line should follow the greater curvature of the stomach parallel to and about 3 to 6 cm. from the attachment of the greater omentum.

Enough sutures should be used to ensure a stable adhesion. The abdominal incision is then closed in the usual manner by starting with the closure of parietal peritoneum on the suture line previously made by joining the stomach and the peritoneal lip of the incision.

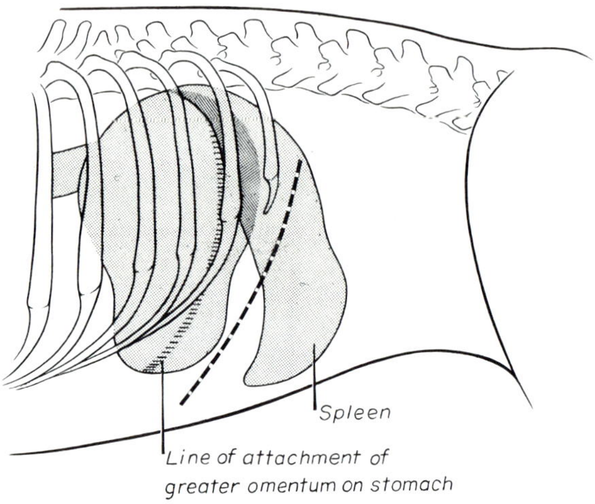

A

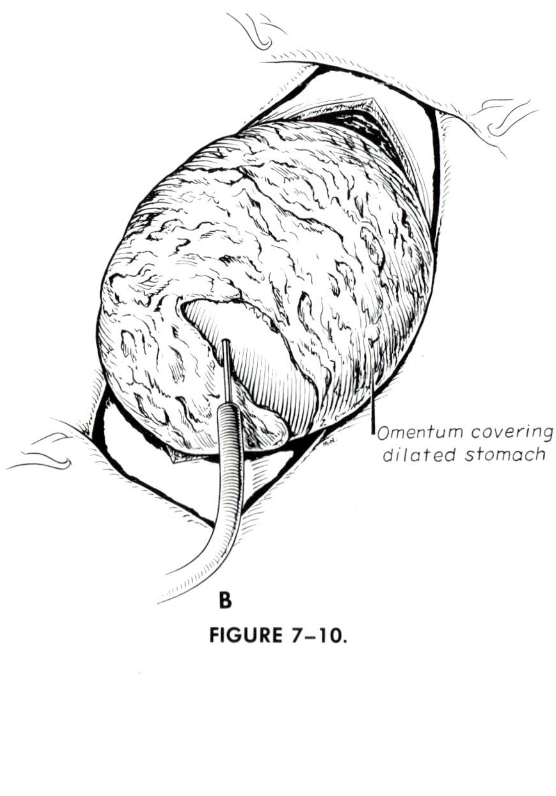

B

FIGURE 7–10.

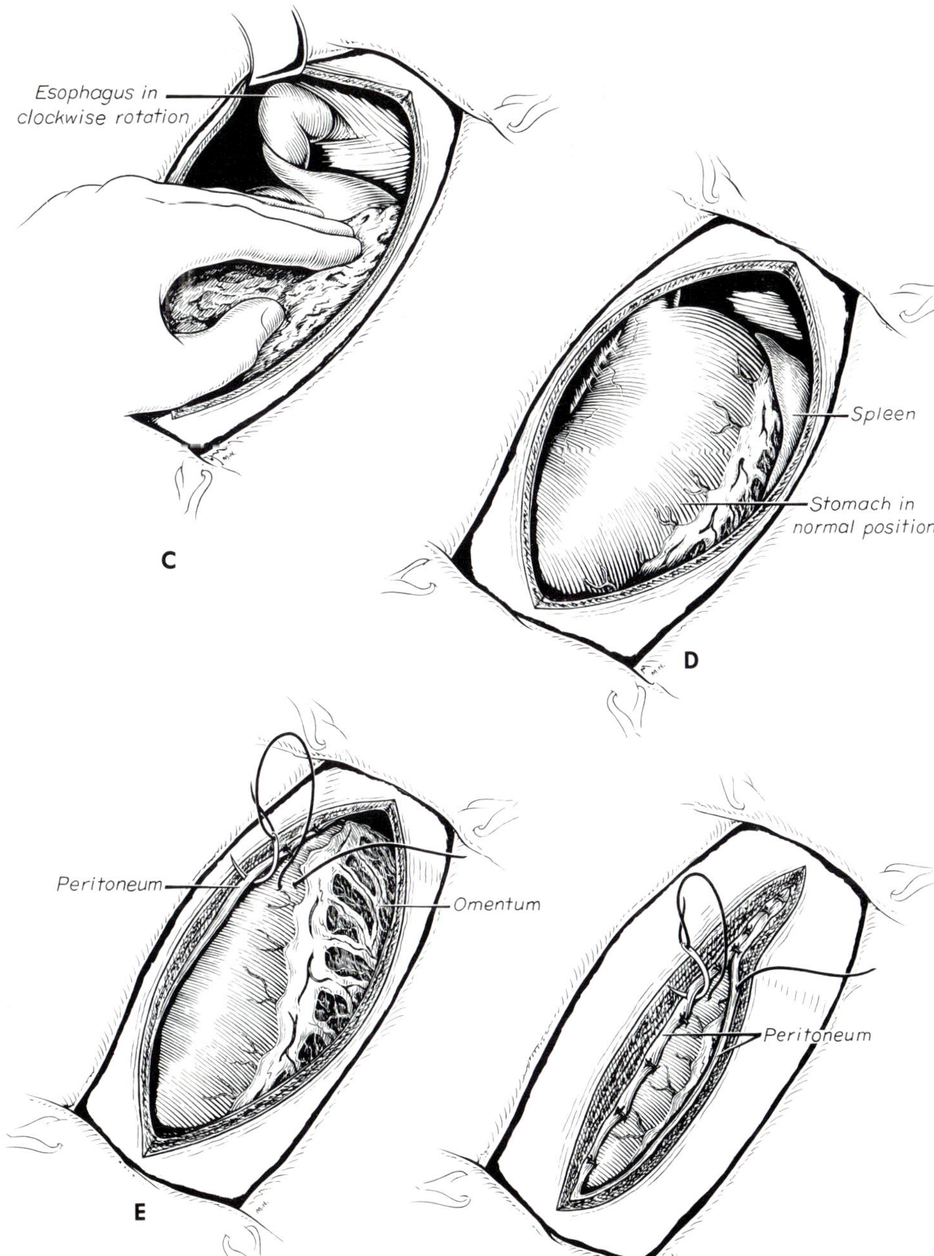

FIGURE 7–10. *Continued.*

ENTEROTOMY

The patient is anesthetized according to the operator's choice with a general anesthetic. Skin preparation is made for a midline incision. Although this is the common incision site for intestinal surgery, other sites may be chosen which will give a better exposure for specific parts of the intestine.

A dorsal recumbent position with the patient held in a positioning frame affords the best access to the abdomen because the muscles are not stretched from the traction of restraining ropes. Lateral expansion of the incision with retractors can easily be accomplished and results in adequate exposure of the surgical site.

The enterotomy is usually performed so that some obstruction can be removed from the gut. Foreign bodies are the most common obstruction. As soon as the abdomen is opened, the involved section of intestine is sought. This is usually fairly easy to find either by sight or by palpation. The segment is examined for viability. If the surface is glistening, moist, and pink to dark red in color, an enterotomy may be performed. If, on the other hand, the surface is dull and dry looking with a dark, almost black color that does not respond to warm saline, then more drastic surgery must be performed.

If possible the loop of intestine is delivered outside the incision and packed off with towels or sponges. Excessive moisture should be avoided because bacterial infection can easily be transferred in this way. Where fluids are to be used, a plastic dam should be laid under the intestinal loop. Dry sponges help to prevent contamination and can be used for packing when excessive fluids are not contemplated. The loop is "milked" gently by placing the thumb and forefinger of each hand over the gut on either side of the obstruction and forcing the ingesta away from the area. Rubber-shod clamps are then placed on the gut just tight enough to prevent any return of ingesta. These clamps are placed with the blades toward the mesentery but not on it. The distance between forceps should be at least three times the proposed length of the intestinal incision.

A longitudinal incision proximal to the obstruction on the antimesenteric aspect of the intestine is begun with a scalpel and completed with scissors (Fig. 7–11). Both should be discarded immediately. Because of the heavy musculature of the dog's intestine, the mucosa rolls outward on being cut. With great care to avoid contaminating the gloves or adjacent tissues, the foreign body is dislodged and withdrawn with Allis forceps. By using dry sponges on forceps or a suction tip, the lumen of the intestine is cleaned and prepared for closing.

Since most of the obstructions occur in the bowel of smallest diameter (jejunum), it is important that the closure not create a stricture. In order to avoid reducing the lumen size, the closure is made transversely. Using 4-0 chromic catgut swaged on a taper point needle, make a transverse bite about 5 mm. from one end of the incision. This bite should include serosa, muscularis, and submucosa. By crossing to the other end of the incision, another transverse bite is taken in the opposite direction to the first. The two ends are then brought together and tied as a simple interrupted stitch. As a result of this stitch, the gut is doubled on itself much in the same manner as a coat sleeve is bent when the elbow is flexed. Interrupted stitches are then placed along the line of contact of the two flexed portions. While the flexion in the gut may cause some concern, it will entirely disappear within six to eight weeks, and during this time, the lumen will actually be larger at this point.

The intestinal clamps are removed. The instruments used in the resection and the packing around the area are discarded. If the gloves have become contaminated, they should be changed. Fresh drapes are applied if necessary, and the usual abdominal closure is made.

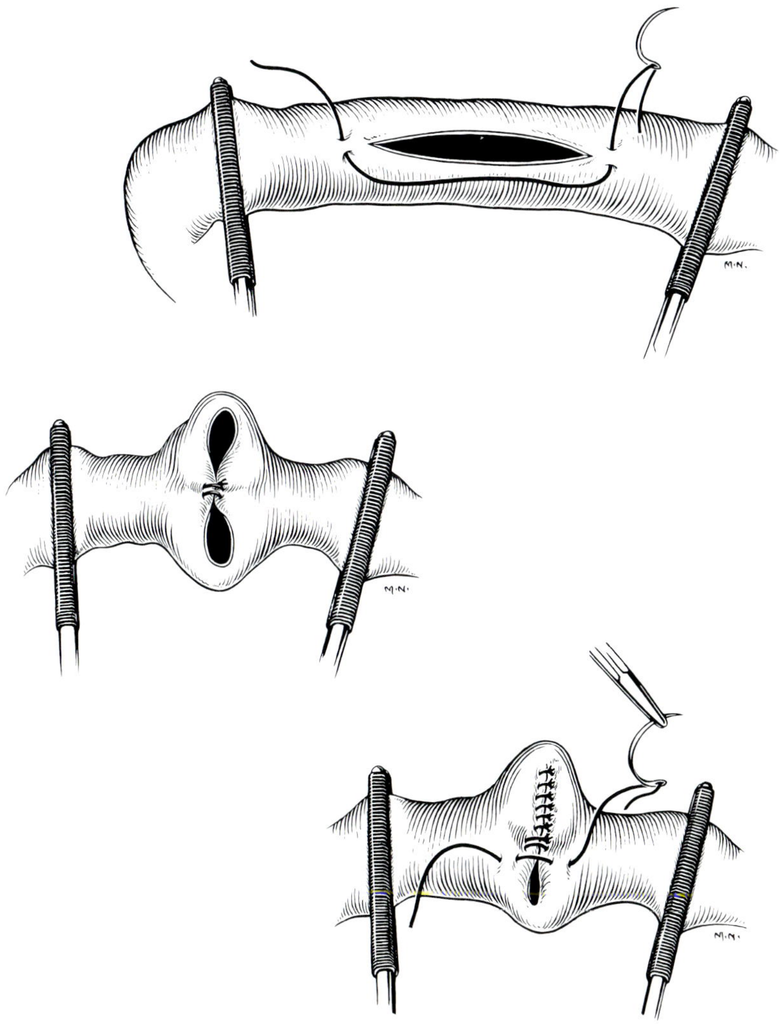

FIGURE 7–11.

INTESTINAL RESECTION

Most of the preliminary steps for intestinal resection are described in the section on enterotomy. There are numerous methods of anastomosing the intestine. Each surgeon has his own method or is looking for a new method. Only four methods will be described, but they should be adequate to cover any situation that might arise. If the surgery is done carefully according to directions, one should have no difficulty in producing a satisfactory result. The decision to resect the intestine is made after an inspection for viability. If the intestine appears dark or black and the surface is dull, it should be tested by bathing with warm saline. If the color does not change within 2 or 3 minutes, a resection should be performed. There are other reasons for resection, such as intussusception, which are discussed in detail in any good text on general surgery.

A generous loop of intestine is packed off outside the incision by placing a sterile plastic sheet under it and surrounding it with towels or sponges (Fig. 7–12). The section is "milked" and rubber-shod intestinal clamps are applied so that they do not involve the mesentery. The devitalized part of the intestine is segregated by placing one Ferguson angiotribe across the bowel proximal and another distal to it but in tissue that is fully viable. The forceps should be so placed that there is no interruption of the circulation to any part of the intestine that is to be anastomosed. It is important to place the forceps in a spot that is clearly supplied from an arterial arcade outside the area to be resected. Blood vessels within the resected area should be ligated by drawing the ligature around the vessel with a mosquito hemostat.

Forceps are clamped inside and in close approximation to the angiotribes. The Ferguson angiotribes are clamped tightly so that they will crush the gut, and a scalpel blade is passed between each set of forceps and as close to each angiotribe as possible. The mesentery is freed with scissors, and the section of intestine is discarded along with the forceps. A dry sponge is used to wipe the cut ends between the blades of the Ferguson angiotribe (Fig. 7–13).

By using the Parker-Kerr method of oversewing a forceps, the transected ends of the intestine are closed (Fig. 7–14). This method, sometimes called the basting stitch method, is actually a continuous Cushing stitch applied over a forceps. Using 4-0 chromic catgut with a swaged on taper-point needle, make the first bite longitudinally and toward the forceps. The next bite is made transversely and parallel to the forceps, and a similar bite is taken in the same direction on the opposite side of the forceps. This is continued until the far side of the intestine is reached.

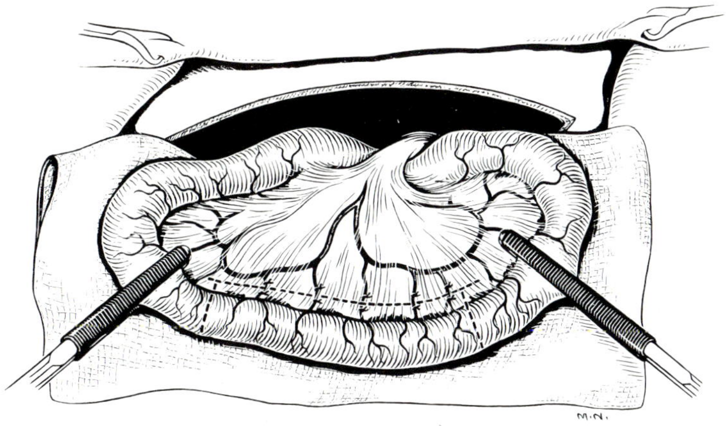

FIGURE 7–12.

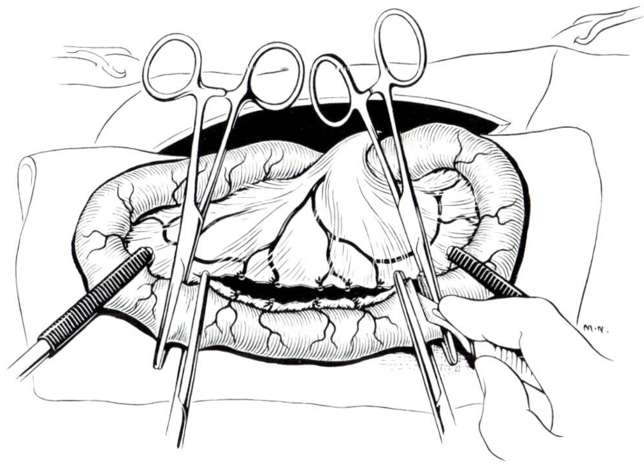

FIGURE 7–13.

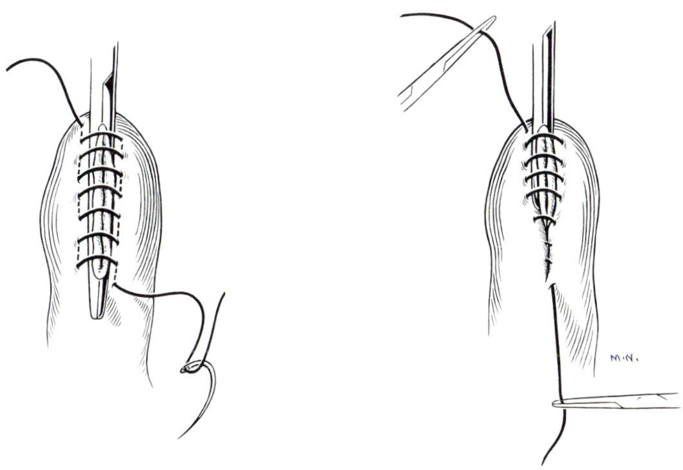

FIGURE 7–14.

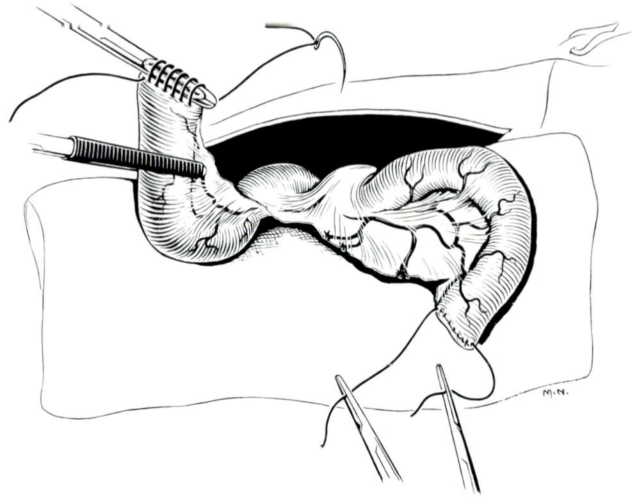

FIGURE 7–15.

The last bite is then made longitudinally away from the forceps. Each bite should be about 2 mm. from the forceps, about 3 to 4 mm. long, and deep enough to catch the submucosa. The surgeon holds the free ends of suture while the assistant releases the rachet on the forceps and gently opens and closes the blades about 5 mm. When the tissue is free of the blades, the forceps are gradually withdrawn while traction is applied to the suture. The ends invert bringing about serosa to serosa contact (Fig. 7–15).

END-TO-END ANASTOMOSIS

An aseptic anastomosis can be performed by joining the closed ends together and then withdrawing the basting stitches. This method can be used to good advantage when both segments are approximately the same size. The two segments are approximated at their mesenteric aspect, and an interrupted Lembert stitch is begun at the mesentery from the under side of the intestine and carried just outside the basting stitch around the circumference of the gut to the mesentery on the upper side (Fig. 7–16).

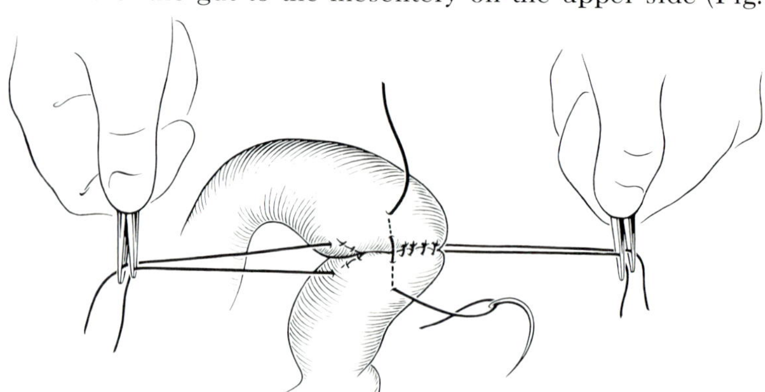

FIGURE 7–16.

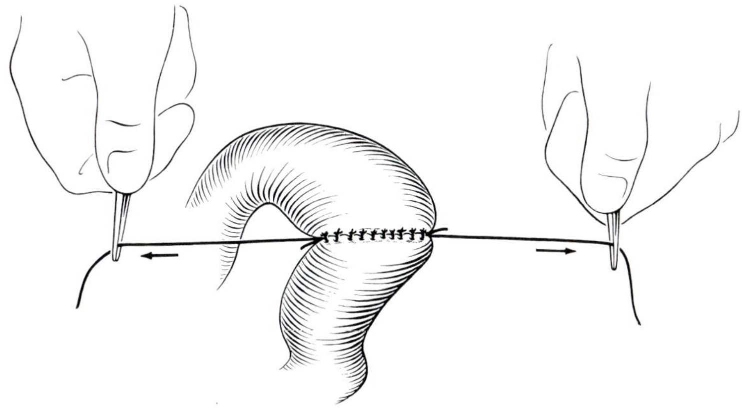

FIGURE 7–17.

Traction is applied to one end of the basting stitch to determine by movement which opposite end is a continuation of that suture. One end of this thread is then cut close to the intestine. The opposite end of the other thread is also cut. By placing the fingers close to the intestine and pulling on the free ends of suture, the basting stitches can be removed without breaking (Fig. 7–17).

The resection is then tested for patency by pushing with the finger or a blunt instrument against the intestinal wall in the direction of the junction (Fig. 7–18). The portion of the intestine crushed by the forceps will slough, so the inverted portion should not be great enough to form a diaphragm or a stenosis. The intestinal clamps are released, and the resection is further tested by "milking" ingesta through it. The mesentery is closed by interrupted stitches that are placed through the overlapped edges. Two or three sutures are usually sufficient, but they should be placed so as to avoid blood vessels in the area (Fig. 7–19).

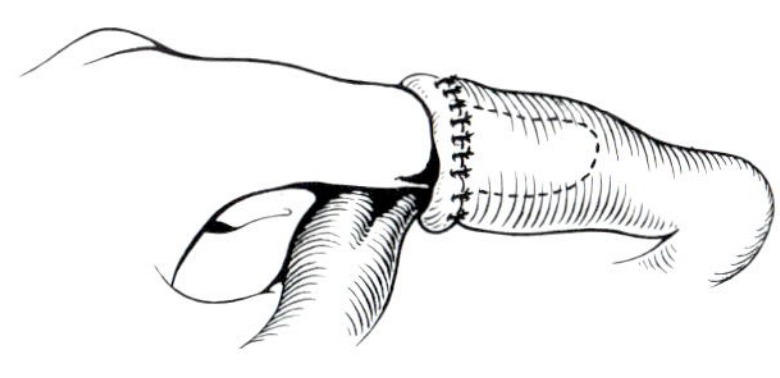

FIGURE 7–18.

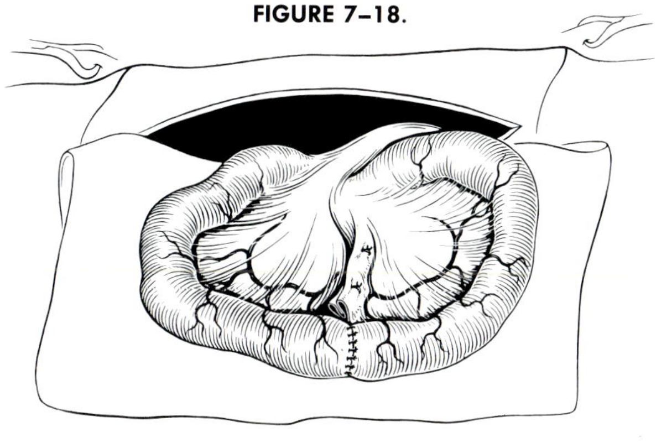

FIGURE 7–19.

END-TO-END OBLIQUE ANASTOMOSIS

The end-to-end oblique method of anastomosing may be used when two intestinal segments of unequal diameter are to be joined end to end (Fig. 7–20). The segment with the smaller lumen is cut obliquely to match the larger lumen. This is accomplished by placing the crushing forceps at an angle to the mesentery so that it covers a distance on the smaller segment equivalent to the transverse diameter of the larger segment. The angle with the mesentery should always be acute so that the antimesenteric side is shorter, thereby avoiding any circulatory problems. The remainder of the procedure is the same as for the usual end-to-end anastomosis.

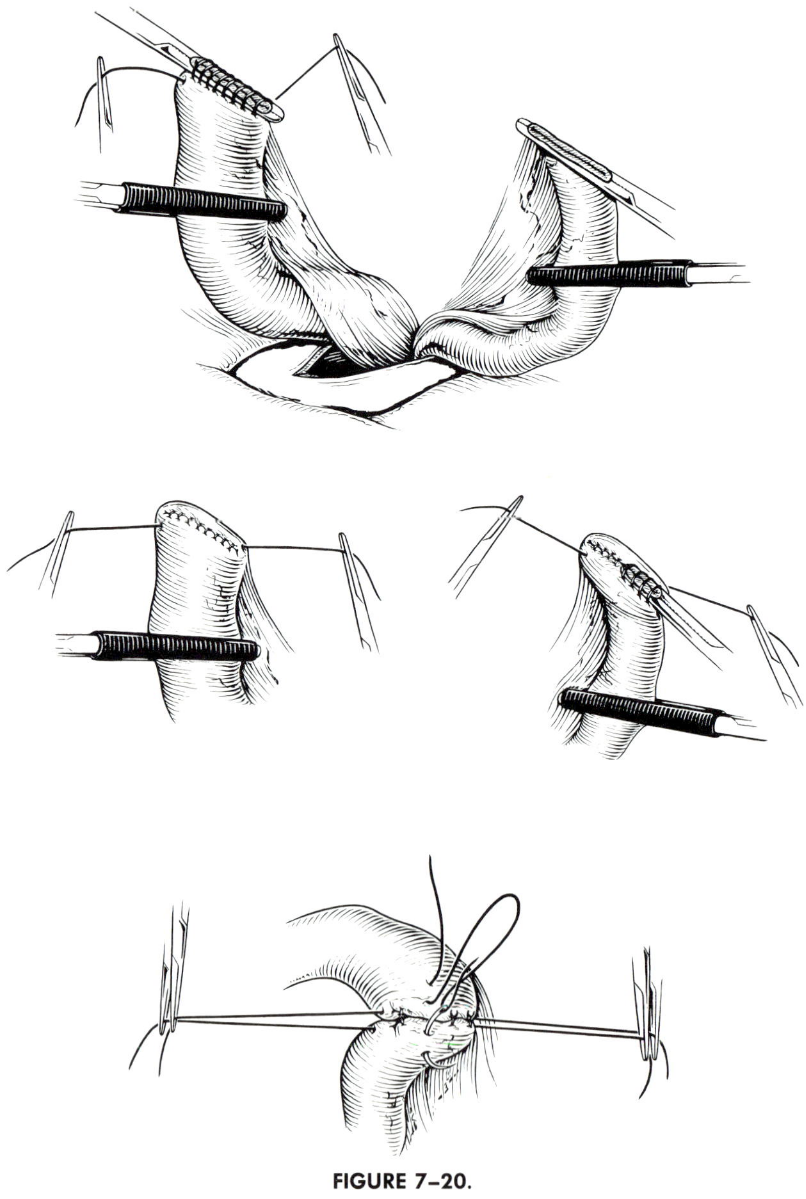

FIGURE 7–20.

SIDE-TO-SIDE ANASTOMOSIS

Side-to-side anastomosis may be used where segments are unequal in size or where there is likely to be a problem with stenosis (Fig. 7–21). It is begun by closing the ends of the segments. In this case the ends will be closed permanently; therefore, after the first suture line has been completed and the gut closed, a second suture line is made. By using one end of the suture, a continuous Lembert stitch is carried back to the other end of the suture and tied.

After both segments are permanently closed, they are overlapped at a distance of about three times the diameter of the larger segment with the mesenteric borders together. By laying the intestine so that the mesentery is underneath, it is possible to suture the two segments to each other fairly close to their mesenteric attachment. When this continuous Lembert stitch reaches from the stump of one segment to the stump of the other, the suture is laid aside until later in the procedure.

An incision is made in both segments so that the openings can be apposed and so that they are equal in length to approximately one and one-half times the diameter of the smaller segment. Beginning at one end of the apposed incisions, place the first bite through both segments and tie the knot outside the opening. Then pass the needle through the gut to the lumen and carry a continuous stitch to the opposite end. At this point the needle is passed back through the gut to the outside, and a continuous Lembert stitch is carried back to the original knot and tied.

The first line of sutures is then continued over the second line back to the starting point and tied. The bowel clamps are then released and the mesentery closed. The abdominal closure is made after the proper precautions are taken as to contaminated drapes and instruments.

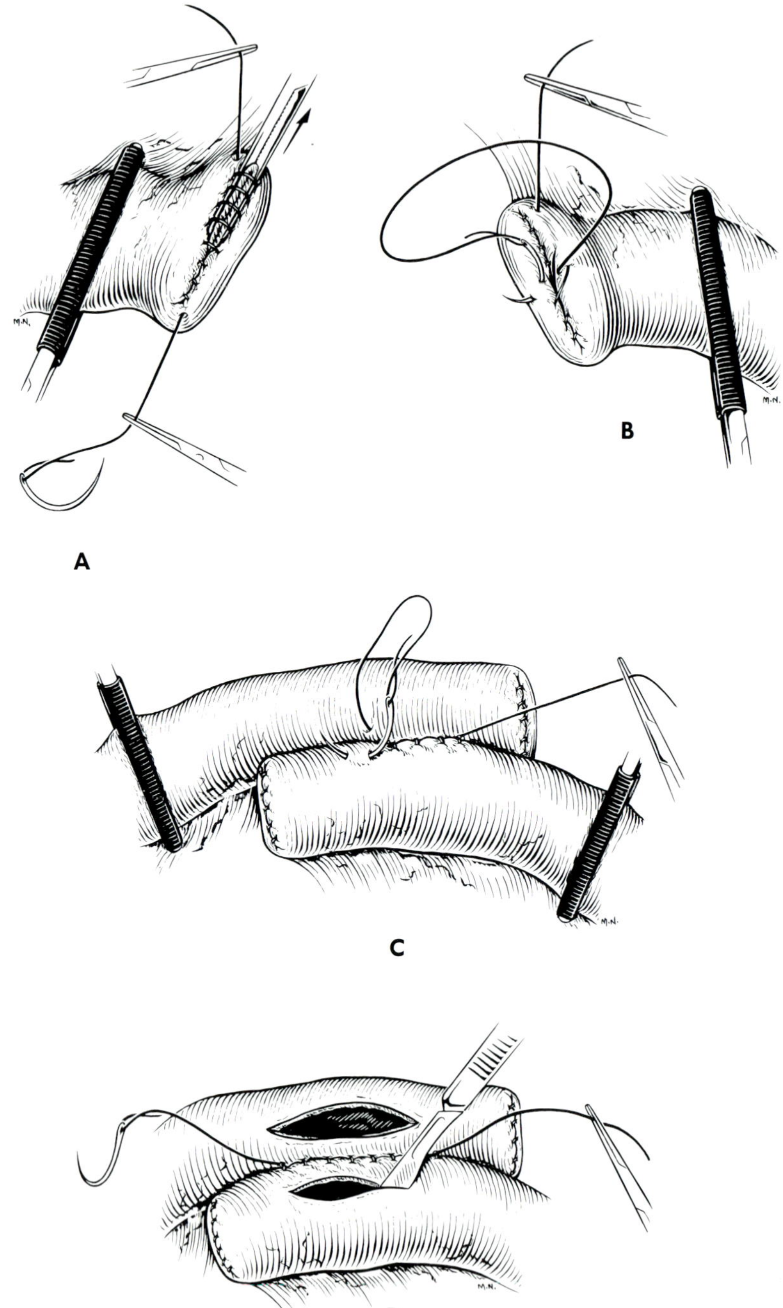

FIGURE 7–21.

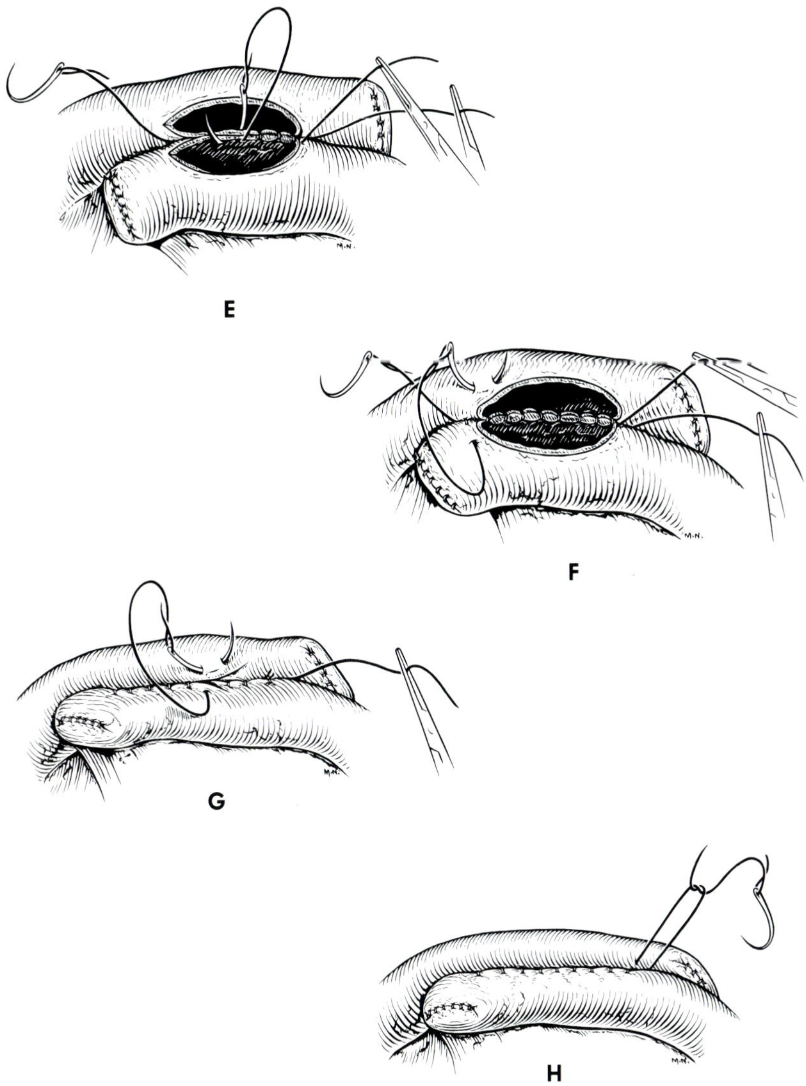

FIGURE 7–21. *Continued.*

END-TO-SIDE ANASTOMOSIS

End-to-side anastomosis can be used wherever one or both segments cannot be joined side to side and where the segments are of unequal diameter (Fig. 7–22). The end of the large segment is closed permanently by a double row of sutures. The small segment is closed with a temporary single row of sutures. The same careful preparation for contamination is made.

An incision is made along the antimesenteric border of the large segment. It should be equivalent to the diameter of the small segment and should begin about 1 cm. from the closed end of the large segment.

The end of the small segment is placed against the opening, with the mesentery on the same side as that of the large segment but at right angles to it. A continuous Lembert stitch is begun at the mesentery and carried around the small segment to the starting point. One end of the basting stitch is cut and the suture withdrawn. The opening is tested for patency and the mesentery closed. The usual precautions are observed regarding sterility before the abdominal closure is made.

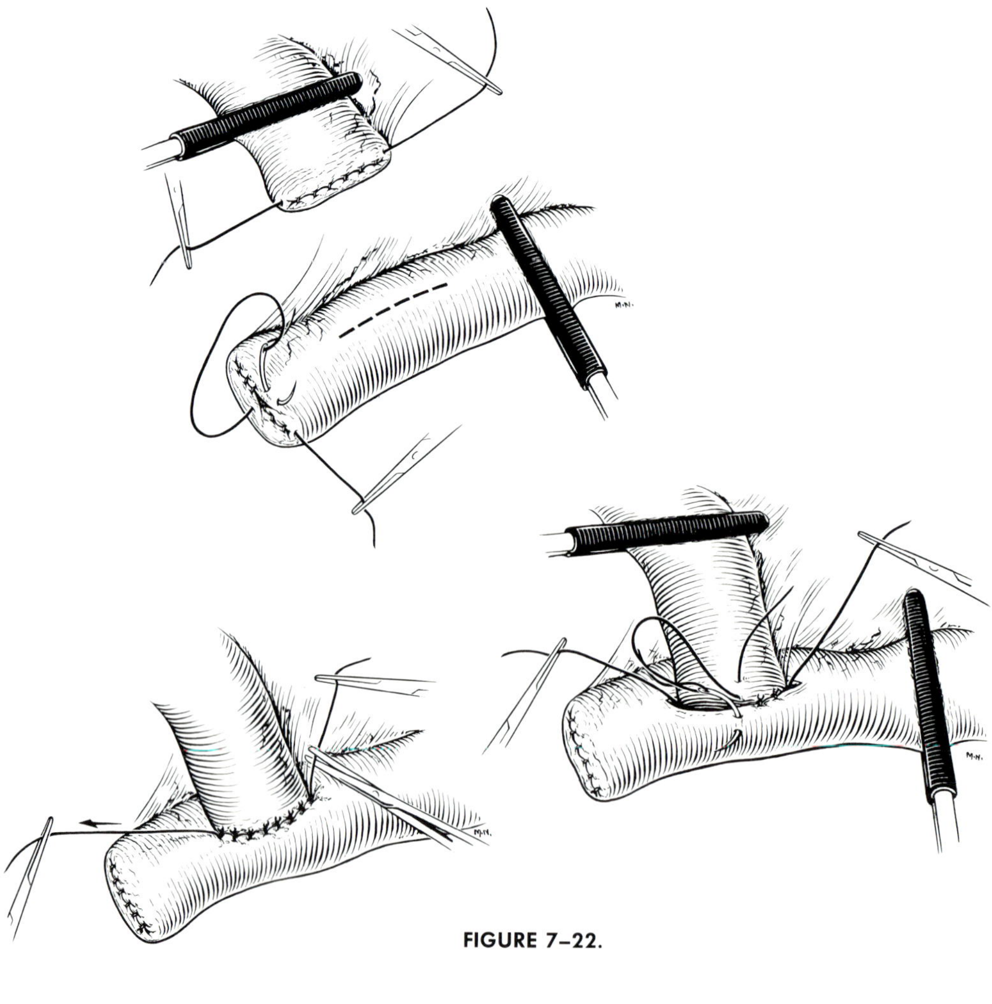

FIGURE 7–22.

TYPHLECTOMY

While the typhlectomy is performed rather infrequently, it is a fairly simple procedure and requires no expertise.

The patient is anesthetized and prepared for a midline or right paramedian incision. The position should be dorsal recumbent and the usual four- or six-drape system of covering the patient is used.

The abdomen is opened in the customary manner. A hand's breadth paramedian incision opposite the umbilicus affords the best exposure, although a midline incision is usually adequate. Sometimes the midline incision does not allow the surgeon to deliver the cecum quite as well without maintaining traction on the colon.

After the cecum has been brought into position for surgery, it is packed off with sponges or towels (Fig. 7–23). The blood supply to the cecum should be examined closely because there may be some slight variation in the pattern of the vessels. In general, all the circulation is derived from the ileocecocolic artery. Since the arteries and veins are visible, it is best to select those branches which cross the ileocecal fold to the body of the cecum and double ligate them. The cecum is then separated from the ileum with scissors. A branch of the ileocecal artery may be uncovered in the process and will require double ligating and dividing.

As soon as the base of the cecum is entirely free, it is clamped with a Ferguson angiotribe about 6 mm. from the colon and with the forceps across the colon (not parallel with it). Another forceps is applied distal to the first and the cecum divided between the forceps with a scalpel. The blade should be against the first forceps. After wiping the cut edges with a sponge, the forceps are oversewn with 4-0 chromic catgut by the Parker-Kerr method.

The two free ends of the basting stitch are tied together. This creates a fold which runs parallel to the long axis of the colon. A row of either continuous or interrupted Lembert stitches are placed along the crease. If the stump of the cecum was originally of proper length, the final row of sutures should make the closure about level with the wall of the colon without decreasing the lumen. Abdominal closure follows the usual routine, and no special aftercare treatment is required.

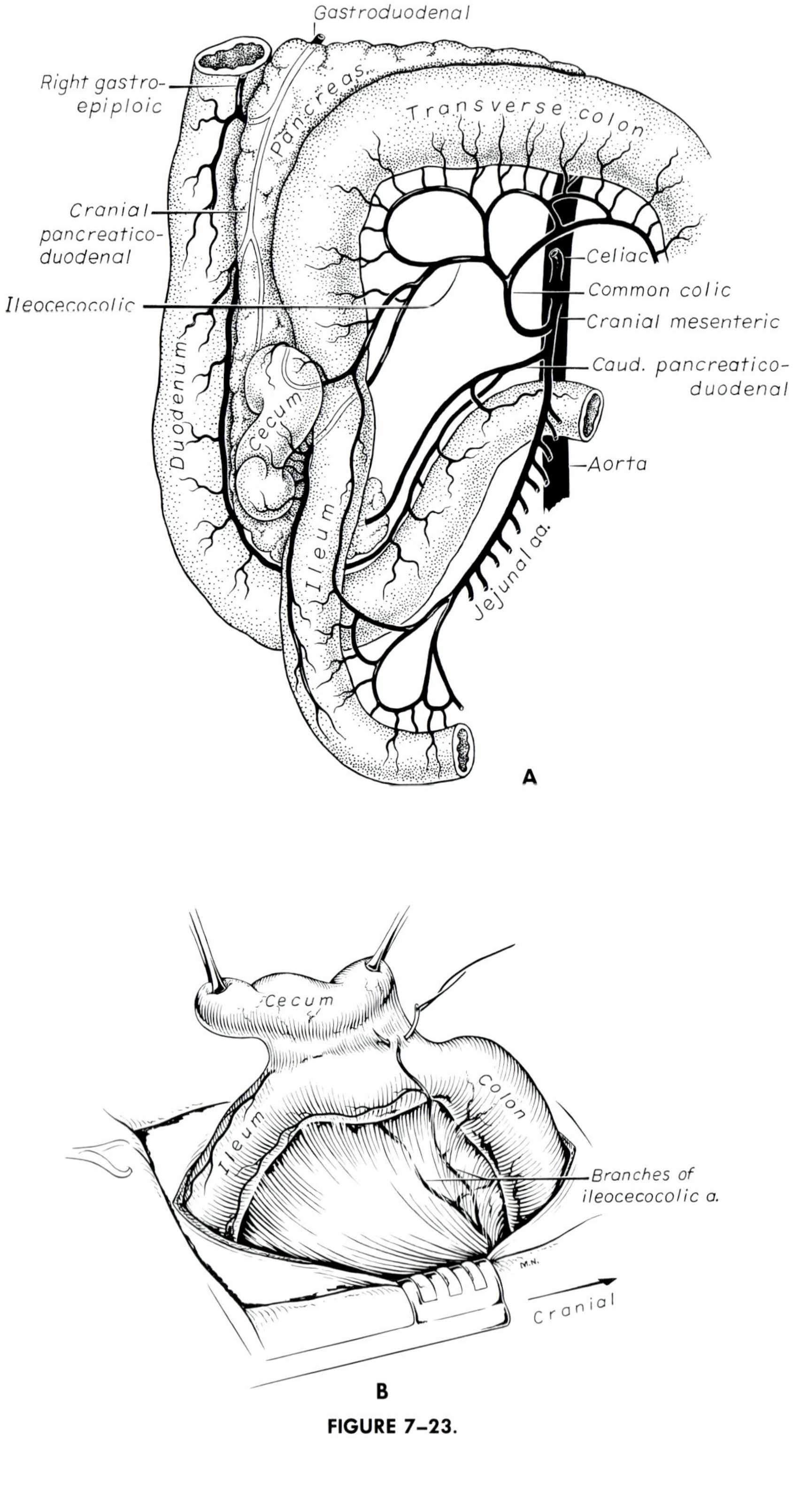
Gastroduodenal
Right gastro-epiploic
Pancreas
Transverse colon
Cranial pancreatico-duodenal
Celiac
Ileocecocolic
Common colic
Cranial mesenteric
Caud. pancreatico-duodenal
Duodenum
Cecum
Aorta
Ileum
Jejunal aa.
A
Cecum
Colon
Ileum
Branches of ileocecocolic a.
Cranial
B

FIGURE 7–23.

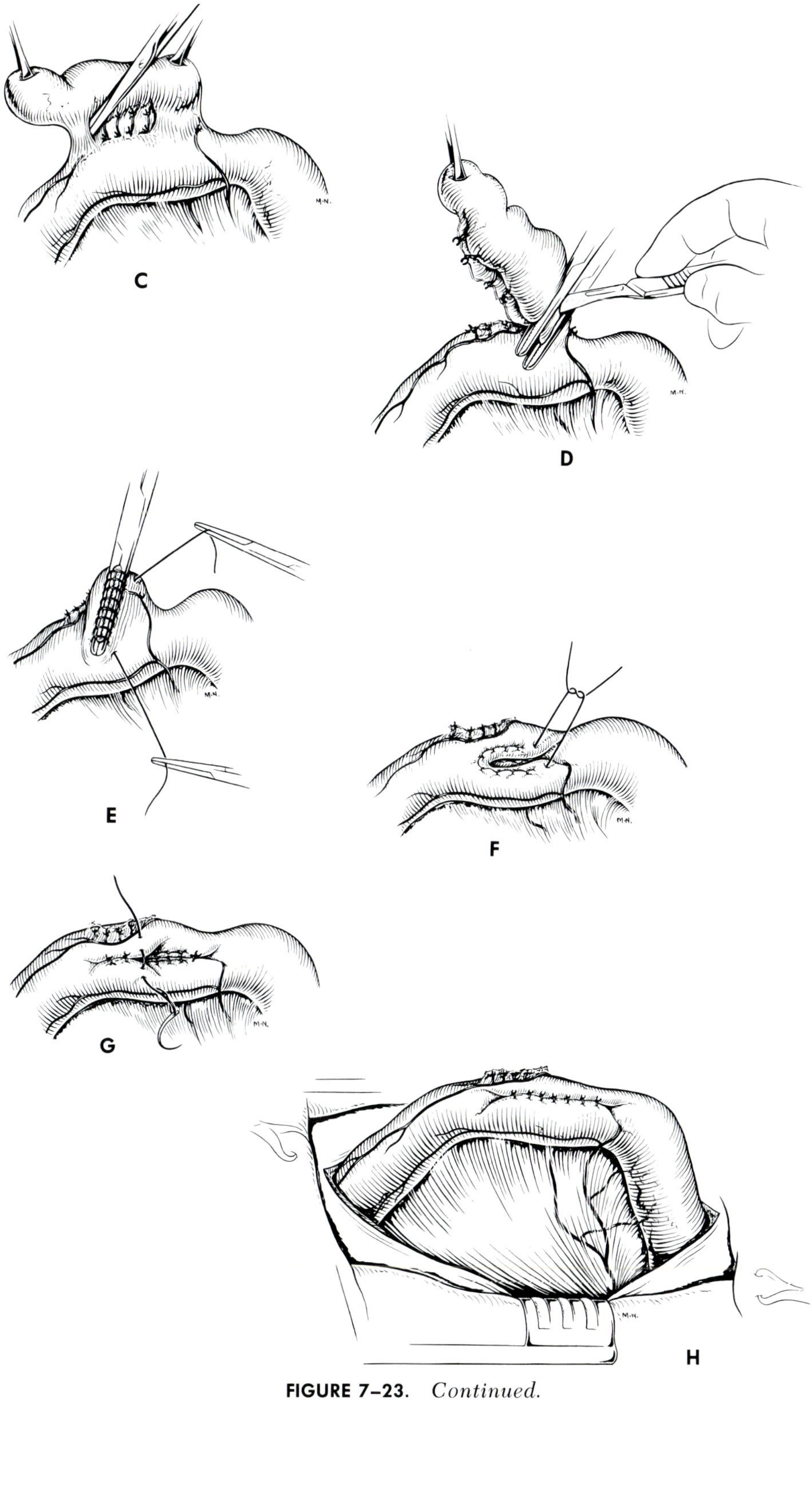

FIGURE 7–23. *Continued.*

COLOPEXY

Whenever a prolapse of the rectum occurs, it should first be examined for viability by using the same criteria as set forth for the intestine. If the prolapse is viable, the best permanent repair can be made by colopexy.

The patient is given a general anesthetic and the abdomen prepared for surgery. The position should be dorsal recumbency, and the draping should be for a left caudal paramedian incision.

An incision of approximately 7 to 8 cm. is made (Fig. 7–24). The descending colon should be immediately beneath the incision. The colon is grasped by a gauze sponge held between the fingers, and traction is applied in the cranial direction. Unless the prolapse is extremely edematous, it should reduce under this treatment. Slight pressure on the prolapsed portion by an assistant with moist sponges may help in stubborn cases.

When the prolapse has been reduced, slight traction on the colon is maintained by an assistant. Using 4-0 chromic catgut and a half circle or five-eighths circle taper-point needle, begin the first suture by placing it through the peritoneum at the caudal end of the incision. A bite is then taken in the colon deep enough to engage the submucosa, and finally the suture is placed through the peritoneum on the opposite side of the incision. The suture is cut long enough to allow about 8 cm. of catgut on either side of the incision. Place at least three or four such sutures about 1 cm. apart, and then, starting with the first suture, which is the caudal one, tie the simple interrupted stitches so that the serosa of the colon is involved with the closure of the peritoneum.

When the fixation sutures are finished, any further opening in the peritoneum is secured, and the incision is closed in the usual manner.

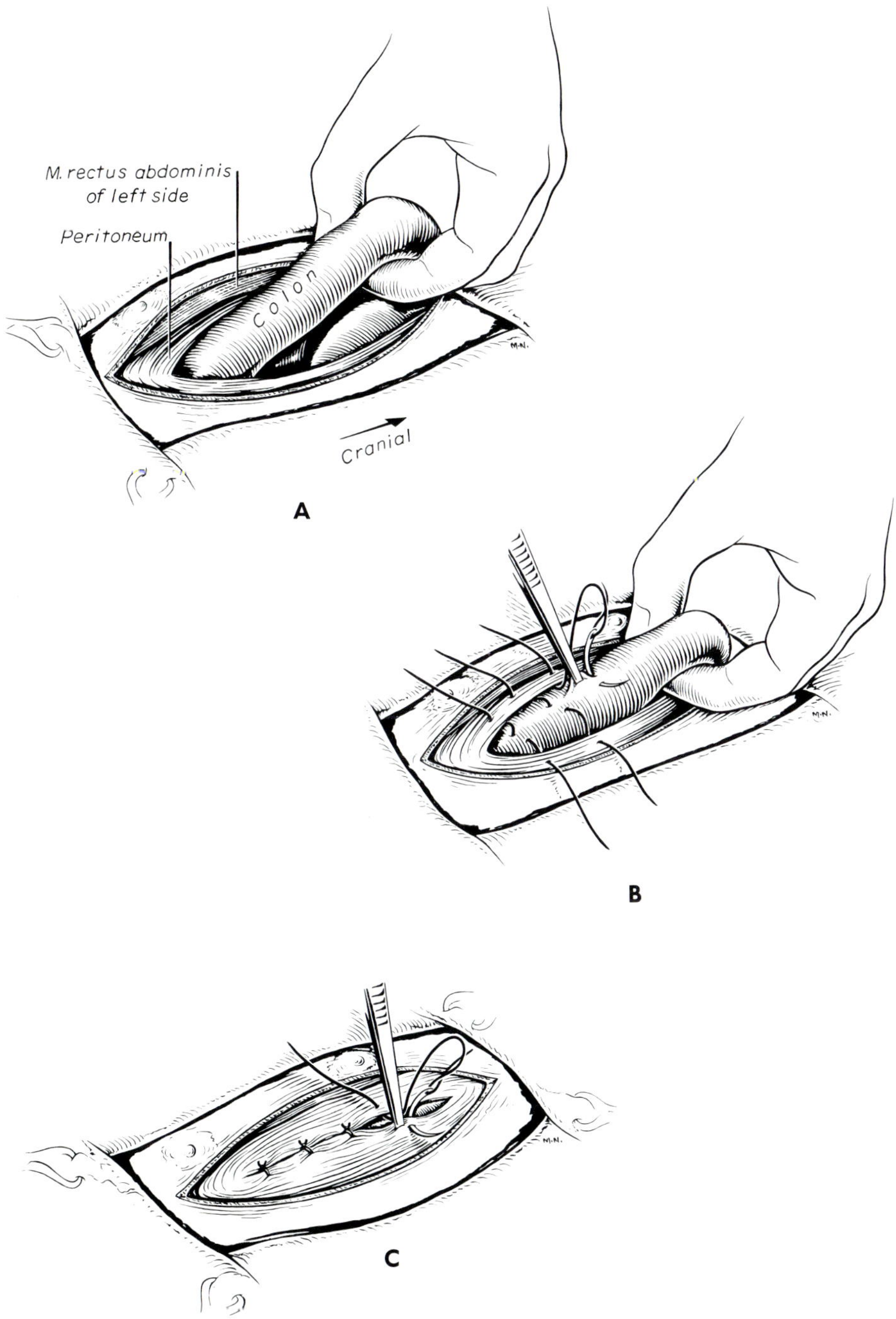
M. rectus abdominis
of left side
Peritoneum
Colon
Cranial
A
B
C

FIGURE 7–24.

AMPUTATION OF THE RECTUM

If on examination a prolapsed rectum is found to be necrotic or badly lacerated, that portion should be amputated.

The patient is given a general anesthetic, and the anal region is prepared for surgery by clipping around the tail head, anus, and perineal region. The area should be thoroughly cleansed with hexachlorophene and water. This is followed by sponging with 70 per cent isopropyl alcohol.

The patient is placed on the table in sternal recumbency with the tail tied over the back. The hind legs are secured to the end of the table, and a sandbag or Flexicast is placed under the thighs to elevate them. The table is tilted slightly so that the rear is higher than the head. A single drape with a center opening can be used. The prolapse is placed on the upper side of the drape and covered with a sterile towel. The drape is secured around the anus and to the tail head with towel clamps.

Very slight traction is applied to the prolapse before surgery is begun to ensure that the tissue will be viable at the suture line. Usually 2 to 3 cm. of fresh tissue will unfold without difficulty. This will probably be part or all of the anal canal. A purse-string suture of heavy silk (3) is placed around the anus and tied fairly tight.

Something should be inserted into the lumen of the everted rectum to indicate the internal mucosal boundary. This may be a glass rod, a test tube, a knife handle, or any smooth-surfaced object that will stretch the tissues slightly.

Using 0 braided silk on a five-eighths circle needle, place a series of horizontal mattress stitches around the circumference of the prolapse about 2 cm. from the anus (Fig. 7–25). Each suture should penetrate from mucosa to mucosa. When the needle strikes the object in the lumen, it is turned so that it returns to the outer mucosa for tying. These sutures should be close together and form a perfect ring around the prolapse.

The prolapse is amputated with scissors about 4 mm. distal to the sutures, and the cut edges are checked for any bleeding vessels. When proper hemostasis has been obtained the purse-string suture is removed. The sutured edges will be retracted within the anus.

Needless to say, the aftercare consists mainly of treating the etiological agent.

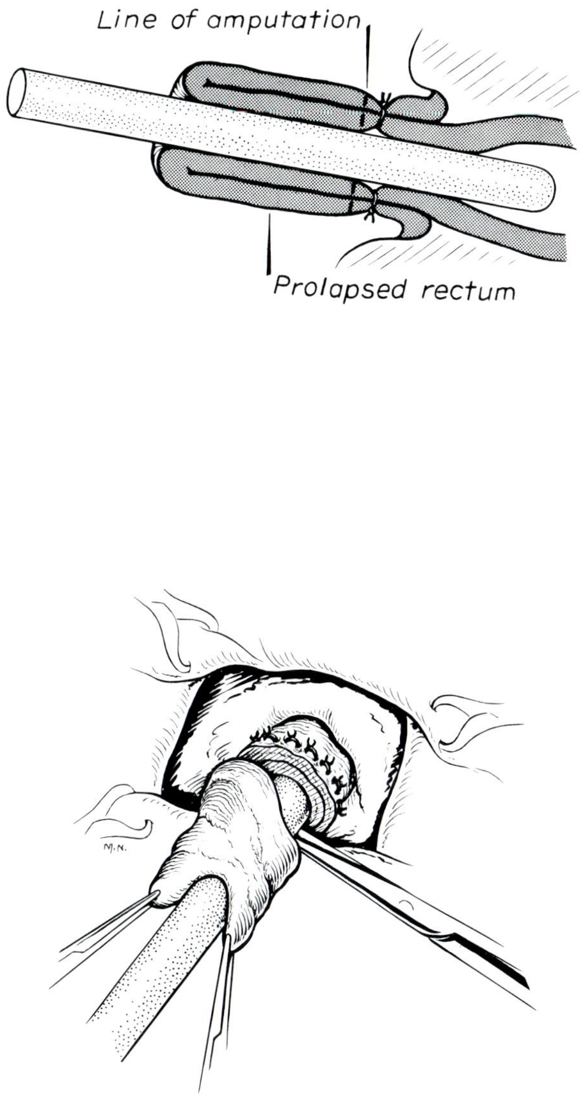

FIGURE 7–25.

RECTAL DIVERTICULUM

As a result of weakening and atrophy of the coccygeus and levator ani muscles, the caudal portion of the rectum bulges to form a pouch or diverticulum. In order to correct this condition surgically, it is not only necessary to obliterate the diverticulum but also to reinforce the repair so that the rectal wall cannot be stretched laterally.

All fecal material should be removed from the rectum and diverticulum by enema two or three hours prior to surgery. Preparation and positioning of the patient is identical to that used for amputation of the prolapsed rectum, except perhaps that the preparation of the skin should extend farther laterally on the side to be operated. A purse string is placed around the anus.

The tail is fastened cranially and laterally away from the incision site. The drapes are placed so that the surgical opening will be lateral to the anus and the base of the tail. The longitudinal opening should extend from the sacrum to the pubis.

A skin incision is begun lateral to the tail head at the point where there is resistance to the touch. It is carried slightly lateral to encircle the protruding sac and then parallel to the midline as far as the ischial arch (Fig. 7–26).

There is usually very little tissue between the skin and the dilated portion of the rectum. Any loose areolar tissue or fat which may be present is pushed aside so that the rectal wall is well exposed. Beginning at the cranial border of the diverticulum and ending at the caudal border, place a series of interrupted Lembert stitches along the lateral surface. The sutures should be 3-0 multifilament stainless steel placed about 5 mm. apart. They should be long enough to invert the dilated rectal wall. The suture ends should be cropped close so that there will be no sharp ends.

It is very important that the suture line be given support. This is best accomplished by suturing the caudal border of the levator ani to the cranial edge of the external sphincter of the anus with 3-0 multifilament stainless steel. Further support can be given by suturing the superficial fascia found in this area. The skin should be reshaped by removing a crescent-shaped piece from the lateral edge of the incision. It should be tailored in such a manner that when the edges are joined the skin surface will be free of wrinkles or bulges. The skin is closed with interrupted stitches. One may use whatever external suture material seems appropriate.

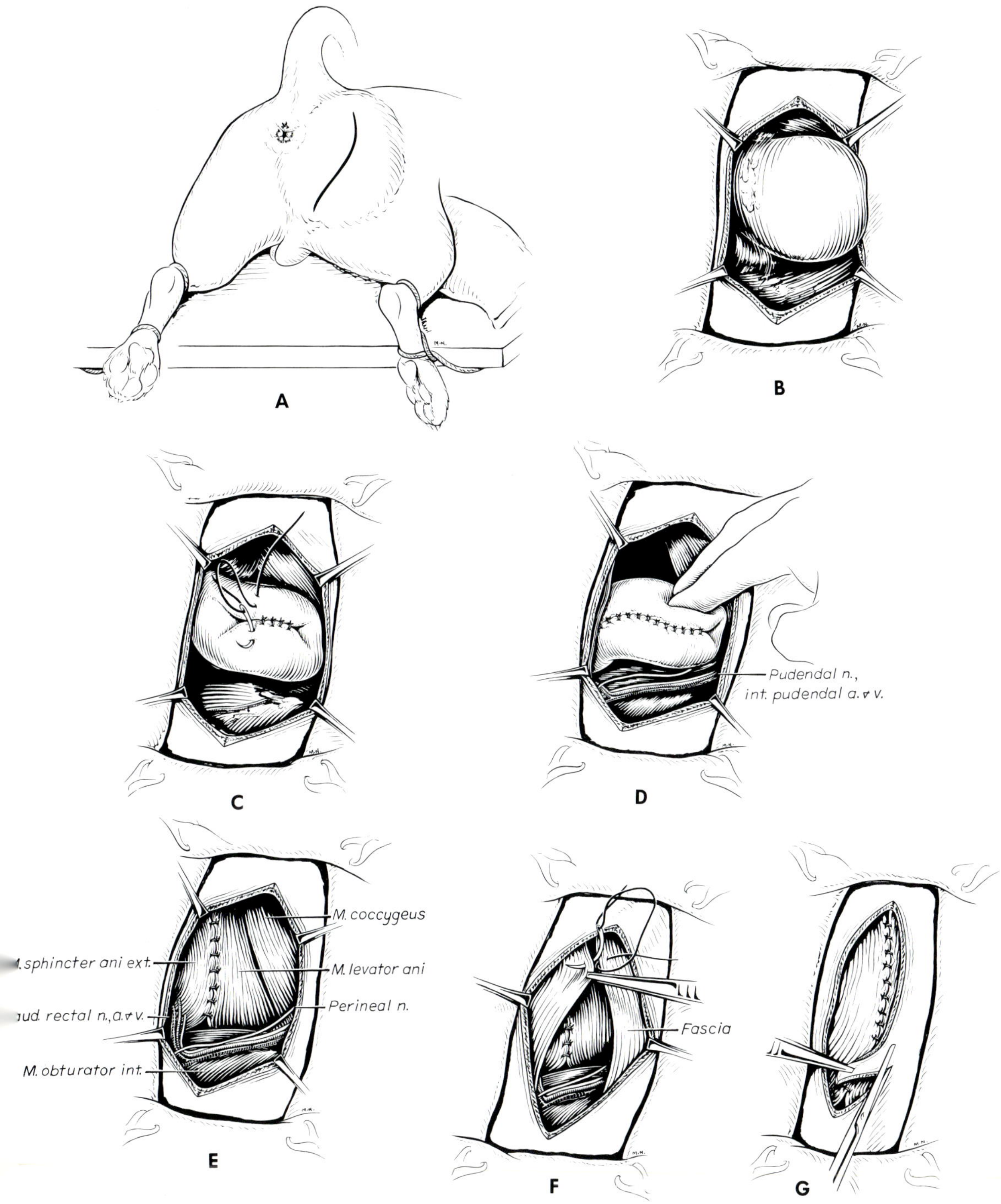
A
B
C
Pudendal n.,
int. pudendal a. & v.
D
M. coccygeus
sphincter ani ext.
M. levator ani
Perineal n.
ud. rectal n., a. & v.
M. obturator int.
E
Fascia
F
G

FIGURE 7–26.

EXTIRPATION OF THE ANAL SACS

Much has been written on the surgical extirpation of the anal sacs. Actually, the surgery is extremely simple and uncomplicated. Presurgical treatment should consist of irrigation of the sacs with saline followed by 2 to 3 days' treatment with antibiotic ointment placed directly into each sac.

The preparation is the same as for any surgery in the anal region. The position is sternal recumbency with the pelvis elevated and the tail restrained cranially. The area may be draped by a single drape having a central opening.

The incision is made by placing one blade of the Metzenbaum surgical scissors into the duct and opening the duct and sac in one stroke (Fig. 7–27).

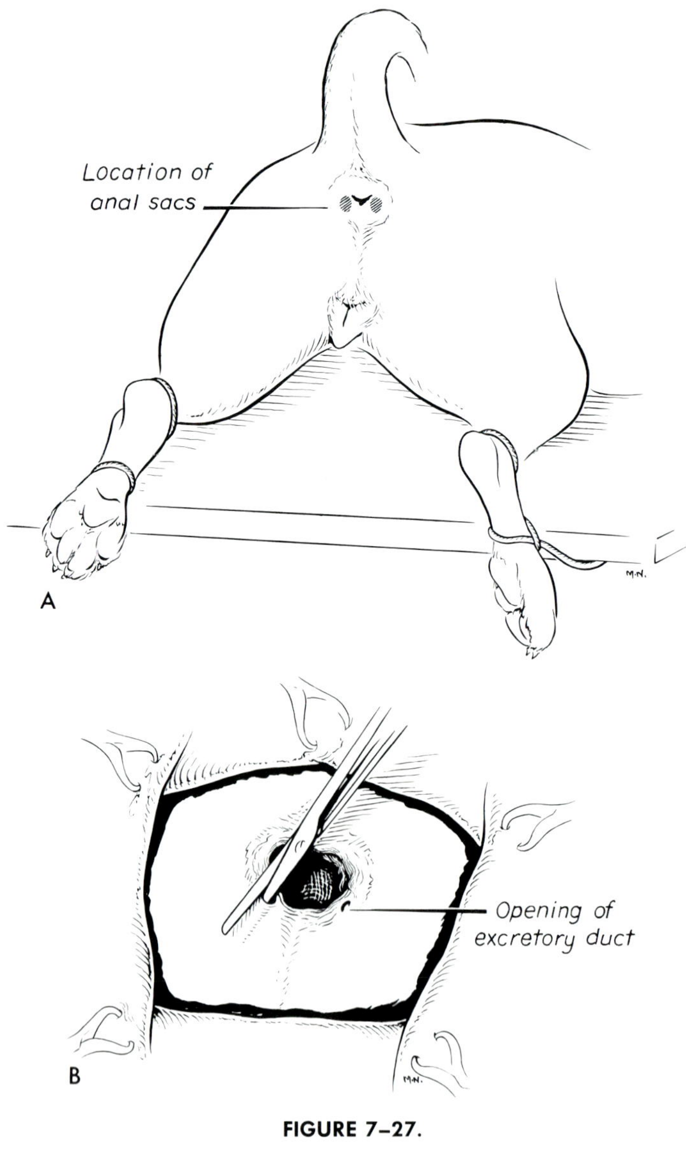

FIGURE 7–27.

If the duct is too small to accommodate the scissors blade, a groove director may be inserted and the incision made with a No. 11 Bard-Parker blade. Once the incision is completed, the sac lies open and exposed so that it can be readily distinguished from the surrounding tissues. It is greyish in appearance, while the surrounding tissues are pink or flesh colored. Laterally the sac is covered by the sphincter ani externus. The caudal third of this muscle is divided when the incision is made. Medial to the sac is the sphincter ani internus. Care must be taken not to disturb this muscle, since it is the involuntary muscle controlling defecation. Between the internal sphincter and the sac are two branches of the caudal rectal artery.

The lateral edge of the sac is lifted with Allis forceps, and the sac is carefully dissected by the use of scissors. Great care must be taken on the medial side to avoid the arteries and the sphincter, but this should present no problem if the scissors blades are always kept close to the sac and the dissection is done bluntly as much as possible. Better exposure at the crucial area can be had by starting on the lateral side and proceeding medially.

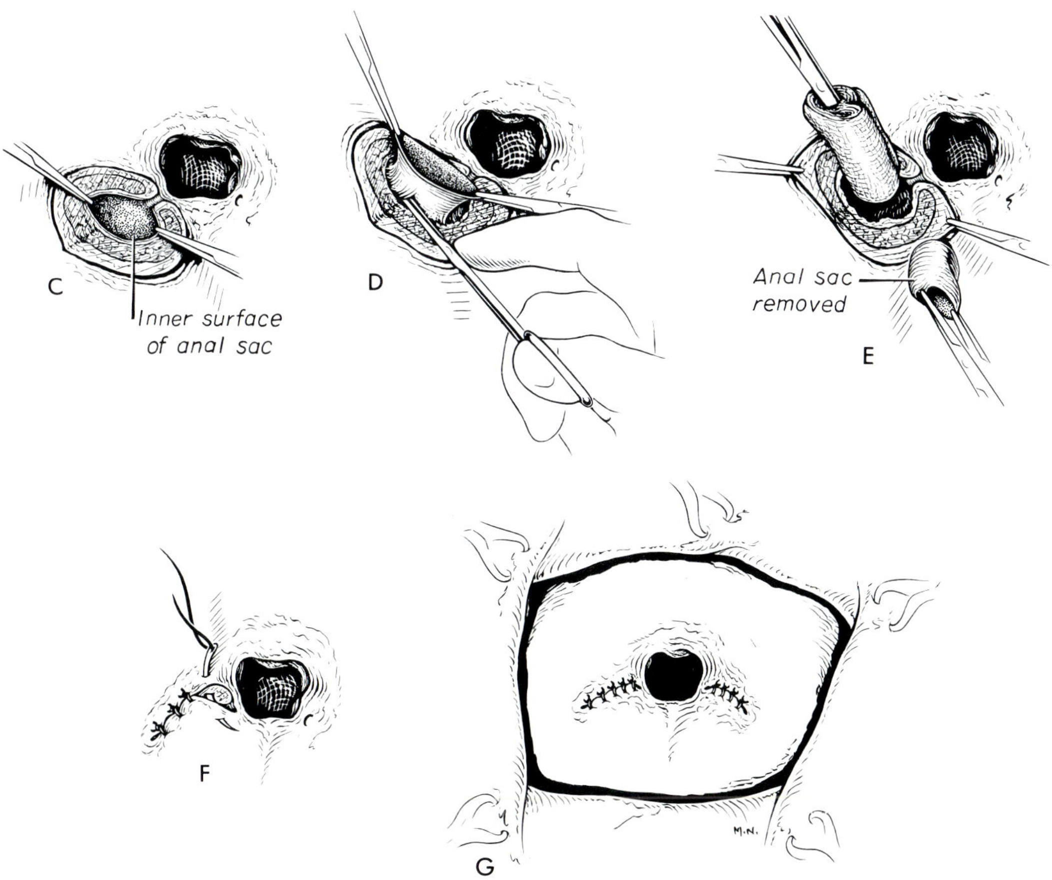

FIGURE 7–27. *Continued.*

After the sac has been removed, the cavity is closed by drawing the sides together with two or three interrupted stitches of 2-0 chromic catgut. The skin is closed with interrupted stitches of 5 silk.

REFERENCES

Berzel, C., and Brinker, W. D. *J.A.V.M.A.* 129:241, 1956.

Blackburn, P. S., and McFarlane, D. *J. Comp. Path.* 54:189, 1944.

Cawley, A. J., and Sorrell, B. *Vet. Med.* 54:247, 1959.

English, O. B. *Aust. Vet. Jour.* 35:41–43, 1959.

Glen, J. B. *Vet. Record.* 78:488–492, 1966.

Hertzler, J. H., and Tuttle, W. M. *Arch. Surg.* 65:398, 1952.

Hoffer, R. E., and Hunt, C. E. *Sm. An. Clin.* 3:75–80, 1963.

Hulland, T. J., and Archibald J. *Canad. Vet. Jour.* 5:109, 1964.

Kealy, J. K. *Vet. Record.* 76:19, 1964.

Knight, G. C. *Vet Record.* 75:264–266, 1963.

Schultz, L. R., Rodrigues-Pereira, C., and Clatworthy, H. W., Jr. *Amer. J. Surg.* 104:843–849, 1962.

Spivack, J. L. *The Surgical Technique of Abdominal Operations.* 4th ed. Springfield, Illinois: Charles C Thomas, 1946.

Spruell, J. S. A., Head, K. W., Wilson, J. C., and Watt, J. G. *Jour. Sm. An. Pract.* 5:63–65, 1964.

Steele, C. *Vet. Record.* 72:1063, 1960.

Swenson, O., and Clatworthy, H. W., Jr. *Surg.* 25:839, 1949.

Tutt, J. B., and Yarrow, T. G. *Vet Record.* 72:1014–15, 1960.

Wynn-Jones, E. *Cornell Vet.* 42:189–92, 1952.

Chapter 8

COMMON SURGICAL PROCEDURES IN SURGERY OF THE UROGENITAL TRACT

The procedures outlined in this chapter are those commonly required for the usual urogenital problems. For the benefit of the student, each step is described in detail. No attempt is made to describe all methods available. Reference material at the end of the chapter is a source of further information for the reader.

NEPHRECTOMY

Some form of general anesthesia is recommended for nephrectomy. The presurgical preparation will largely depend on the existing condition which requires this type of surgery. Surgical preparation consists of clipping and preparing the skin over the side involved so that a high paracostal incision can be made. This should cover an area from the dorsal midline to the ventral midline and from the middle of the chest caudally to the pelvis.

The patient is positioned in lateral recumbency, with slight elevation of the trunk at the thoracolumbar junction. The usual four-drape system is applied, with an opening about 5 cm. wide and 20 cm. long running approximately parallel to the thirteenth rib and just caudal to it.

A skin incision 20 cm. long is made, beginning at the epaxial musculature 3 cm. caudal to the thirteenth rib and running grossly parallel to the rib (Fig. 8–1). Two drapes or towels are then used to drape to the incision. The incision is continued by separating and dividing with scissors the externus obliquus and internus obliquus abdominis, as well as the transversus abdominis muscles. At this point the abdomen may be opened by dividing the peritoneum, or the approach may be retroperitoneal from the dorsal end of the incision. The decision depends on the condition and size of the kidney. Greatly enlarged kidneys will have displaced the abdominal contents until they occupy most of the incision site.

The Frazer laminectomy retractors are placed near the middle of the incision and expanded fully. The position of the kidney will vary slightly, depending upon whether it is right or left and whether it is enlarged and how much. The right kidney is usually opposite the thirteenth rib, with less variation in position except when greatly enlarged. It then becomes more pendulous. The left kidney will be near the midline of the incision or slightly caudal. Its position is more variable, and when enlarged it can reach to the ventral edge of the incision. In the cat, the position of the left kidney is even more variable. Usually when nephrectomy is required there is no problem in locating the kidney.

Very little packing off is required with the paracostal incision, and frequently the approach to the kidney can be made retroperitoneally even though the peritoneum has been separated during the abdominal invasion. The caudal pole of each kidney is devoid of peritoneum on the dorsal surface, so the retroperitoneal fat can be separated in this region to expose the kidney and free it from its attachments.

No attempt should be made to deliver the kidney through the incision until the renal artery and vein are safely ligated. The artery, a direct branch of the aorta, is short and sometimes double. The right artery is somewhat longer than the left but neither allows for much manipulation. The vein is likewise short, the left being longer than the right, and empties directly into the posterior vena cava. When the blood vessels have been uncovered, they should be ligated by using the three-hemostat method. If possible, the two vessels should be separated, but where they are small, both may be handled together. If the vessels are large, the ligature should be fixed.

Once the artery and vein have been ligated and divided, the kidney may be manipulated freely so that the ureter can be divided between two hemostats and ligated beyond the distal hemostat.

The peritoneum is closed with a continuous stitch by using 2-0 chromic catgut. Using the same material, close the fascial layers and muscle sheaths by the use of interrupted stitches. Care should be taken to avoid the thirteenth thoracic nerve on the caudal side of the incision. The skin incision is closed with interrupted stitches. A suture material of the surgeon's choice may be used.

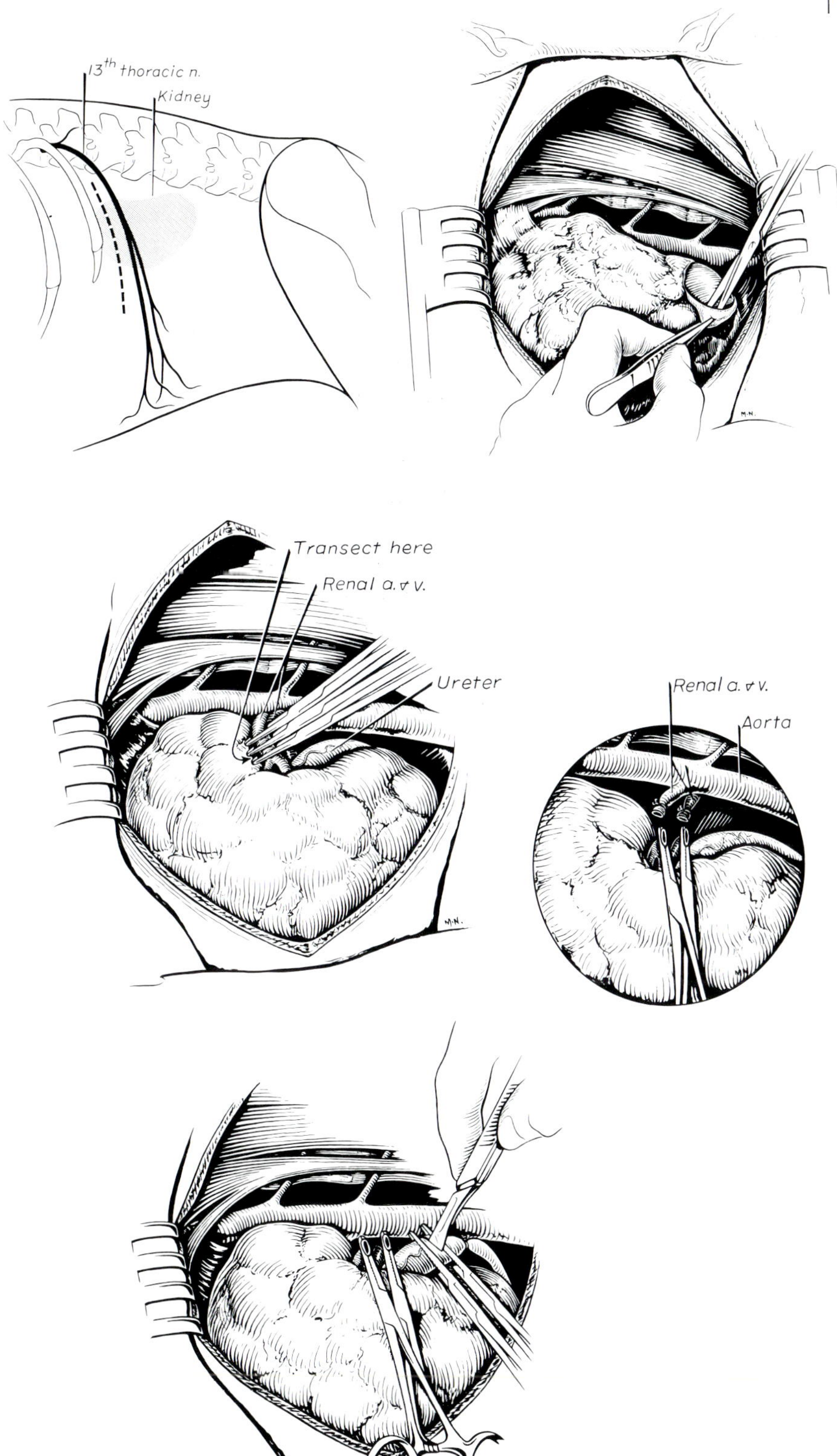
13th thoracic n.
Kidney
Transect here
Renal a. & v.
Ureter
Renal a. & v.
Aorta

FIGURE 8–1.

CYSTOTOMY

A general anesthetic is used, and the entire abdomen is prepared for surgery.

Whenever possible the patient should be catheterized during the preparation and the catheter left in position. In the male, a Bard x-ray catheter with a rubber adaptor can be taped by passing the tape around the body. In the female the metal catheter can be held in place by clamping it across the vulva with a towel clamp. The patient is placed in dorsal recumbency. The hind legs are tied to the table, and the foreparts may be held in a frame or tied. The table is tilted about 1° so that it slopes downward from head to tail. A six-drape system is used, leaving an opening for a caudal midline incision.

The skin incision is at least a hand's breadth and begins at the pubis (Fig. 8–2). This is followed by draping to the incision.

In the male the skin incision is made lateral to the prepuce (Fig. 8–3). Directly beneath the skin will be seen the branches of the external pudendal artery or the caudal superficial epigastric arteries. These usually cross the incision near the caudal and cranial ends of the prepuce. These vessels are double ligated and divided. The prepuce and penis can be reflected by blunt dissection to expose the linea alba. The deep incision follows the linea alba. As the peritoneum is opened, the middle umbilical ligament of the bladder will be encountered. This ligament can be broken without difficulty, thereby permitting the bladder to be reflected caudally as it is delivered through the incision. In this position the fundus is most accessible. It should be slightly caudal to the incision and tilted toward the tail. The incision should be well packed with sponges. If, for any reason, the bladder contains urine, it should be withdrawn by means of the catheter or with a syringe and 20 gauge needle before proceeding.

The incision into the bladder is made at the fundus (Fig. 8–4). A large incision is not required. If the incision is 3 cm. long, the opening can easily be dilated to whatever size is required. The incision can be held open with an eyelid retractor unless an exceptionally large incision is required (Fig. 8–5).

If the cystotomy has been performed for the removal of cystic calculi, they can be removed with forceps or a demitasse spoon. Fine particles will cling to a dry sponge wrapped around a sponge forceps and gently swabbed over the mucosal surface of the bladder (Fig. 8–6). Irrigation will help to flush small stones, but it must be done cautiously to avoid spillage. Other conditions of the bladder, such as tumors, must be dealt with according to the circumstances.

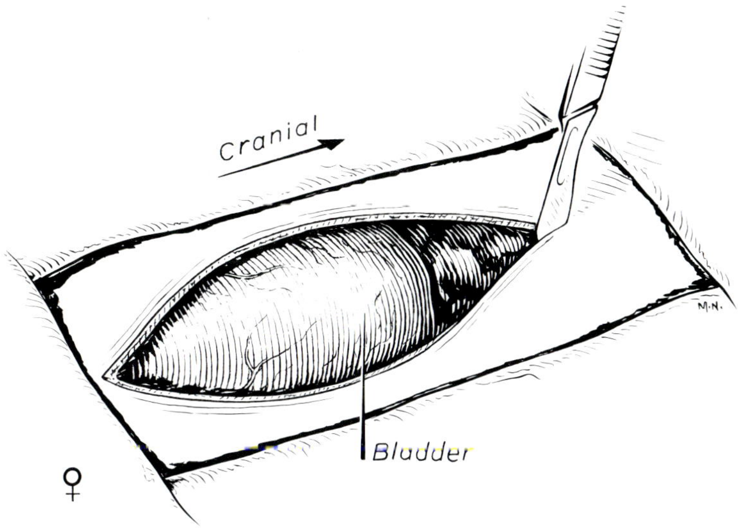

FIGURE 8–2.

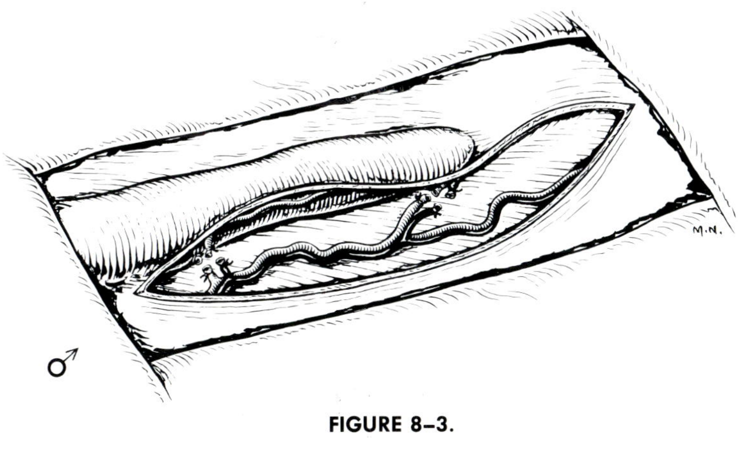

FIGURE 8–3.

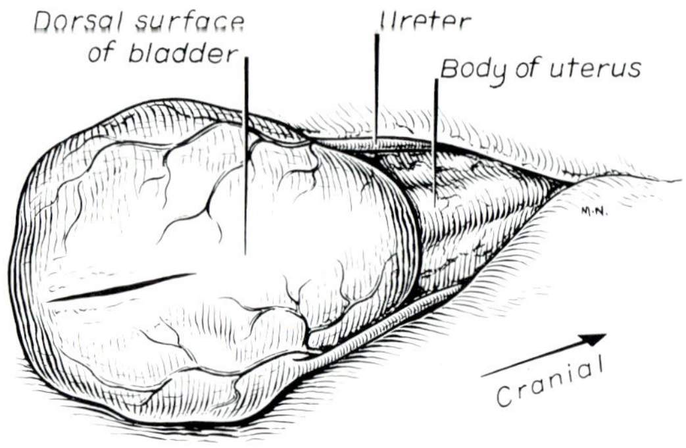

FIGURE 8–4.

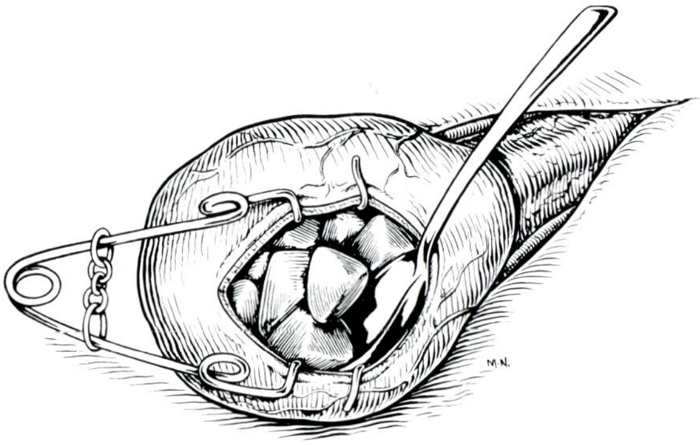

FIGURE 8–5.

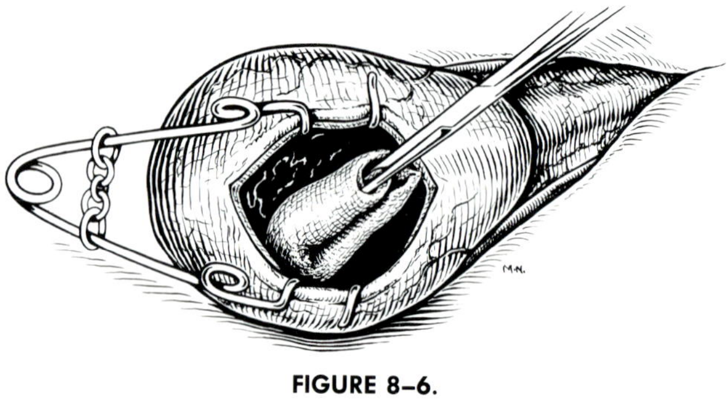

FIGURE 8–6.

When the bladder is contracted, the wall is relatively thick and does not lend itself well to inversion. For this reason the bladder is frequently closed by apposing the wound edges rather than inverting them. Simple interrupted stitches of 4-0 chromic catgut are placed through the three muscular layers of the wall and into the submucosal layer. They should be placed about 5 mm. apart but should not penetrate the mucosa. Remnants of suture material lying in the bladder are likely to be the nidus for further calculi formation. A second row of chromic catgut sutures is used to appose the serous covering of the bladder. This row may be either interrupted or continuous (Fig. 8–7).

The bladder is returned to its normal position, and the abdomen is closed in the usual way. Ordinarily the catheter is removed at the conclusion of the surgery.

In the cat the surgery is approximately the same except that a 17 gauge tomcat catheter is passed in both sexes, and the caudal abdominal midline incision is the same in both sexes. Since the bladder wall is thinner in the cat, it is normally possible to close it with a single continuous Lembert stitch.

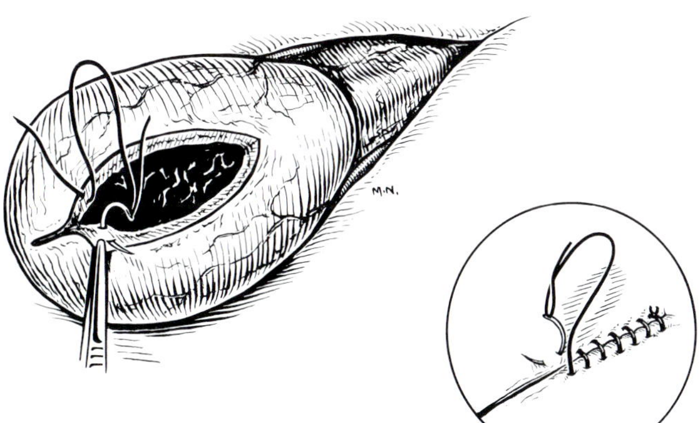

FIGURE 8–7.

URETHROTOMY

Urethrotomy is performed principally on the male dog for the relief of obstructing calculi in the cavernous urethra. The area involved is usually at the base or caudal to the base of the os penis (Fig. 8–8).

A general anesthetic is used, and a generous area cranial to the scrotum and laterally over the abdomen is prepared for surgery. The dog is placed in dorsal recumbency, and the legs are tied to the table to prevent rolling. A catheter or probe is passed into the urethra as far as the obstruction.

Either a single-drape or a multiple-drape system may be used. An opening must be left on the midline from the scrotum cranial about two-thirds the length of the prepuce.

The skin incision is made directly on the midline and over the obstructed area, which can be determined by palpation (Fig. 8–9). The bulbus glandis lies directly beneath this incision. With careful dissection, the urethra can be exposed and located by moderate pressure on the catheter or probe (Fig. 8–10). (This can be manipulated by the operator by grasping it with the drape, which is used as sterile covering). The urethra is incised longitudinally with a sharp scalpel or scissors.

Ordinarily there will be sufficient pressure from urine to dislodge the calculi lying caudal to the incision. Those cranial to the incision will be dislodged by the probe or catheter. The urethra is thoroughly flushed with saline and the catheter is then passed into the bladder.

Suturing of the urethra is not recommended, because of its small size and its friability. If left alone, the incision will gradually heal by granulation and without stenosis. For a number of days following surgery, there will be some bleeding following micturition, but this will gradually subside and is seldom of serious proportions. The patient should be kept quiet, and excitement should be avoided.

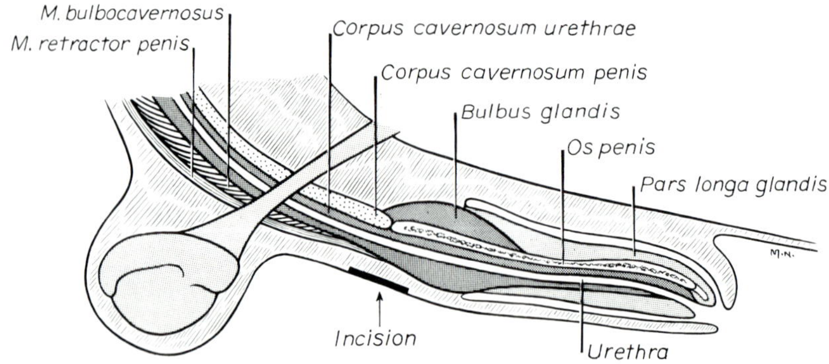

FIGURE 8–8. Diagram of male genitalia showing site of incision.

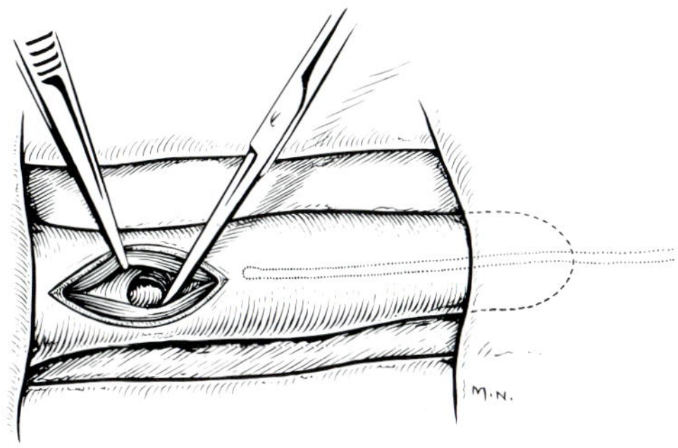

FIGURE 8–9.

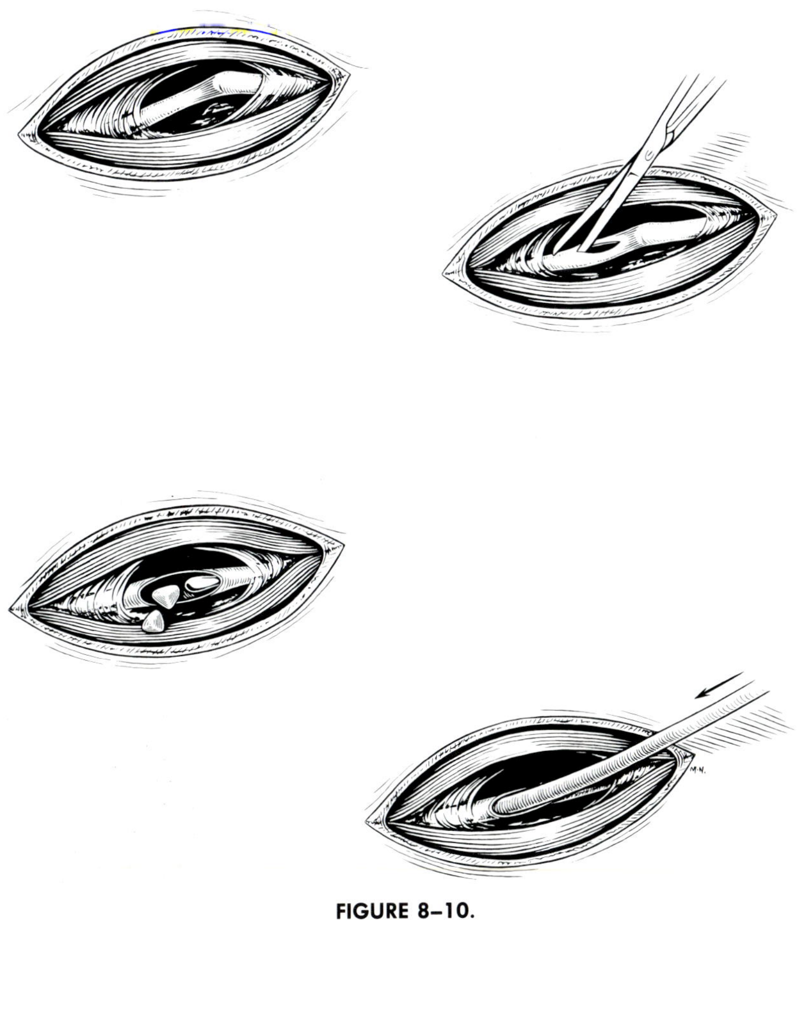

FIGURE 8–10.

ORCHIDECTOMY

When properly executed, an orchidectomy is relatively simple to perform and requires no aftercare. It may be done as the second stage in other surgery or as a simple sterilizing technique.

A general anesthetic is used, and an area cranial to the scrotum, including the prepuce, is prepared for surgery. The position should be dorsal recumbency with the hind legs fastened to the table. A single drape with a small central opening is usually sufficient. This drape should cover the scrotum but expose the area immediately cranial.

With his free hand, the operator gently presses on the drape over one testicle with his middle finger, at the same time guiding it with his forefinger and thumb so that it is displaced to the midline cranial to the scrotum (Fig. 8–11). This procedure should never be forceful or rough, because of the after effect from bruising. An incision is then made through the skin on the midline directly over the testicle. The incision should be about 5 to 6 cm. in length. When the spermatic fascia has been opened, the

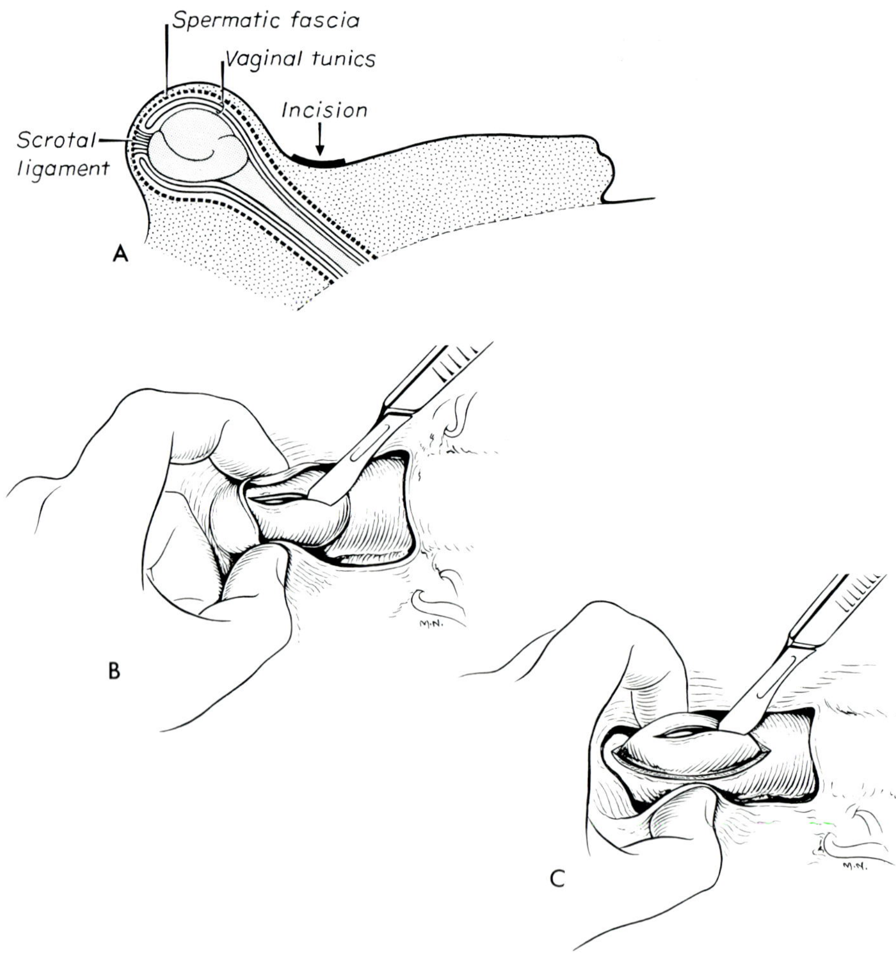

FIGURE 8–11.

testicle and its covering will appear. The tunica vaginalis communis is incised to expose the testicle. A small amount of fluid may escape at this point. The testicle should be lifted so that it unfolds the mesorchium into a thin triangular sheet, with the testicle as the base of a right angled triangle. The spermatic cord becomes the side along which the altitude is measured, and the reflected tunica vaginalis becomes the hypotenuse. Starting at the right angle, the mesorchium is divided close to the testicle as far as the scrotal ligament. If this ligament is divided along the border of the epididymis, there should be only minor bleeding, but some operators prefer to ligate as a precaution.

As soon as the scrotal ligament is divided, the testicle and spermatic cord can be retracted farther and a three-forceps ligature applied. As an added safeguard, the ligature may be fixed by passing the needle through the ductus deferens and tying it before passing it around the cord.

The opposite testicle is then pushed forward toward the same incision until the median septum is in position to incise. The procedure is then repeated.

Three or four simple interrupted stitches are placed in the skin to close the incision. No special aftercare is required.

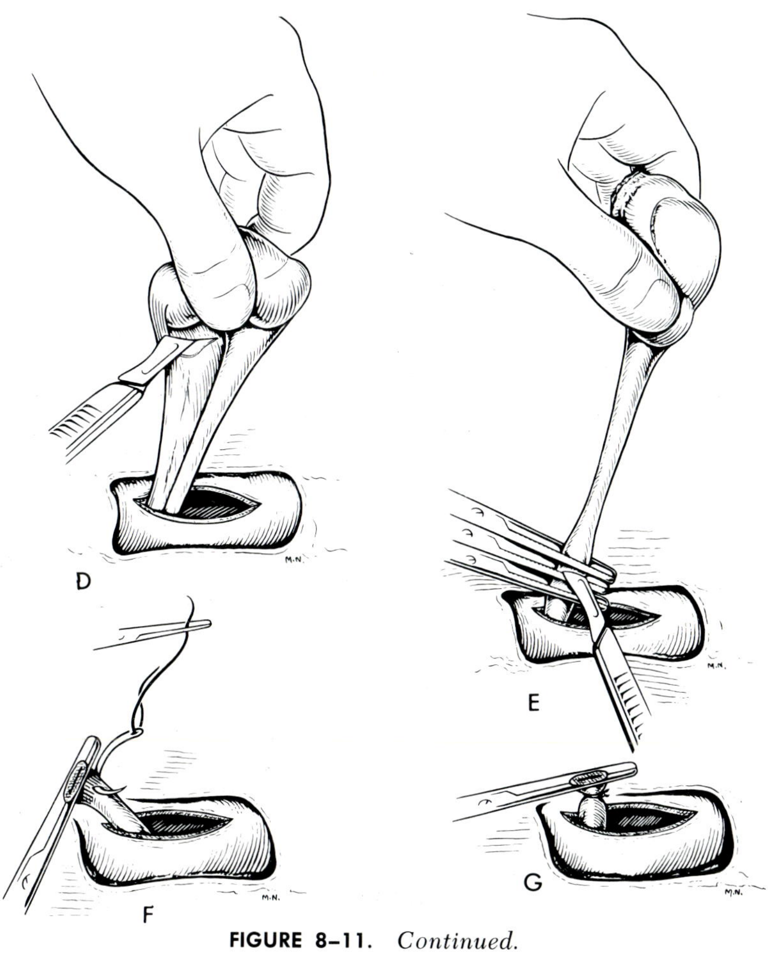

FIGURE 8–11. *Continued.*

PROSTATECTOMY

The conditions met with in cases where prostatectomy is required are far different and far more difficult to contend with than those found in the surgical laboratory, where the prostate is normal or nearly normal. Hyperplasia and prostatic cysts often produce a prostate many times its normal size. Blood vessels are greatly enlarged, the neck of the bladder is deeply embedded in the prostate, and the normal landmarks are distorted. The prostatectomy, therefore, will not be an easy, straightforward procedure. It may require ingenuity and some change in the routine in each individual case.

General anesthesia is recommended for this procedure. Preparation begins with catheterization and evacuation of the bladder. The catheter is left in place so that it can be utilized during the surgery. The entire abdomen, from the scrotum to the costal arch, is prepared in the usual way.

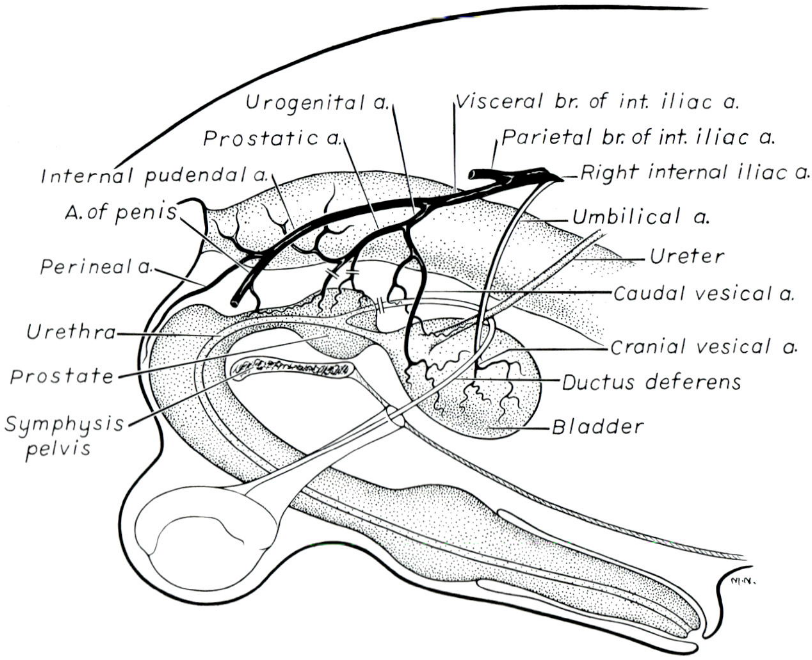

FIGURE 8–12. Plan of arterial supply to prostate and bladder. Points for ligation and transection of arteries and ductus deferens are shown.

The patient is placed in dorsal recumbency with the hind legs tied to the table and the foreparts held in a frame in such a manner as to ensure relaxation of the abdominal muscles. The catheter is fastened on the side away from the operator and coupled to tubing which leads to a receptacle. A rubber-shod clamp is used on the sheath. A six-drape method of draping to the incision is used.

A skin incision is made just lateral to the prepuce (Fig. 8–13). It should curve to the midline cranial to the prepuce. When completed, it will extend from the pubis to the umbilicus or even a few centimeters beyond. The superficial blood vessels lying lateral to the sheath are branches of the external pudendal or the caudal superficial epigastric artery and should be double ligated and divided. By blunt dissection with scissors, the sheath and penis are reflected so that the entire incision can be completed on the midline (Fig. 8–14).

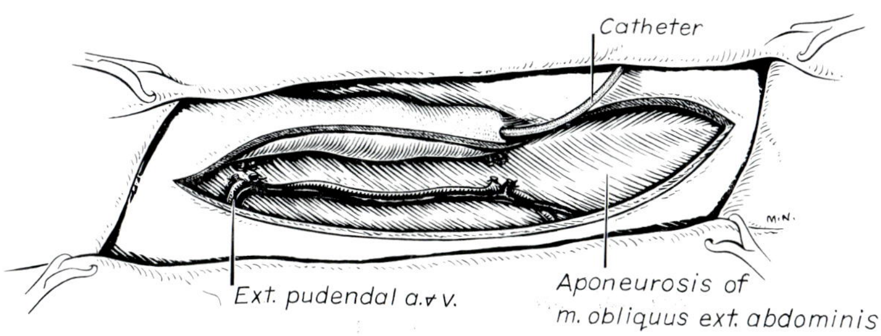

FIGURE 8–13.

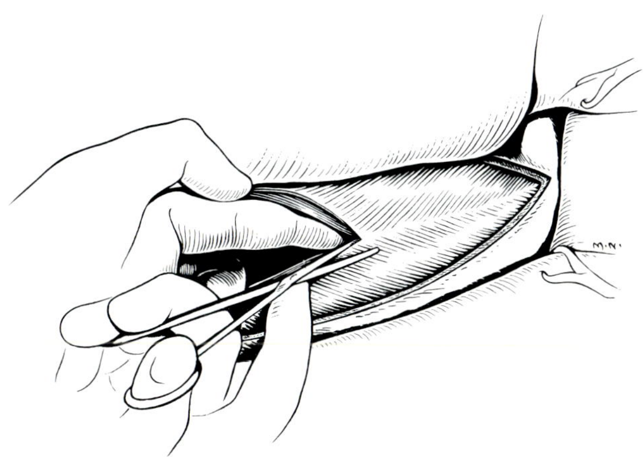

FIGURE 8–14.

The middle umbilical ligament is separated from its attachment along the midline and the retractor is inserted so that the incision can be widely spread (Fig. 8–15). Whenever the prostate is grossly enlarged, the bladder should be examined first so that the lateral ligaments of the bladder can be identified and the ureter located in the fold of each ligament. This is a precautionary measure which is taken so that the ureters will not be injured during surgery. While the bladder is reflected caudally, the ductus deferentes can be double ligated with chromic catgut and separated (Fig. 8–16).

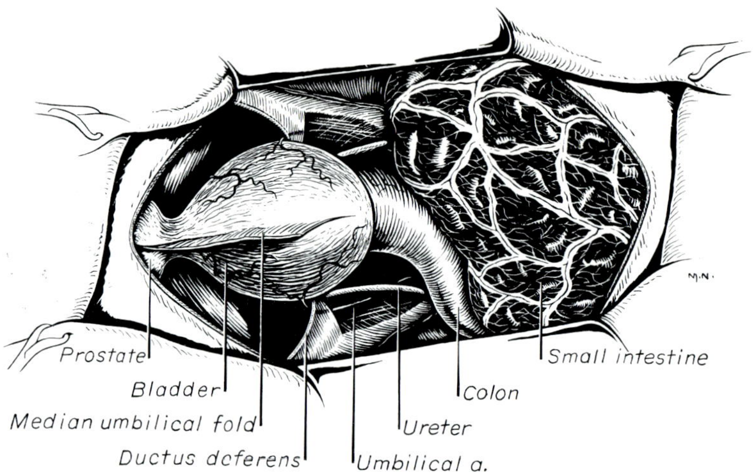

FIGURE 8–15.

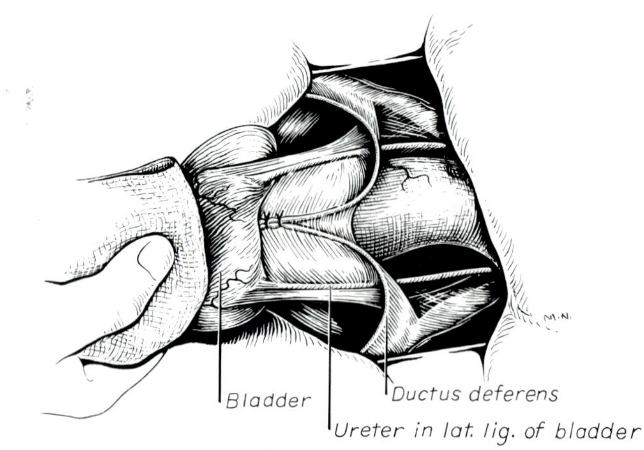

FIGURE 8–16.

The next step is the ligation of all blood vessels supplying the prostate (Fig. 8–17). Do not interfere with those that supply the bladder and the urethra. The urogenital artery branches are frequently relatively large. Fortunately they can be seen easily, and by careful ligating, the supply to bladder and urethra will not be interrupted. Double ligate and divide on both sides of the prostate.

Careful dissection with scissors around the neck of the bladder is undertaken next in order to preserve as much of the bladder sphincter as possible (Fig. 8–18). This dissection should be carried as far caudal as possible. The catheter will help in locating the urethra. Before transecting the urethra, the suction apparatus should be connected to the catheter tubing, and the ureters should be clamped with rubber-shod serrefines or "bulldog" clamps (Fig. 8–19).

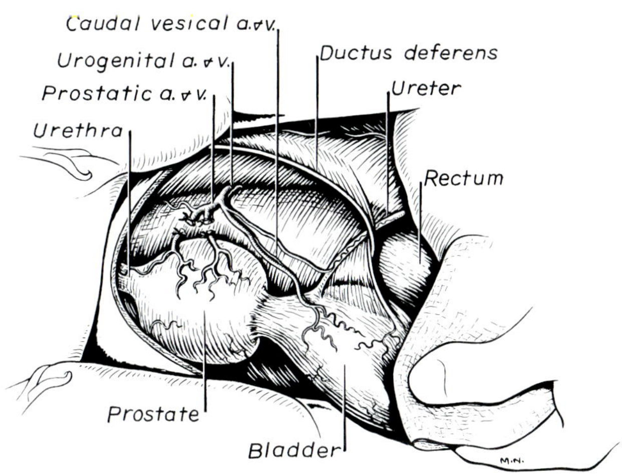

FIGURE 8–17.

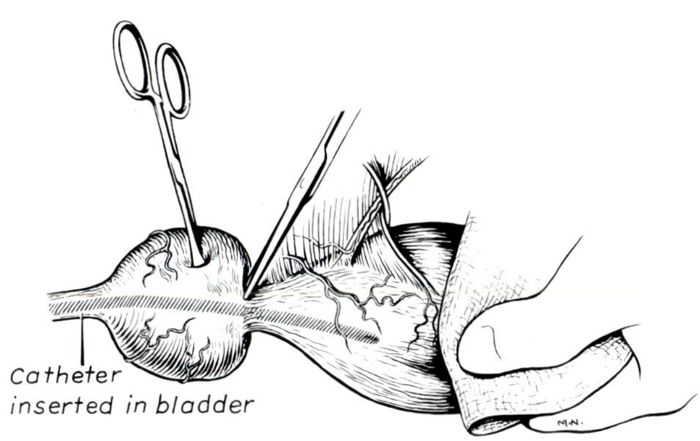

FIGURE 8–18.

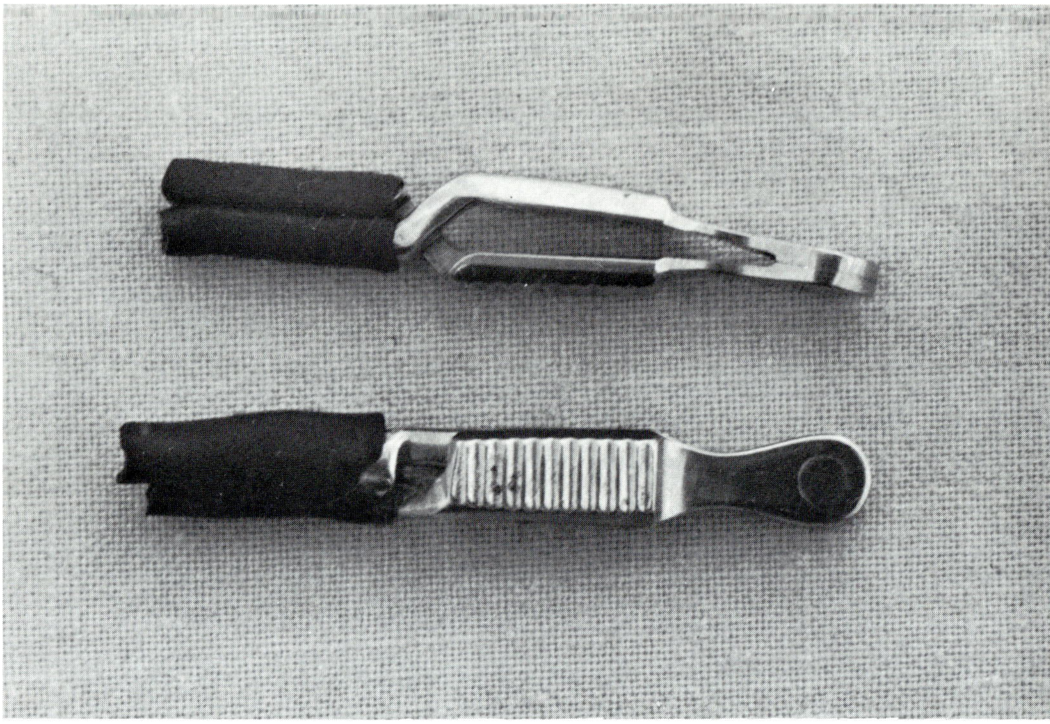

FIGURE 8–19.

The urethra is cut close to the prostate both cranially and caudally as the catheter is withdrawn (Fig. 8–20). The urethra may require a rubber-shod forceps to prevent it from slipping too far into the pelvis. The prostate must finally be freed from its peritoneal attachment to the rectum. In some cases there may be small blood vessels which require ligating before the prostate can be entirely separated.

Suturing of the urethra to the bladder is begun by placing a simple interrupted stitch (Fig. 8–21) through all layers on the dorsal side while holding the two ends with rubber-shod clamps. These clamps should be placed transversely at a point about 1 cm. from the cut ends. After two or three sutures have been placed, the clamps are removed and the catheter, without suction, is passed into the bladder. Suturing is continued by placing small interrupted stitches of 4-0 chromic catgut about 2 mm. apart (Fig. 8–22). The serrefines are removed, and the abdominal incision is closed in the usual manner.

In order to keep the catheter in place for four or five days until healing of the urethra is begun, it should be cut flush with the tip of the penis and a silk suture placed through the ventral side of catheter and the mucous membrane of the penis (Fig. 8–23). When this is tied and the knot cut short, there will be no problem due to the patient tugging at the catheter.

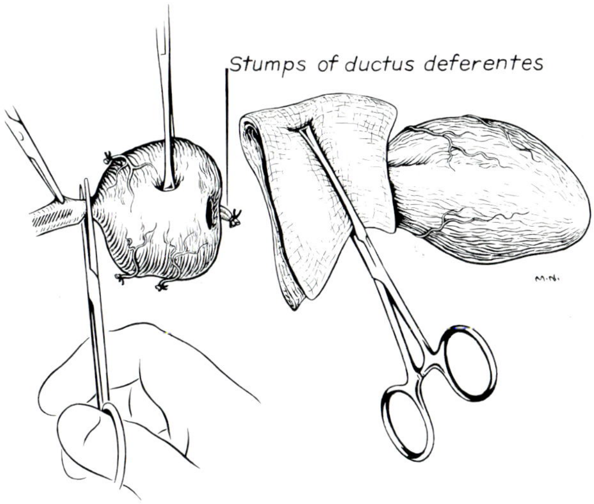

FIGURE 8–20.

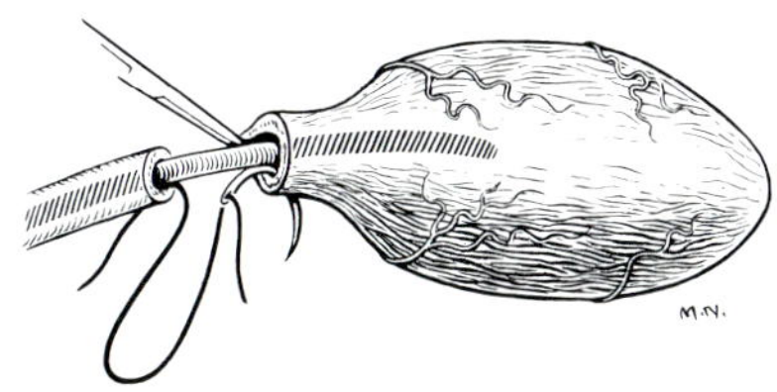

FIGURE 8–21.

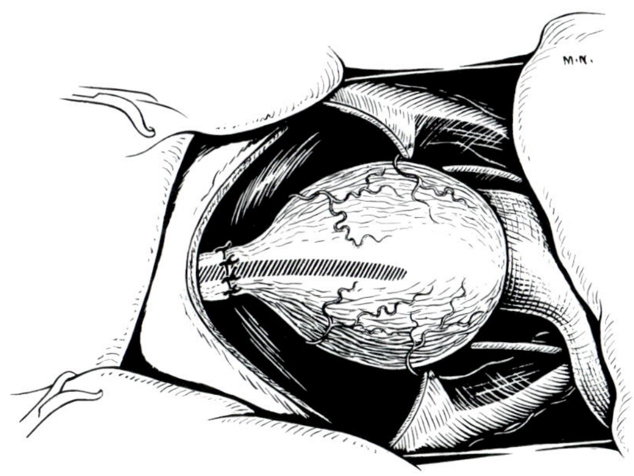

FIGURE 8–22.

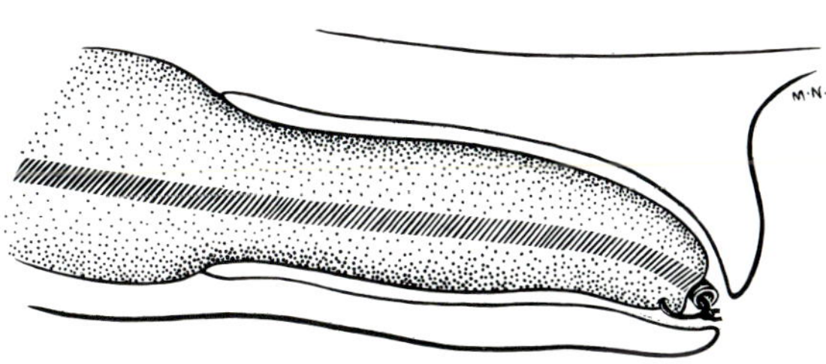

FIGURE 8–23.

OVARIOHYSTERECTOMY

OVARIOHYSTERECTOMY FOR STERILIZATION

This operation, commonly called spaying, is performed more frequently than any other in canine and feline surgery (Fig. 8–24). It is accomplished under general anesthesia. The skin preparation should include the abdominal area from pubis to costal arch and be wide enough to include the breasts. The patient is positioned in dorsal recumbency with the legs fastened to the table firmly enough to maintain the body position. A single drape is applied, with the central opening positioned to expose the umbilicus at the cranial end.

The operator takes a position in which the patient's head is to his right. The incision is begun at the umbilicus and carried caudally 6 to 12 cm., depending on the skill of the operator. If the incision is kept on the midline, the aponeurosis and peritoneum can easily be penetrated with scissors, and very little hemorrhage will result. At this point, one should tilt the table 45°, elevating the pelvis so that the abdominal contents will gravitate cranially. This will facilitate the surgery to a considerable degree.

A small retractor (an aneurysm hook works extremely well) is inserted in the center of the incision, and traction is applied in the direction of the operator. At the same time, an ovariectomy hook is gently slipped along the left abdominal wall, with the loop pointing cranially until it reaches the region of the spine (Fig. 8–25). The loop is then turned in the transverse direction and lifted. When it emerges from the incision, it should bring with it either a fold of the broad ligament or the left horn of the uterus (Fig. 8–26). The retractor is discarded and the uterine horn grasped between the thumb and forefinger (Fig. 8–27). The hook is discarded and the horn elevated far enough to disclose the left ovary. By placing a finger beneath the ovary, the supensory ligament can be felt as a taut band running cranially. Enough pressure with the finger should be exerted on the ligament to separate it, but care should be taken not to tear the mesovarium covering the ovarian artery and vein. When the suspensory ligament separates, the ovary can be elevated at least another 2 to 3 cm. Further traction should cease at this point. A pedicle is formed by breaking a small opening in the mesovarium, caudal to the ovarian vessels, and a Ferguson angiotribe is clamped across the pedicle (Fig. 8–28). A fixed ligature of 2-0 chromic catgut may be placed around the pedicle, beneath the angiotribe leaving space for another angiotribe to be clamped between the ligature and the first angiotribe, or a three-forceps method of ligating may be used. The ovary is then separated from the mesovarium and the stump allowed to return to its normal position, after carefully checking for any hemorrhage.

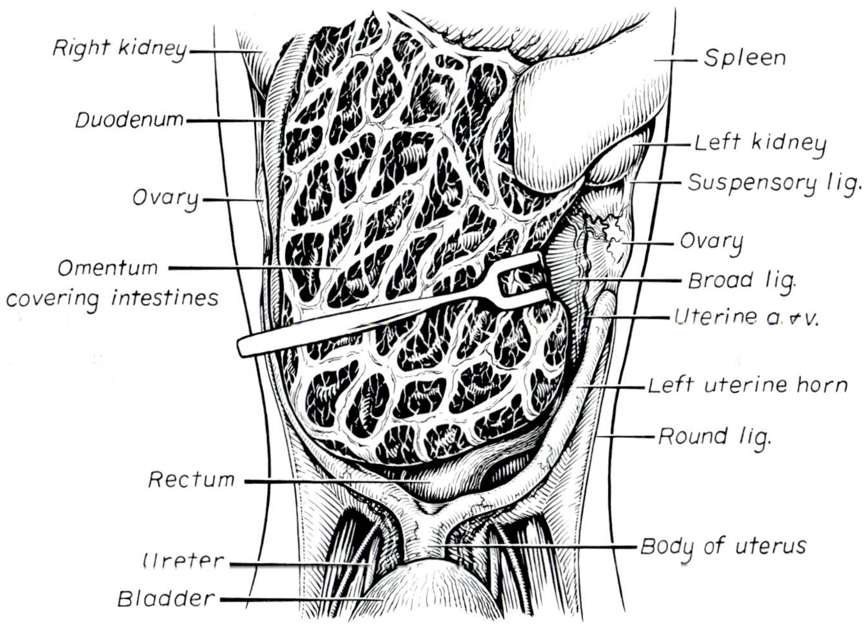

FIGURE 8–24. Anatomy of the abdominal region.

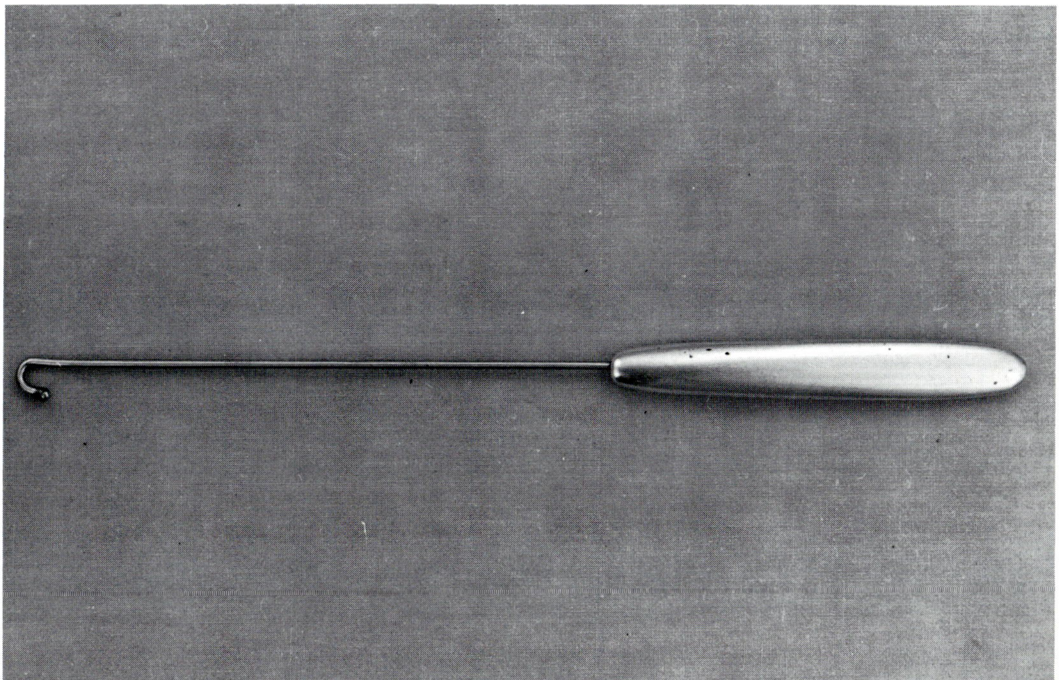

FIGURE 8–25.

The broad ligament is separated caudally along the left horn but at a sufficient distance from it to avoid damage to the uterine artery and vein (Fig. 8–29). At about the midpoint of the broad ligament, a band will be found which is the round ligament of the uterus. Traction is applied to this ligament until it breaks free (Fig. 8–30). A retractor is then placed in the caudal commissure of the incision and retracted caudally to expose the bifurcation of the uterus. Sometimes slight traction in a cranial direction on the left uterine horn is necessary. From the bifurcation, the right horn is traced to its cranial end and the right ovary elevated. Frequently it is necessary to reach through the incision with the index finger and break the suspensory ligament before the right ovary can be delivered. Ligation of the ovarian vessels and separation of the broad ligament is repeated.

Both horns are elevated and a Ferguson angiotribe is placed across the uterus at the cervix (Fig. 8–31). A fixed ligature is applied to the stump, and the uterus is separated between angiotribes cranial to the ligature (Figs. 8–32 and 8–33).

Closure of the abdominal incision is made with several simple interrupted stitches of 2-0 chromic catgut through fascia and peritoneum and two or three interrupted stitches in the skin of whatever material seems best suited. When spaying older bitches, it is wise to use continuous stitches in the peritoneum, followed by interrupted in the fascia and skin.

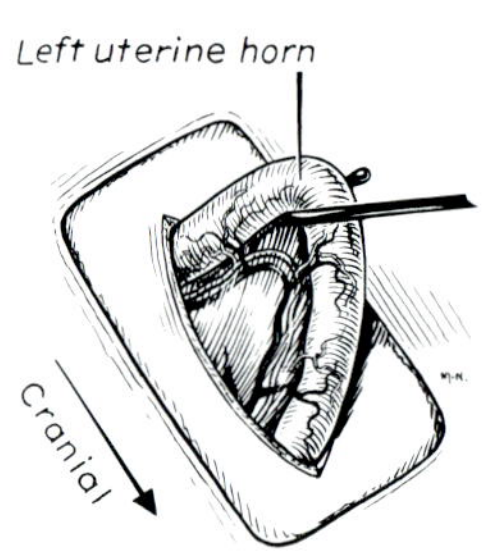

FIGURE 8–26.

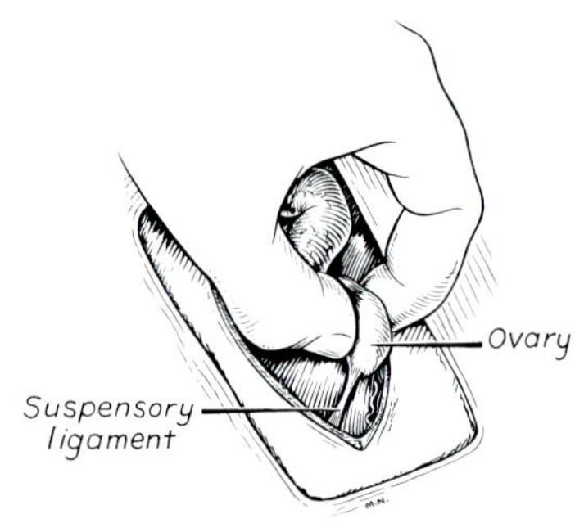

FIGURE 8–27.

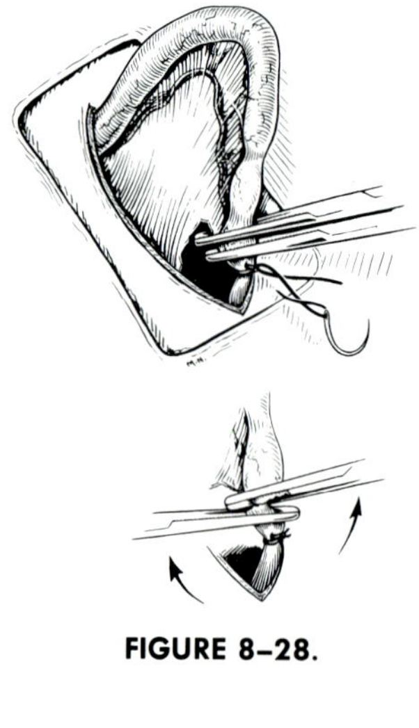

FIGURE 8–28.

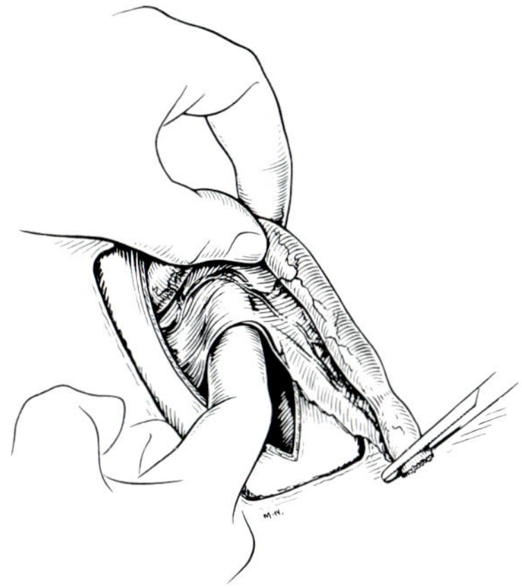

FIGURE 8–29.

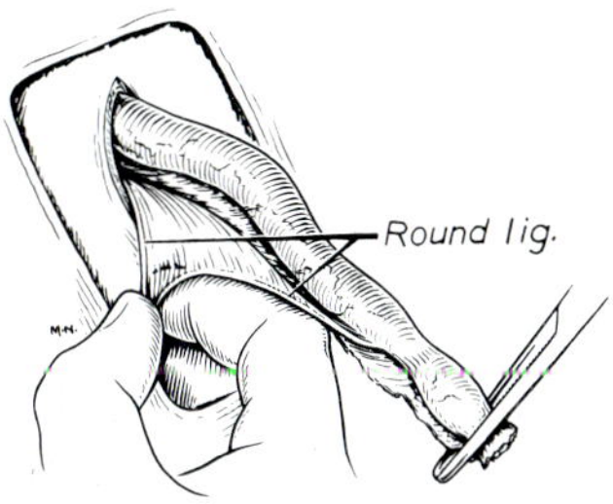

FIGURE 8–30.

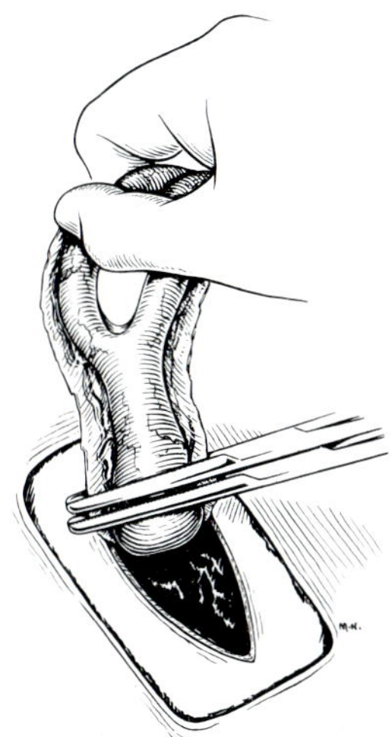

FIGURE 8–31.

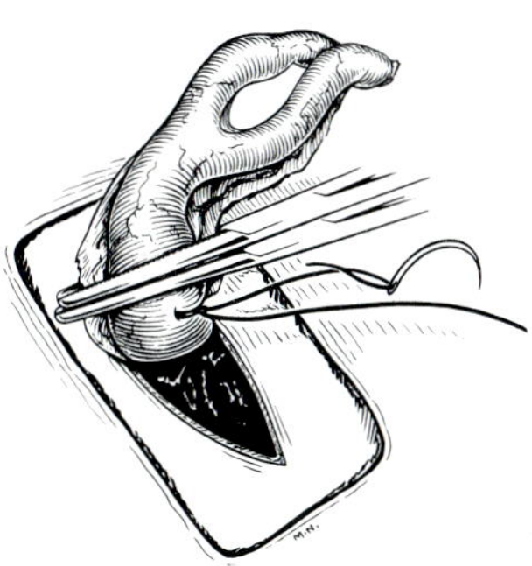

FIGURE 8–32.

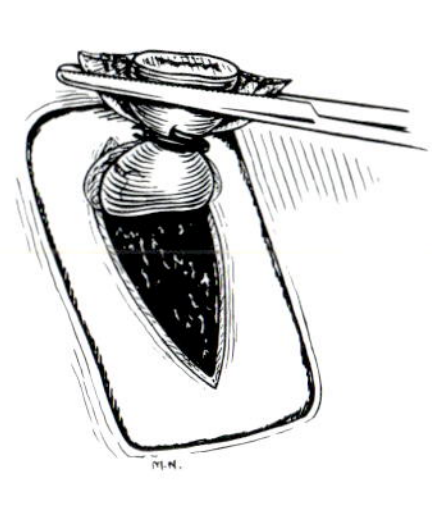

FIGURE 8–33.

OVARIOHYSTERECTOMY FOR DISEASE

The selection of an anesthetic is far more important when the surgery is performed for disease (pyometra, etc.) than when it is a sterilizing procedure. General anesthetics such as halothane and methoxyflurane are frequently used. Selection must be based on the age and condition of the patient. An ultrashort-acting barbiturate is given prior to intubation.

Preparation requires that a good soap-and-water bath be given to remove all discharges from the skin, especially the hind parts. Prepare the abdomen in the usual manner, making certain that the area prepared extends laterally at least 6 cm. beyond the breasts. Even in cases where an endotracheal tube is not required for anesthesia, it is well to intubate as a precautionary measure. The patient is placed in dorsal recumbency, with the rear legs tied and the foreparts in a frame.

A six-drape system is used for covering the abdomen. The opening runs along the caudal midline from the pubis to a point 6 cm. cranial to the umbilicus. After draping, a generous incision covering at least the caudal midline is made and the horns of the uterus are gently delivered to the outside (Fig. 8–34). These horns are often quite friable and therefore should be carefully placed on either side of the incision. The incision is packed with a towel to prevent contamination of the abdomen in the event of seepage from the uterus.

If the incision has been carried far enough cranial, the ovaries and suspensory ligaments should be well exposed. The ligaments are broken, and the pedicles are ligated with 2-0 chromic catgut as described in the spay operation. As the broad ligament is separated, it may be necessary to ligate some of the vessels, since they are much larger than those encountered during a normal ovariohysterectomy. Separation of the broad ligament is continued caudally as far as the cervix.

On either side, the uterine artery and vein are ligated at a point opposite the caudal end of the cervix (Fig. 8–35). Hemostats may be applied to these vessels somewhat cranial to this point. A pile clamp is placed across the uterus at a point just cranial to the ligatures, with the grips toward the assistant, and a second clamp is placed cranial to the first and as close to it as possible, with the grips toward the surgeon (Fig. 8–36). With a scalpel, the uterine stump is divided between the clamps by holding the blade tight against the caudal clamp. The scalpel is discarded, and the uterus is carefully lifted away from the operative site. A sponge is used to wipe the end of the stump between the pile clamp blades while an assistant holds it so that it faces upward.

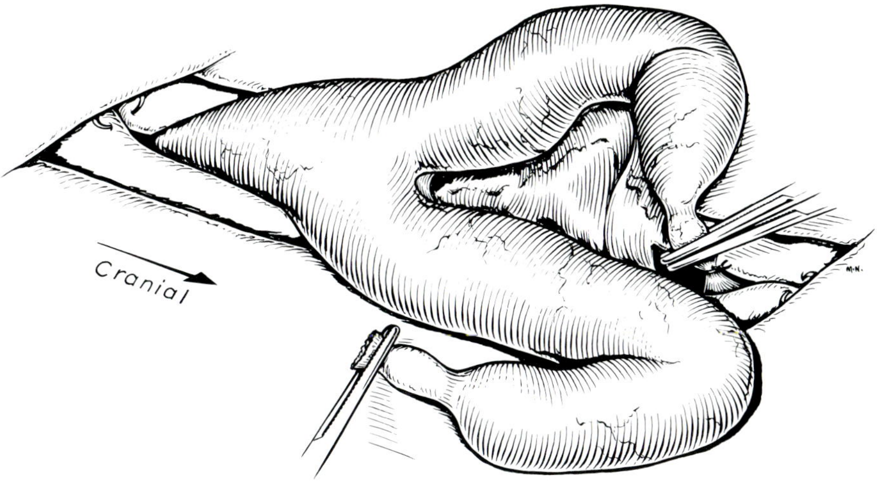

FIGURE 8–34.

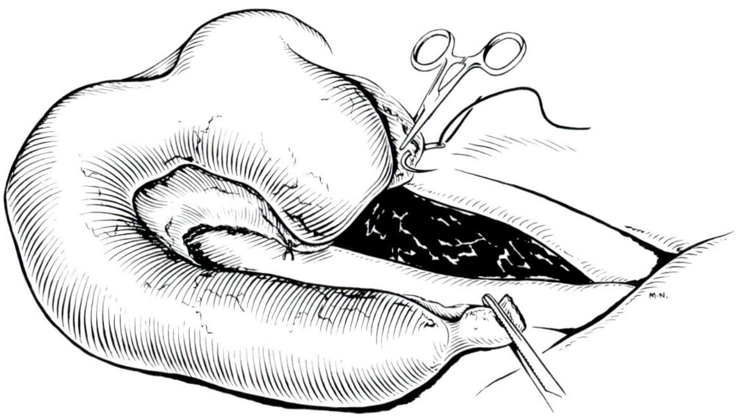

FIGURE 8–35.

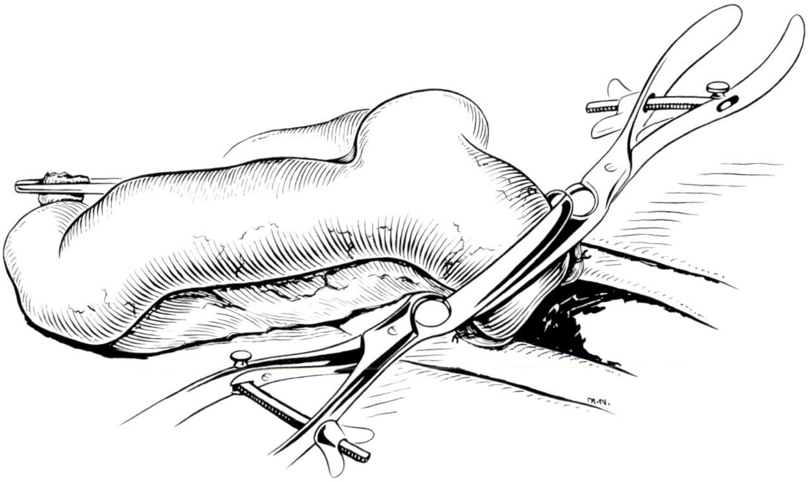

FIGURE 8–36.

The pile clamp is oversewn by the Parker-Kerr method (Fig. 8–37). This tissue is very sturdy and does not lend itself to inversion as easily as the intestine. It also requires a stronger needle and somewhat coarser catgut. After the stump has been inverted (see section on intestinal resection in Chapter 7) and before any knots are tied, the needle is passed through the flap of broad ligament adjacent to it and then a tie is made with the opposite end of the suture (Fig. 8–38). This is repeated by picking up the broad ligament on the other side and tying so that the stump is covered by two layers of broad ligament.

Because bitches with pyometra are notoriously slow in healing, it is a good precautionary measure to suture the peritoneum with a continuous stitch of 2-0 chromic catgut, but the remainder of the incision should be closed with interrupted stitches of 3-0 multifilament stainless steel. The choice of suture material beyond that for the peritoneum is largely optional. It is recommended that the abdomen be supported by a bandage for one week postoperative.

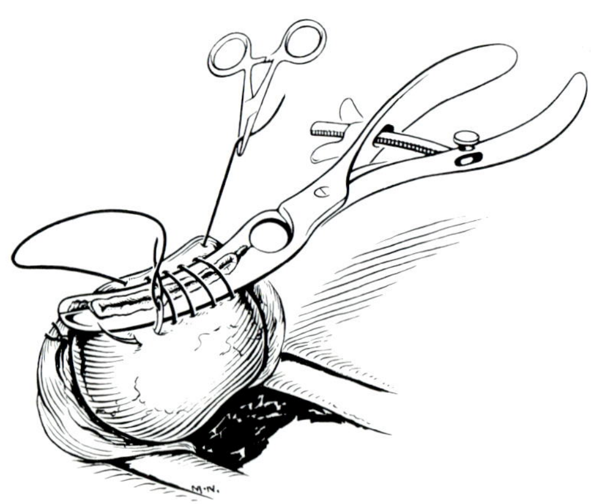

FIGURE 8–37.

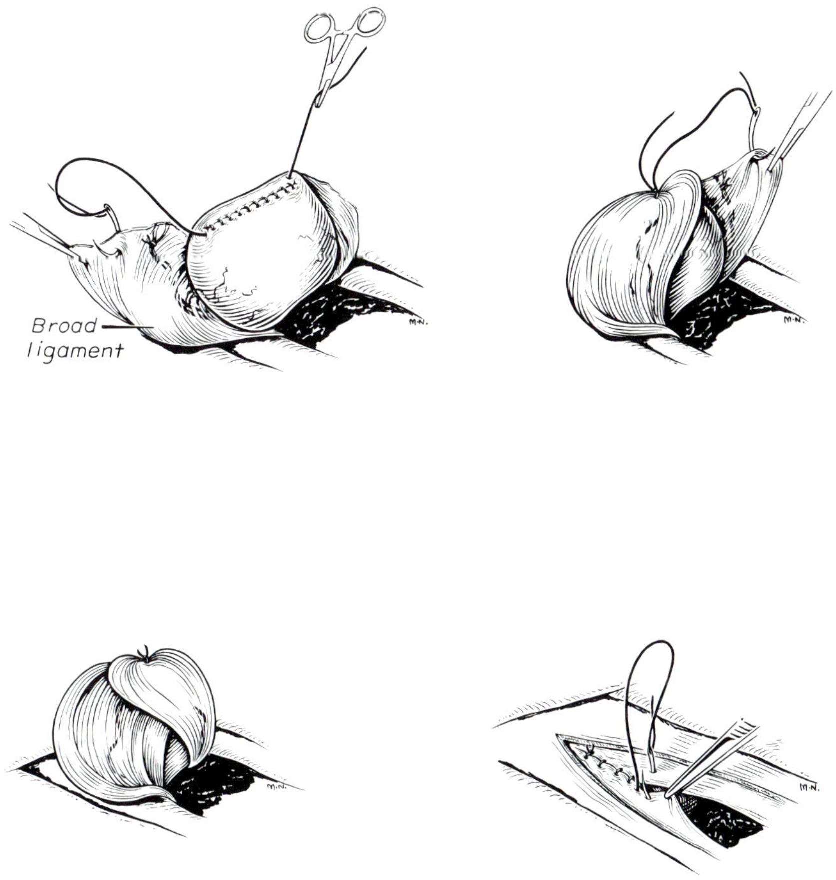

FIGURE 8–38.

CESAREAN SECTION—HYSTEROTOMY

This procedure should not be undertaken until the first stage of labor is well under way. The patient is premedicated with 15 mg. of morphine sulphate intramuscularly and allowed to defecate and regurgitate before continuing with the preparation. If a mask or cone is to be used, 0.6 mg. (1/100 gr.) of atropine sulfate should be given to control excessive salivation. The atropine should not be used if the patient is to be intubated.

Skin preparation is the same as described for ovariohysterectomy for disease. The patient is placed in dorsal recumbency with all four legs tied to the table. The caudal end of the bitch should be somewhat lower than the cranial end. In addition to the normal surgical setup, there should be an additional stand with a number of turkish towels, a few sterile hemostats, a pair of sterile scissors and a few 6 inch strands of external suture material.

The patient is draped with a six-drape system, the final two drapes being applied after the skin incision is made. The skin incision should extend from the umbilicus to the pubis. Because of the abdominal distention, the aponeurosis is usually thin and easily penetrated once the skin is opened. Both uterine horns are carefully delivered by placing the hand beneath each one and rolling it lateral to the incision. In so doing, the dorsal aspect of the uterine body is presented just caudal to the caudal commissure of the incision. The incision is then packed off by placing a towel between the two horns (Fig. 8–39).

A longitudinal incision long enough to permit passage of a fetus without tearing the uterine wall is made in the dorsal aspect of the body. The pup that is presenting is withdrawn with one hand while the other hand exerts pressure over the placental zone by gentle squeezing. The fetal membranes are removed from the pup's head before dropping it into a towel held by an assistant. By gentle pressure on the horns at the placental sites, the pups are "milked" from the uterus. Finally the entire uterus is checked to be certain that no pups are retained, and 1 ml. of Pitocin is sprayed over it to hasten involution. The incision in the uterine body is

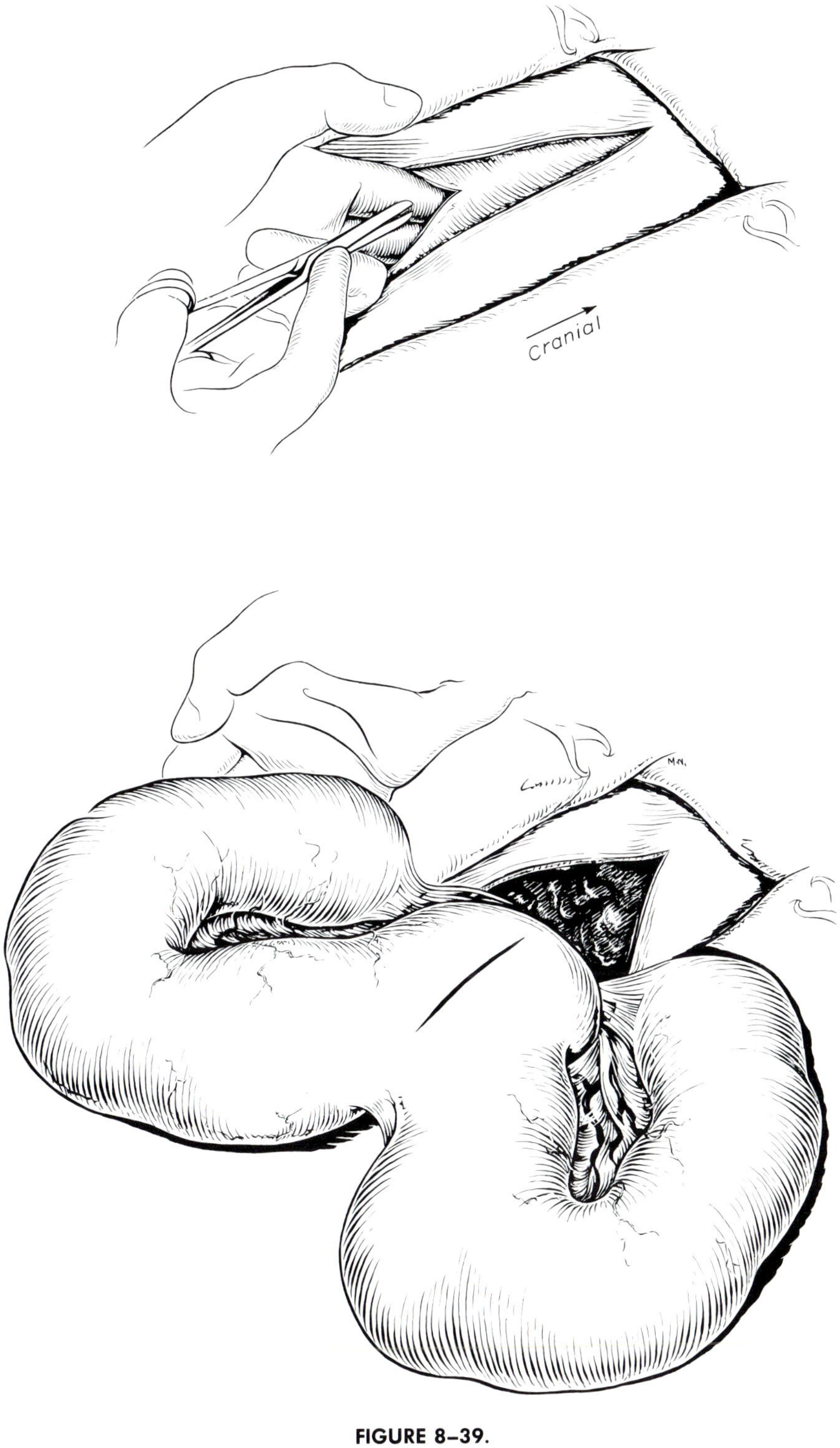

FIGURE 8–39.

closed with two rows of continuous Lembert stitches by using 3-0 chromic catgut and a taper-point needle. The uterus is sponged clean, the packing towel is removed, and the uterus is placed in its normal position in the abdomen.

Closure of the abdominal incision is begun with a continuous stitch of 2-0 chromic catgut in the peritoneum. This is followed by at least two rows of carefully placed interrupted stitches in the fascia and muscle sheaths. Another row of interrupted stitches may be required in the subcutaneous fascia to bring the skin close to apposition. Finally, a row of interrupted stitches is placed in the skin.

The closed incision is covered by several layers of adhesive tape laid longitudinally between the breasts. This is further supported by placing strips of adhesive tape around the body between the breasts in a circumferential direction. This allows the pups to nurse without interfering with the incision. Often this bandage will become too tight on the following day. It can be loosened by cutting along the spine, allowing the bands to gape, and retaping the openings with short strips. The bandage should be kept in place for one week. Meanwhile, the care of the puppies has been carried out by an assistant.

As the pup is received from the surgeon, the umbilical cord is clamped with a hemostat at a point about 2 cm. from the abdomen. The cord is cut just distal to the hemostat, the fetal membranes are discarded, and the pup is rubbed briskly with the towel while both it and the hemostat are supported in the hands. As soon as the pup is breathing normally, the hemostat may be removed. If the cord shows signs of bleeding, the hemostat is reapplied, and a length of suture material is tied between the hemostat and the abdomen.

Puppies that do not respond to rubbing, may be helped by mouth to mouth breathing, alternate dipping in hot and cold water, or an injection in the umbilical artery of 0.25 to 0.5 ml. of Coramine (Ciba). They should be kept in a warm place away from the bitch until she has entirely recovered from the anesthetic.

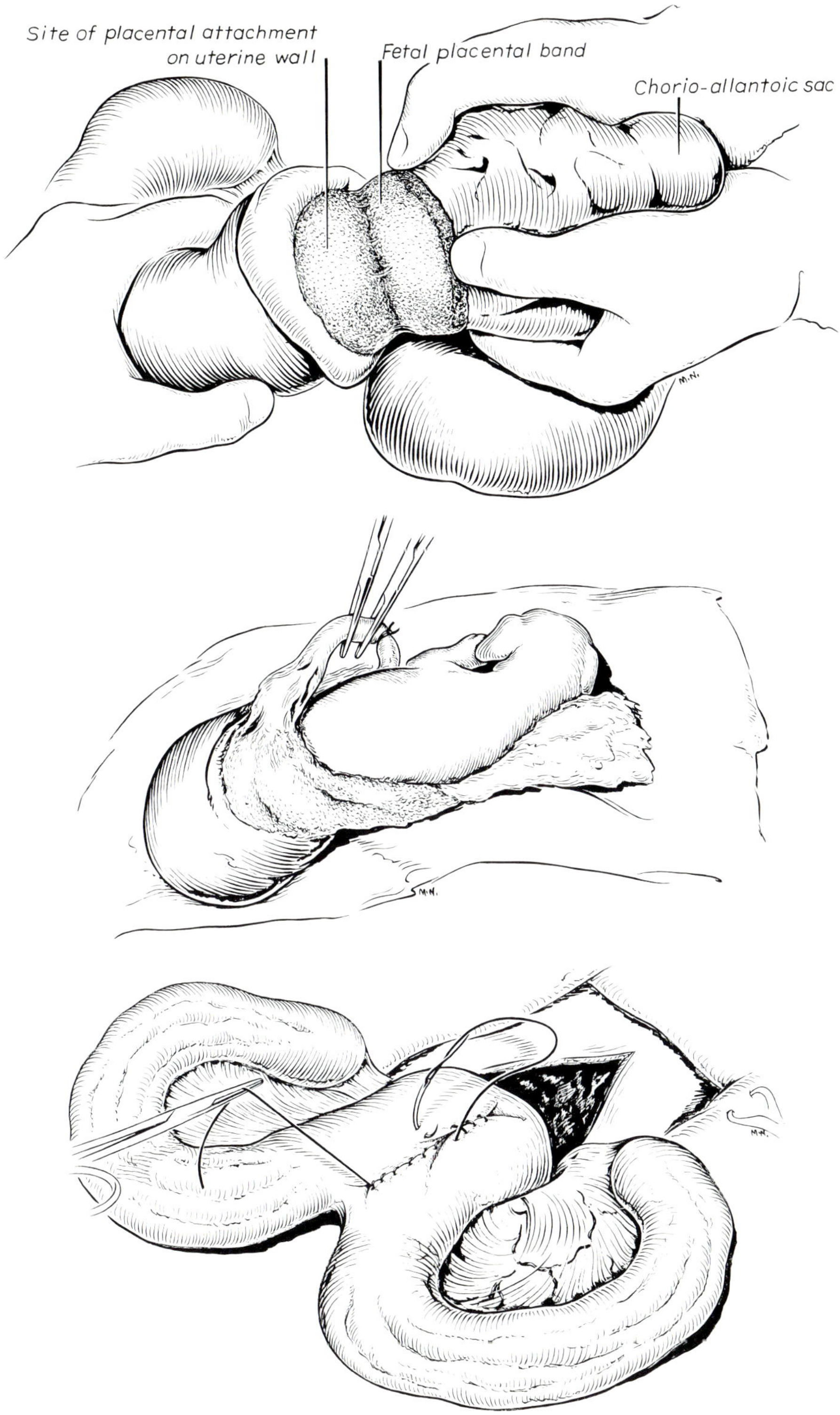

FIGURE 8–39. *Continued.*

VAGINAL PROLAPSE

Two types of prolapse are recognized: the true vaginal prolapse, in which the entire vaginal wall is everted, and the hyperplasia of the vaginal floor, in which only the edematous ventral mucosa is everted.

VAGINAL RESECTION

The patient is given a general anesthetic and the perineal region is clipped. The tail is bandaged and fastened forward over the back. The entire area, including the prolapse, is thoroughly cleansed with soap and water. Antiseptics are applied to the skin of the vulva and the perineal area.

The most convenient position is sternal recumbency with the hind legs extended caudally and sandbags or Flexicast under the thighs to elevate the pelvis. The table is tilted forward, and the operator takes a position at the end of the table. A single drape can be used. Only the vulva and the prolapse are exposed through the central opening.

The prolapse is lifted, and a metal catheter is inserted into the urethral meatus, which usually lies on the ventral side of the prolapse close to the lips of the vulva (Fig. 8–40). With the catheter in place, there is less likelihood of injuring the urethra during surgery (Fig. 8–41).

Unless the vagina is badly mutilated, the surgery can be done on the protruding mass. If the eversion is necrotic or otherwise unfit for surgery, it will be necessary to evert a few extra centimeters to obtain normal tissue. A blunt instrument such as a scalpel handle is inserted through the center of the eversion. If great care is taken, the index finger may be used, but this usually results in a torn glove during the suturing.

Mattress stitches are placed close together around the circumference of the prolapse. The inner layer is sutured to the outer layer. These sutures are usually size 3 to .5 silk. The suture line is so placed as to encircle the prolapse just caudal to the urethral meatus in the prolapsed position. When the prolapse is reduced, the suture line will be cranial to the meatus. The sutures should not be wide. They can be placed with a five-eighths circle needle from outside to inside to outside and tied.

When the suture line is completed, the prolapse is amputated with scissors at a point just caudal to the sutures. The stump is held with Allis forceps until it has been inspected for bleeding. Extra sutures are placed if there are bleeding vessels. When released, the stump will retract inside the vulva. At this point, the catheter is removed. The sutures will eventually slough, and the swelling will subside in 10 days.

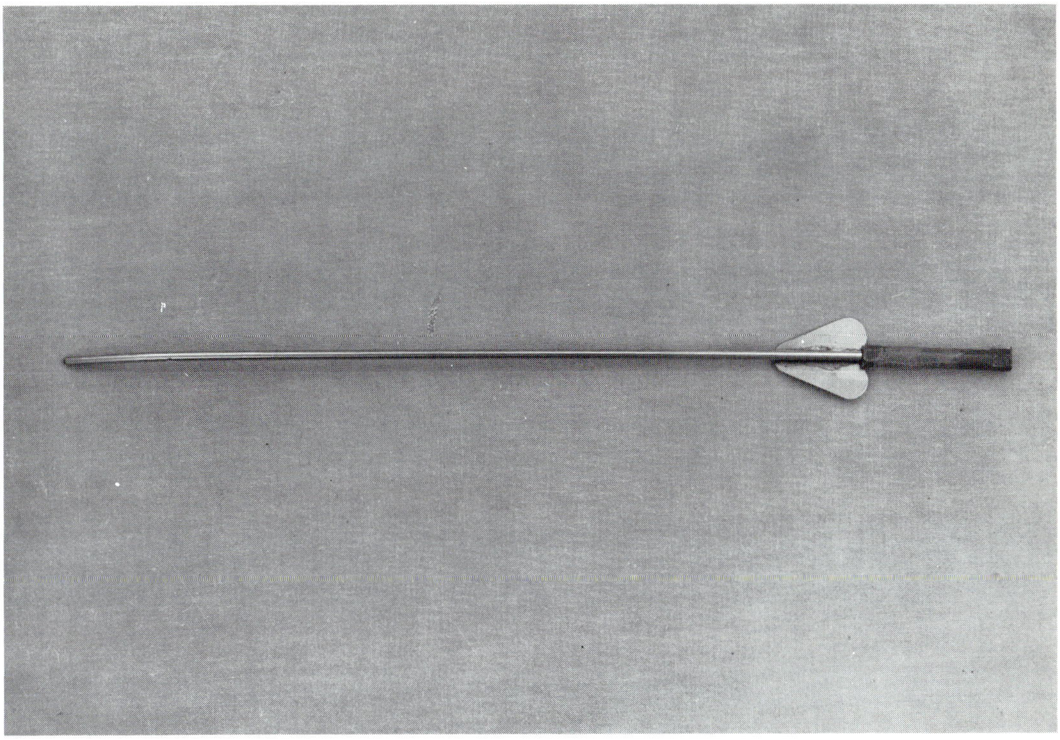

FIGURE 8–40.

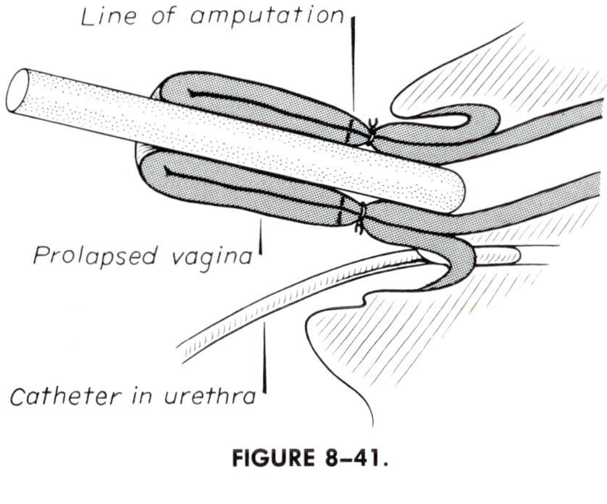

FIGURE 8–41.

SUBMUCOSAL RESECTION

Hyperplasia of the vaginal floor is seen more frequently than the true prolapse. It can be identified by the dome-shaped mass protruding from the vulva. It lacks a central orifice.

Anesthesia, preparation, and positioning are the same as for a true prolapse. The drapes are laid so that the median raphe between the vulva and the anus is exposed. The anus should be covered. A purse-string stitch in the anus is optional.

A skin incision is made from the dorsal commissure of the lips of the vulva to a point opposite the dorsal wall of the horizontal vagina. The episiotomy is completed with scissors (Fig. 8–42). The heavy fibrous tissue should be cut cleanly. By placing one blade of the scissors in the vulva and the other externally on the midline, the cleavage may be made in a single stroke. Hemorrhage is usually easily controlled with a few hemostats.

Following the episiotomy, the edematous mass should be fully exposed. An elliptical incision is made with a scalpel and begins at the cranial border of the mass. This incision should be the depth of the mucosa and approximately the width of the mass. As the incision is made, the mucosa is peeled away from the submucosa. Because of the profuse capillary bleeding, it is well to close the incision directly behind the dissection as it proceeds caudally. Simple interrupted stitches of size 1 silk are used to approximate the cut edges of the mucosa.

The episiotomy is closed by placing interrupted silk stitches in the mucosa so that the knots are tied in the vagina. Several rows of 3-0 multifilament stainless steel sutures are buried in the fibrous layers, and the skin is closed with interrupted stitches.

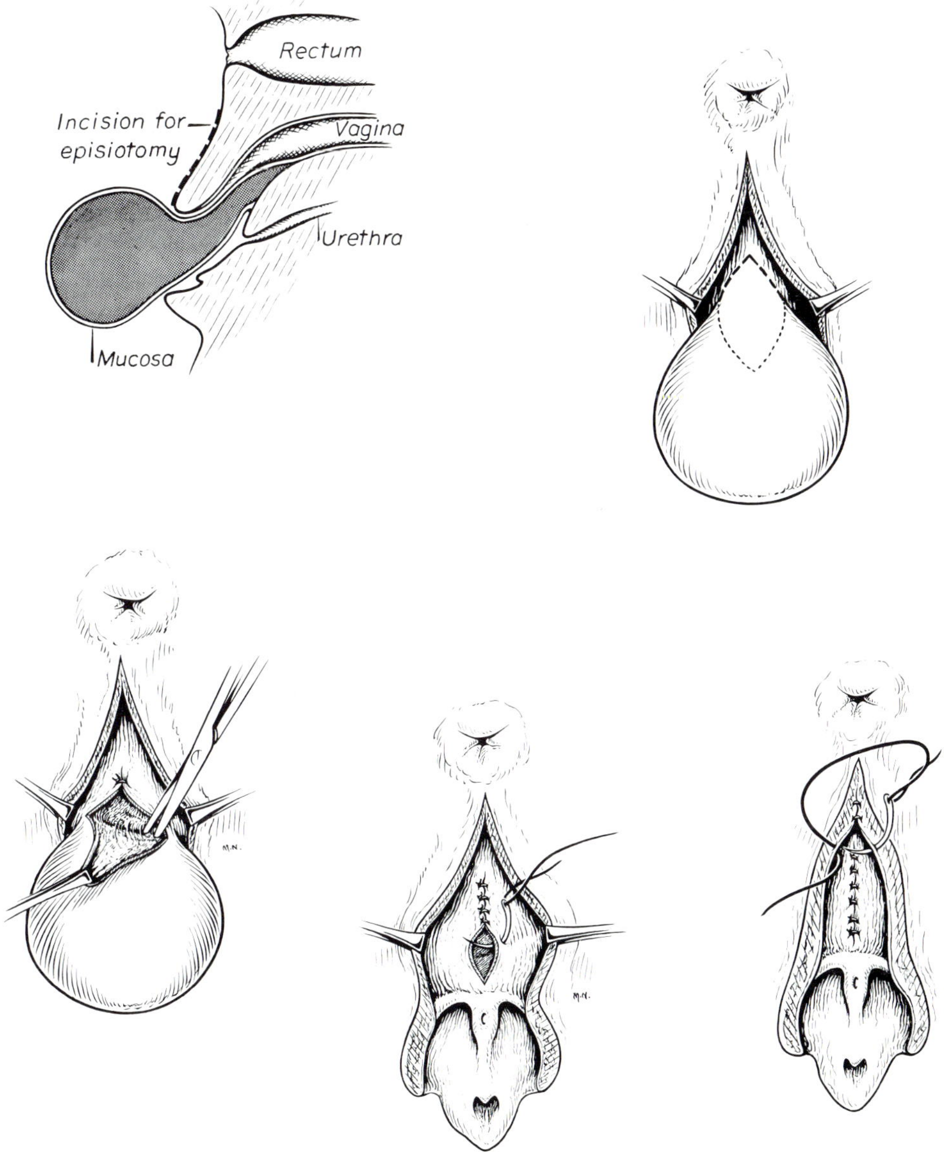

FIGURE 8–42.

REFERENCES

Brodey, R. S. *J.A.V.M.A.* 140:1339, 1962.
Christensen, G. C. *Am. Jour. Vet. Res.* 13:236–245, 1952.
Gordon, N. *J.A.V.M.A.* 136:215–221, 1960.
Joshua, J. O. *Vet. Record.* 77:642–646, 1965.
Kwaak, W. E. *Vet. Med. & S. A. Clin.* 59:691, 1964.
Leach, J. L. R. *Jour. Sm. An. Pract.* 4:285–288, 1963.
Nakamura, Y., and Hirose, T. *Jour. Jap. Vet. Med. Assoc.* 12:163–167, 1959.
Pettit, G. D. *J.A.V.M.A.* 136:486–490, 1960.

Chapter 9

COMMON HERNIORRHAPHY PROCEDURES

Some hernias are so simple that their repair requires very little explanation. The umbilical hernia is an example. Some are so variable in location and extent that each case is a problem in itself and requires ingenuity and a proper knowledge of body closure. Such is the case with the ventral hernia. The femoral hernia presents more of a problem in diagnosis than in treatment. It is seen more frequently in cats than in dogs. The common hernias dealt with in this chapter are the diaphragmatic, the inguinal, and the perineal.

DIAPHRAGMATIC HERNIORRHAPHY

While there are several approaches to repair of the diaphragm, a simple, commonly used method will be described. Under certain circumstances other methods may be more appropriate and convenient, but as a general rule the abdominal approach can be adapted to most situations.

If a presurgical examination reveals transudate in the thorax, the fluid should be withdrawn the day before surgery. It is also helpful to predetermine which side of the chest is involved so that the opposite side can be kept uppermost during the induction of anesthesia. Herniated organs lying on the lungs can cause respiratory embarrassment.

A general anesthetic is used, preferably pentobarbital sodium. As soon as the patient is anesthetized, an endotracheal tube is passed and the cuff inflated. The oxygen tank and some type of ventilation apparatus is kept at hand in case artificial respiration is required.

An area covering the cranial two-thirds of the abdomen and the caudal third of the thorax is prepared for surgery. A frame is used to hold the patient in dorsal recumbency, and the hind feet are tied to the table. A six-drape system is used. Assuming that the location of the hernia is unknown, lay the first four drapes in the usual manner, leaving a hand's breadth opening just caudal to the xiphoid process. This is to allow for a 6 cm. midline opening for exploratory purposes. If the location of the hernia is known to be on a particular side, the drapes are laid for a paracostal incision on that side. When the hernia is centrally located, the drapes are laid for a midline incision from xiphoid to umbilicus.

The appropriate incision is made and the edges draped (Fig. 9–1). Various abdominal organs will be found in the thorax. Of these, the omentum, a lobe of the liver, the stomach, and the spleen are most commonly present, either singly or collectively. Less frequently the intestine is found. When the rent is large, these organs will move freely between abdomen and thorax. A small tear frequently incarcerates a lobe of the liver. This usually results in a large accumulation of transudate in the thorax.

The surgical procedure will vary according to the conditions found in each individual case. However, the next step is the retrieval of abdominal organs from the thorax. The liver is usually the most difficult because of its friability. If the diaphragmatic opening is small, enlarge it toward the periphery with scissors. Avoid cutting deeper into the tendinous portion, because this is more difficult to close properly. The liver should be lifted gently by at least two fingers. Retractors can be dangerous, particularly if the lobe has been incarcerated. It will be swollen and extremely friable. In such a case, there will be fluid in the thorax, and this should be removed with the suction apparatus even though paracentesis has been performed prior to surgery. If one does not have suction equipment, a natural sponge can be autoclaved beforehand and kept in readiness for such cases. (*Note:* When the natural sponge is autoclaved in sterilizing tubing, it will shrink to the size of a walnut and appear useless; however, it will return to its normal size and shape when placed in fluid.)

Other organs are ordinarily replaced without too much difficulty. A problem may arise in finding space for them in the abdomen. When large amounts of abdominal viscera are moved to the thorax for a period of time, the abdominal muscles contract and limit the space. Since the operator must have room in which to make the diaphragmatic repair, it is sometimes necessary to place some of the more mobile organs, such as intestine, omentum, and spleen, on the drape and cover them with moist sponges or a towel.

For the purpose of discussing closure of the diaphragm, the perforations may be classified as those in the tendinous portion, those in the muscular portion, and those along the periphery. Closure of tears in the central tendon is the most difficult because the tissue is thin and the sutures leave small openings through which air can leak into the chest. A simple continuous stitch is used to close the rent while the liver is gently displaced caudally. The respiratory movement of the diaphragm is watched closely so that the needle will not inadvertently puncture the liver. When

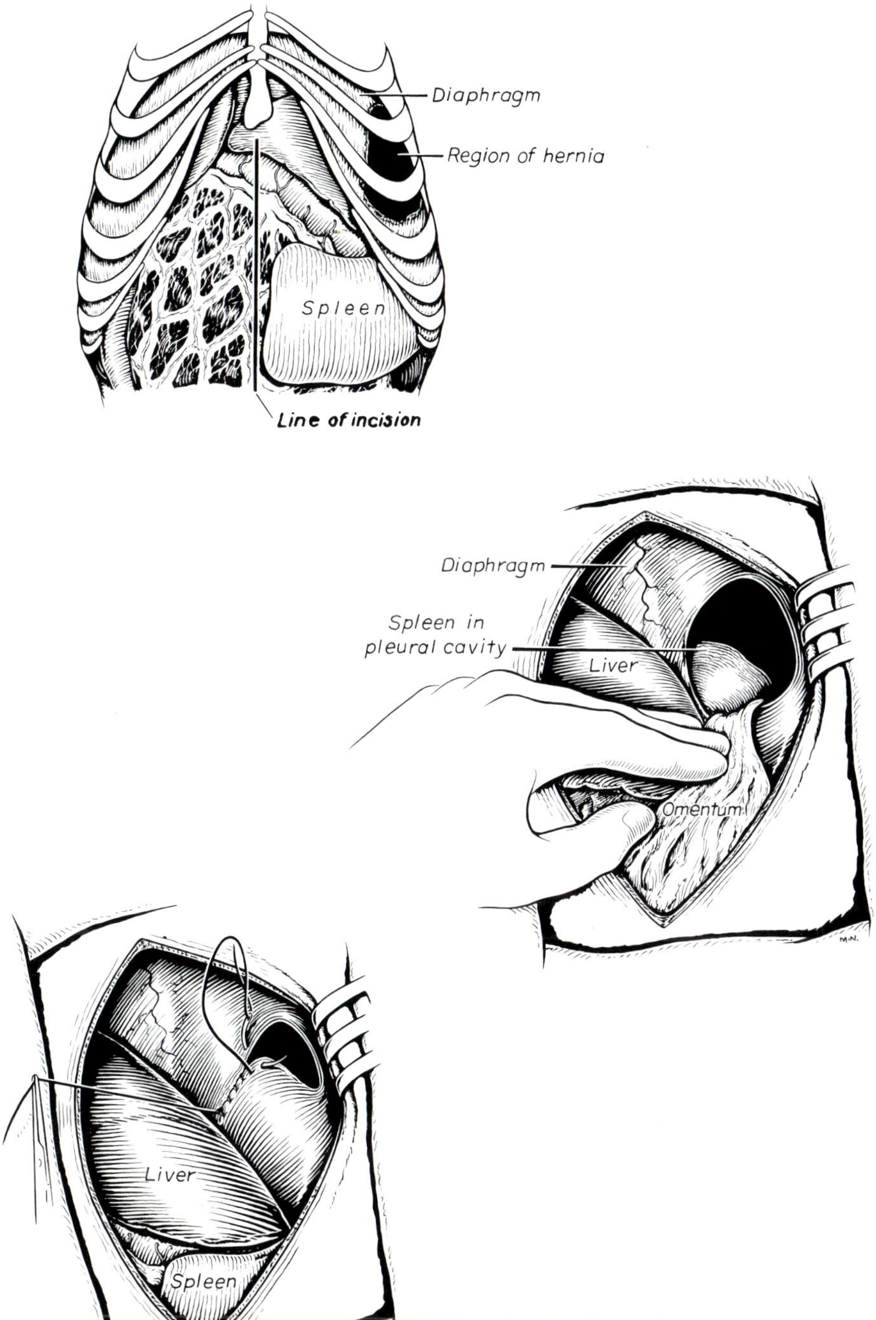
Diaphragm
Region of hernia
Spleen
Line of incision
Diaphragm
Spleen in pleural cavity
Liver
Omentum
Liver
Spleen

FIGURE 9–1.

the opening is about to be closed with the last stitch, pressure is applied to the lungs to fully expand them. This may be done by pressure on a rebreathing bag, by direct manual closure of a T valve, or by increasing the valve pressure to 30 cm. of water in the PR-3 type of resuscitator. At the same time, the last stitch is held apart with a hemostat until the lungs are fully expanded. The hemostat is then withdrawn and the stitch tied. The liver is immediately pressed against the diaphragm to seal the openings made by the sutures. Fortunately a seal will form rapidly and will be maintained by the pressure of viscera against the liver. Replace the organs that were exteriorized during surgery, making certain that they are returned to normal position, and close the abdominal incision in the usual manner. If the closure is difficult because of the crowding of abdominal organs, an assistant can elevate the incision by placing an index finger at each commissure and pulling upward. This will allow peritoneal closure without interference from the viscera.

The easiest closure is one made following a rent in the muscular portion of the diaphragm. If the rent is large, it may be held in apposition by Allis forceps. Otherwise, the tear requires no special treatment during the suturing. A continuous Cushing stitch of 3-0 chromic catgut will produce an airtight seal. The final stitch is made in the same manner as described in the previous paragraph. A second row of sutures is placed for reinforcement after the thorax has been sealed.

When the tear is along the periphery, the torn edge may be sewed to the peritoneal edge of the incision with a simple continuous stitch of 3-0 chromic catgut. A single row of sutures is usually sufficient. The same method of sealing the thorax is used. In this case the abdomen is closed by suturing the peritoneum on the caudal edge of the incision to the suture line produced by suturing the diaphragm and peritoneum of the cranial edge.

PERINEAL HERNIORRHAPHY

The perineal hernia is seen almost exclusively in males and may be unilateral or bilateral. The surgery consists of a herniorrhaphy and an orchidectomy. If the hernia is bilateral, it is expedient to make the correction in two stages. One side is repaired and the orchidectomy performed at the first stage. One month later the opposite side is repaired.

The patient is anesthetized with a general anesthetic, and the area covering the perineum, the base of the tail, and the caudal half of the pelvis is clipped and prepared for surgery. A purse-string stitch is placed around the anus and tied with a large bow so that it can be removed readily. The tail is tied over the back. A sternal positioning with the hind legs over the end of the table and a Flexicast under the hips to elevate the pelvis provides the best access to the perineal region.

A four-drape system is used, with an opening lateral to the tail and over the hernia and extending from the sacrum to the ischial arch. This should be well fastened with towel clamps to avoid slipping.

The skin incision is begun lateral to the tail head and cranial to it at about the level of the sacrum (Fig. 9–2). It is carried caudoventrally, curving slightly lateral at the hernial bulge and returning to its original course ventral to the hernia until it reaches the ischial arch. A thin layer of subcutaneous fascia has to be separated with scissors in order to expose the hernial contents.

Frequently the bladder and the prostate are herniated. The bladder may be distended with urine as a result of strangulation (Fig. 9–3). In

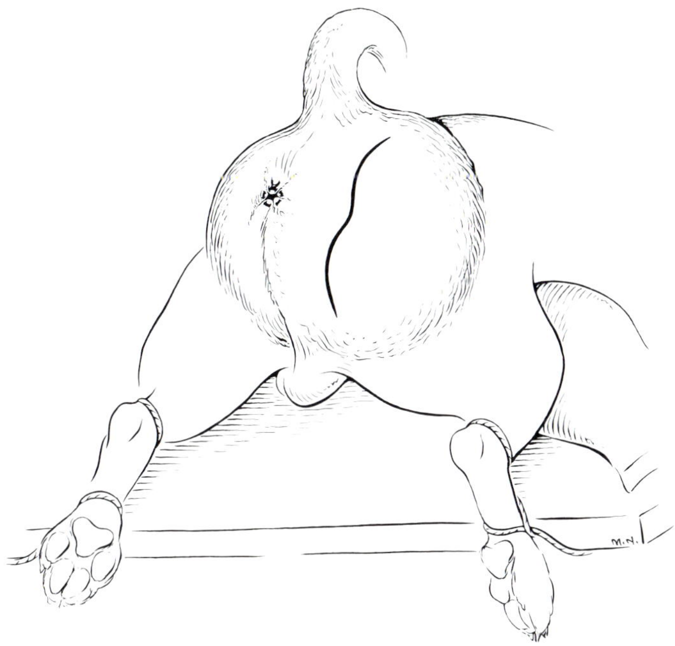

FIGURE 9–2.

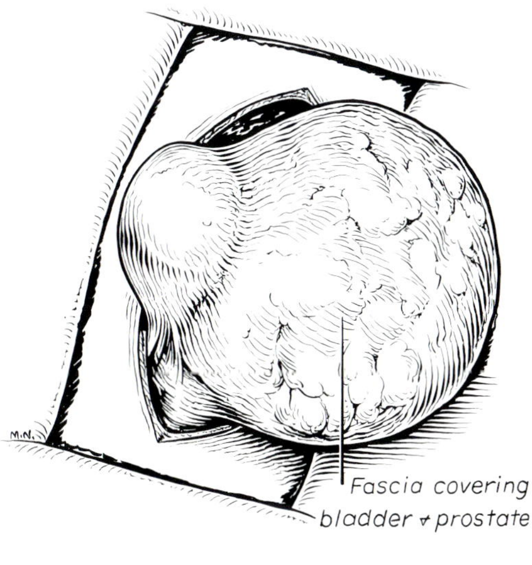

FIGURE 9–3.

such cases it is impossible to catheterize, and the bladder must be reduced by tapping with a 20 gauge needle and a 20 ml. syringe (Fig. 9–4). A sterile kidney basin should be held tightly to the bladder beneath the needle to avoid spillage and to serve as a collecting receptacle. Large cysts may also be present in the prostate. These will also require tapping in the same way.

Nearly every perineal hernia contains retroperitoneal fat retained in a lace-like fibrous net. It is not uncommon to find small spherical nodules dispersed throughout this tissue. These nodules vary in color from white to a reddish brown. These are hematomas produced by the forceful straining of the patient. The variation in size and color represents the various stages of healing.

The organs are returned to the abdominal cavity and the area surveyed for the closure (Fig. 9–5). Theoretically the hernial opening is bounded medially by the rectum and the external anal sphincter, laterally by the coccygeus, the sacrotuberous ligament and the levator ani, and ventrolaterally by the obturator internus. Traversing the ventral third of the opening and running from lateral to medial is the internal pudendal artery with its satellite vein and the perineal nerve (Fig. 9–6).

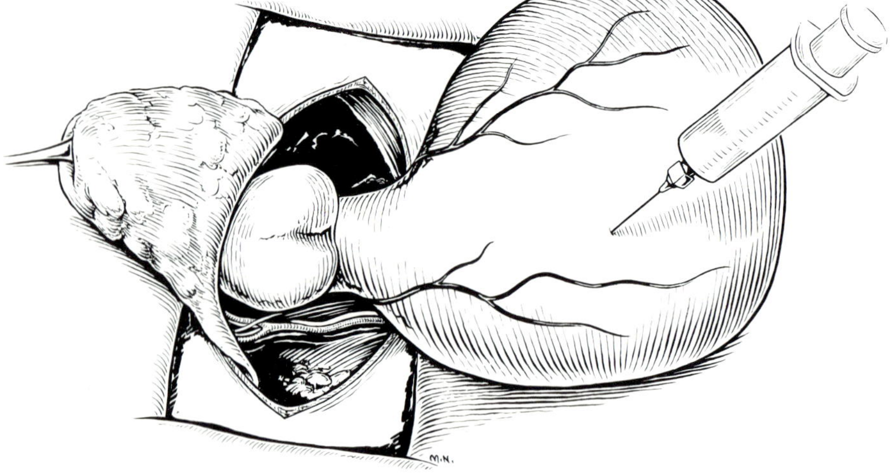

FIGURE 9–4.

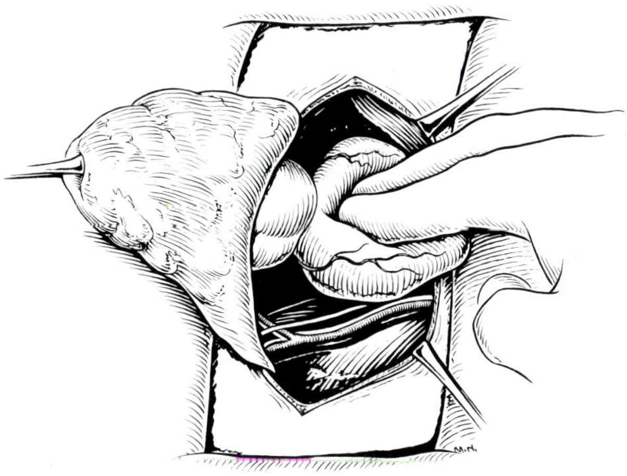

FIGURE 9–5.

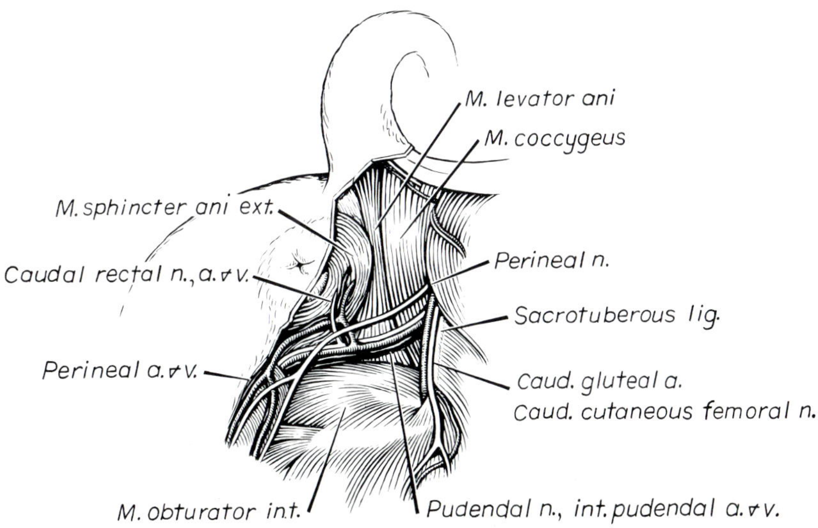

FIGURE 9–6. Perineal area in a normal dog.

If all of these structures can be uncovered and identified, the closure should not be difficult. Beginning dorsally, suture the caudal edge of the coccygeus and levator ani muscles to the cranial edge of the external anal sphincter using interrupted stitches of 3-0 multifilament stainless steel (Fig. 9–7). As the suturing continues ventrally, the levator ani will no longer be available, but the coccygeus muscle and the sacrotuberous ligament may be used as far ventral as the point where the blood vessels cross. Great care should be taken not to disturb the artery, vein, and nerve. The ventral part of the opening is closed by suturing the cranial edge of the external anal sphincter to the obturator internus (Fig. 9–8). This closure should be further supported by dissecting a flap of perineal fascia on either side of the incision and closing this fascia over the first suture line with simple interrupted stitches.

Often the coccygeus muscle is so atrophied that it cannot be identified or used. In such cases it becomes necessary to suture whatever tissue is available. Pelvic fascia and the sacrotuberous ligament may be utilized, and these may be sutured to the wall of the rectum. Such a closure should also be fortified with a fascial closure (Fig. 9–9).

When the underlying tissues have been closed, the redundant skin should be trimmed with scissors so that the skin closure will be even and smooth (Fig. 9–10). Most of the trimming should be done on the lateral side so that the suture line will not be too close to the anus. The skin is closed with interrupted stitches of stainless steel.

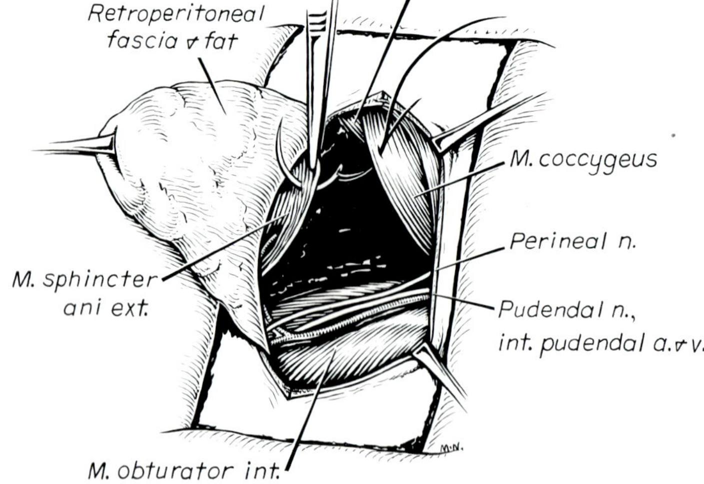

FIGURE 9–7.

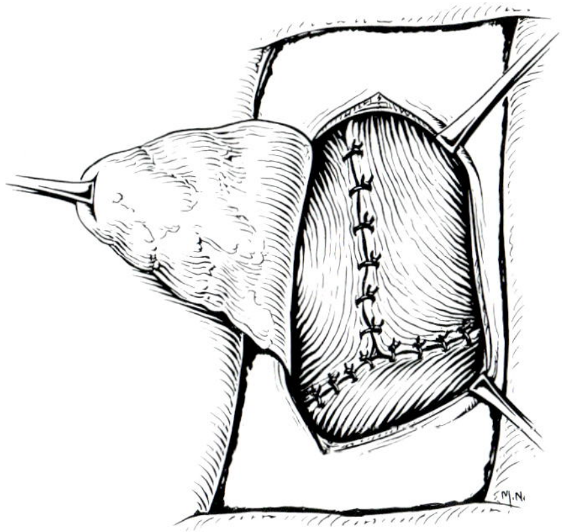

FIGURE 9–8.

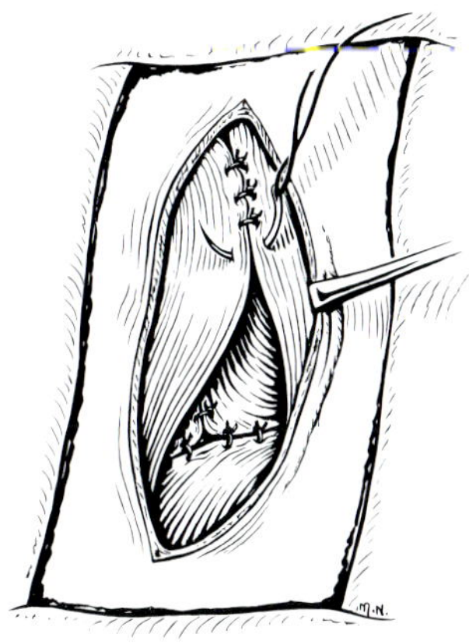

FIGURE 9–9.

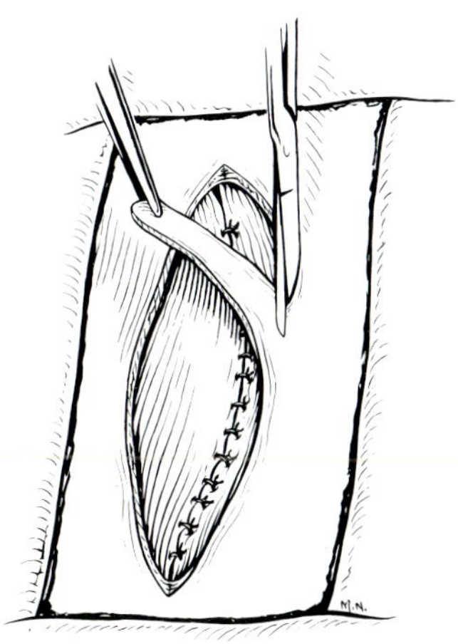

FIGURE 9–10.

INGUINAL HERNIORRHAPHY

The inguinal hernia is most commonly seen in the female (Fig. 9–11). It may be unilateral or bilateral. A general anesthetic is required, and the usual skin preparation is made over the entire abdomen as well as the medial sides of the thighs. The patient is placed in dorsal recumbency with the hind feet tied to the table and the foreparts supported in a frame.

A four- or six-drape system is used, leaving a midline opening from pubis to umbilicus. The skin incision is made from the pubis craniad and is at least a hand's breadth in length. By blunt dissection in a lateral direction beneath the breast, the external inguinal ring can easily be exposed. The skin incision is retracted in the direction of the hernia, and the sac is examined (Fig. 9–12). It frequently contains omentum, intestine, and a uterine horn.

In some cases, where the hernial ring is large and there are no adhesions, the hernia can be readily reduced. In other cases, the hernia may be irreducible because of adhesions or because the sac contains a gravid horn of the uterus. Sometimes, if the hernial sac is opened, the hernia can be reduced. At other times, it may require dilation of the ring by placing a finger in the cranial end. It is also possible to assist reduction by continuing the midline incision into the abdomen and applying careful traction to the herniated viscera. This should be a last resort maneuver and is seldom required.

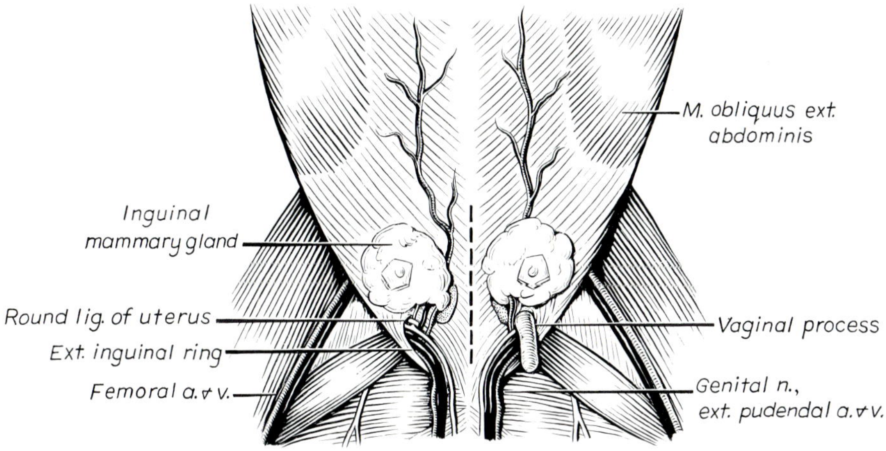

FIGURE 9–11. Area of external inguinal rings. The vaginal process is not shown on right side. Dotted line indicates skin incision.

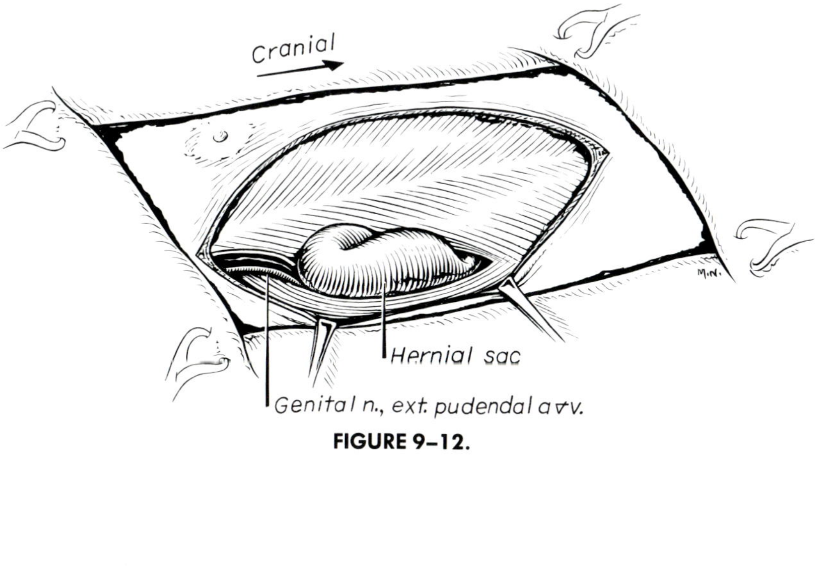

FIGURE 9–12.

The sac should be inverted or removed before the inguinal canal is closed (Fig. 9–13). If possible the internal ring should be closed with the first row of sutures and the external ring with a second row. In small dogs this is not always feasible. The suturing should begin at the cranial end of the ring. Use interrupted stitches of 2-0 chromic catgut placed about 5 mm. apart. This row of sutures should unite the inguinal ligament with the caudal border of the obliquus internus abdominis and the lateral border of the rectus abdominis (Fig. 9–14). As the caudal commissure is approached, it is necessary to allow for the external pudendal artery and vein. The suturing should be done very carefully so that the vessels will not be injured, and the last suture should not be close enough to interfere with circulation. If a hemostat is laid beside the blood vessels as the closure is made and then removed after the last suture is tied, it will usually provide sufficient space. A similar row of sutures uniting the aponeurosis of the obliquus externus abdominis will close the external ring. Again, the external pudendal vessels must be treated with great care.

The opposite side should be examined and repaired if necessary. The mammary tissue should be sewn to the abdominal wall. This can be accomplished by placing interrupted stitches of 2-0 chromic catgut through the submammary fascia and the muscle sheath of the rectus close to the midline. No dead space should be allowed to remain, because this space will enlarge when the patient stands. The skin incision on the midline is closed with a row of subcutaneous sutures and interrupted skin stitches of whatever material seems appropriate.

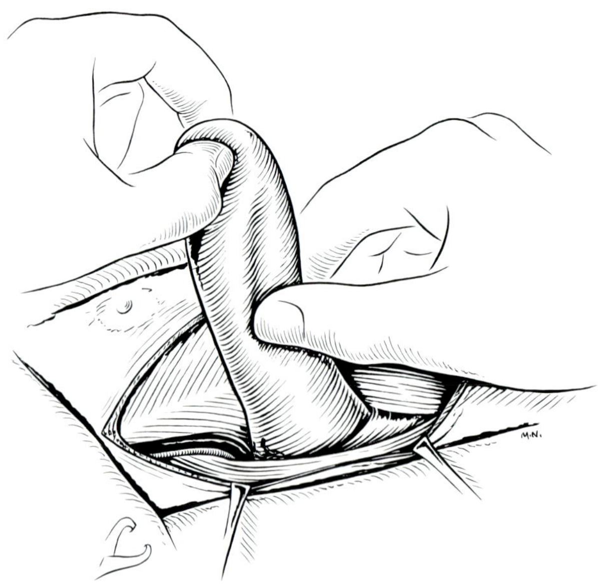

FIGURE 9–13.

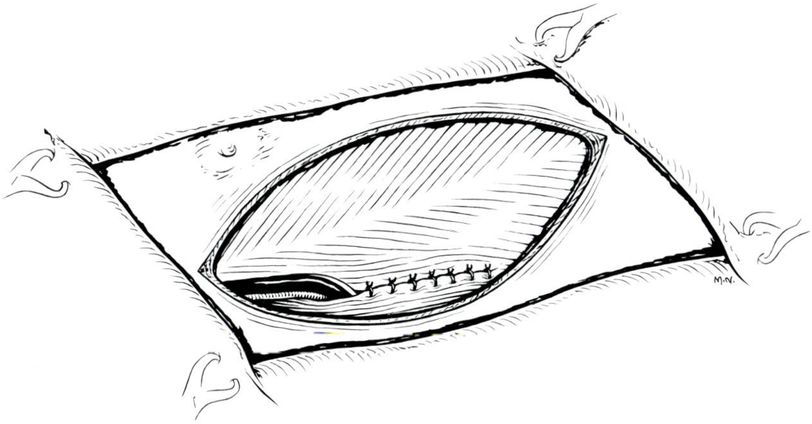

FIGURE 9–14.

REFERENCES

Archibald, J., and Cawley, A. J. *Sm. An. Clin.* 1:73–76, 1961.
Archibald, J., Reed, J. H., and Cawley, A. J. *Mod. Vet. Pract.* 41 (No. 10): 28–36, 1960.
North, A. F., Jr. *Cornell Vet.* 49:379–383, 1959.
Pettit, G. D. *Cornell Vet.* 52:261–279, 1962.
Walker, R. G., and Hall, L. W. *Vet Record.* 77:830–837, 1965.
Wright, J. G. *Vet. Record.* 75:1352–67, 1963.

Index